THE IMMUNOGLOBULIN A SYSTEM

ADVANCES IN EXPERIMENTAL MEDICINE AND BIOLOGY

Recent Volumes in this Series

THE IMMUNOGLOBULIN A SYSTEM

Edited by
Jiri Mestecky
Institute of Dental Research
Departments of Microbiology and Medicine
University of Alabama in Birmingham
Birmingham, Alabama

and
Alexander R. Lawton
Departments of Pediatrics and Microbiology
University of Alabama in Birmingham
Birmingham, Alabama

PLENUM PRESS • NEW YORK AND LONDON

Library of Congress Cataloging in Publication Data

International Symposium on the Immunoglobulin A System, Birmingham, Ala.,
    1973.
    The immunoglobulin A system.

    (Advances in experimental medicine and biology, v. 45)
    Includes bibliographical references.
    1. Immunoglobulin A—Congresses. I. Mestecky, Jiri, 1941·   ed. II. Lawton,
Alexander R., 1938·   ed. III. Title. IV. Series. [DNLM: 1. IGA—Congresses.
WI AD559 v.45 / QW570 I324 1974]
QR186.8.A2157   1973   616.07'9'3   74-8720
ISBN-13: 978-1-4613-4552-7   e-ISBN-13: 978-1-4613-4550-3
DOI: 10.1007/ 978-1-4613-4550-3

Proceedings of the International Symposium on the Immunoglobulin A
System held in Birmingham, Alabama, October 23-25, 1973

© 1974 Plenum Press, New York
Softcover reprint of the hardcover 1st edition 1974
A Division of Plenum Publishing Corporation
227 West 17th Street, New York, N.Y. 10011

United Kingdom edition published by Plenum Press, London
A Division of Plenum Publishing Company, Ltd.
4a Lower John Street, London W1R 3PD, England

PREFACE

The International Symposium on the Immunoglobulin A System was organized in observance of the twenty-fifth anniversary of the School of Dentistry of the University of Alabama in Birmingham. Immunoglobulin A was chosen as the subject of the Symposium because of its broad scope in relation to all biologic sciences, as well as for its particular relevance to prevention of the most common human disease—dental caries. More than 500 scientists, from 13 countries, met in Birmingham, Alabama to review critically past and current research on IgA and to outline goals for integrating future investigations of the many facets of the IgA system.

It is our pleasure to express sincere appreciation to the following, whose efforts made the Symposium possible: to Dr. Sidney B. Finn, Chairman, and all members of the Twenty-fifth Anniversary Planning Committee for their advice and assistance; to Dr. Charles A. McCallum, Dean of the School of Dentistry, for his enthusiastic approval and support; to Dr. Frederick W. Kraus, Symposium Chairman, for the countless hours of meticulous planning that ensured the smooth execution of the Symposium; to Ms. Tonnia C. Maddox whose unstinting dedication was indispensable to the organizational success of the meeting; to those who assisted with the transcription of manuscripts and discussions: Ms. Shirley Snow, Ms. Jan Allen, Ms. Janice Buchanan, Ms. Joy Fisher, Ms. Pam Honeycutt, Ms. Mary Huckabee, Ms. Charlotte Hughes, Mr. Stephen Miles, Ms. Wanda Sales, Ms. Ima Jean Stephens, and Mr. George Weatherly; to Ms. Marjorie Campbell for her able editorial assistance with the printed programs; to Mr. Edward J. McDevitt and his capable crew for monitoring and recording the entire proceedings; and to Mr. Joe Kidd for the superior performance of his Educational Services staff.

THE EDITORS,

Jiri Mestecky
Alexander R. Lawton, III

CONTENTS

SESSION A

Developmental and Cellular Aspects

Chairman: Lars A. Hanson

SESSION B

Structure, Biosynthesis, and Genetics

Chairman: J. Claude Bennett

SESSION C

Structure

Chairman: Jiri Mestecky

SESSION D

Function

Chairman: Frederick W. Kraus

SESSION E

Clinical Considerations

Chairman: Max D. Cooper

SESSION F

The IgA Antibody Response Implications
for Oral Health

Chairman: Alexander R. Lawton

CONCLUSION

SESSION A

DEVELOPMENTAL AND CELLULAR ASPECTS

CHAIRMAN: LARS A. HANSON

THE IgA SYSTEM IN CONNECTION WITH LOCAL AND SYSTEMIC IMMUNITY

Joseph F. Heremans

Department of Experimental Medicine, Université Catholique de Louvain, 4 Avenue Chapelle-aux-Champs, B-1200 Brussels, Belgium

1. A MODEL FOR THE STRUCTURE AND BIOSYNTHESIS OF IgA

The polymerization pattern of the IgA produced by a given plasma cell tumor line is characteristic and constant. Polymerization obviously occurs through intermolecular disulfide interchange between labile SS bonds, but how this is regulated is not clear. Hypothetical sulfhydryl-blocking agents such as cysteine (disulfide-bonded to the crucial cysteinyls of stable monomers) have not clearly been shown to play a role. The J-chain, which is also made by IgA-producing cells, probably contributes by stabilizing the polymers but does not seem required for their formation, since IgM may polymerize without its help. In the IgA dimer the J-chain is held by disulfide bonds and occupies a hidden position (Fig. 1), as shown by antigenic analysis (1). Its incorporation occurs concomitantly with polymerization (2). All this could be the work of a disulfide-rearranging enzyme, whose activity might be the factor regulating polymerization.

The model for the $(IgA)_2.J.SC$ complex proposed in Fig. 1 is based on the following considerations (3).

The geometry of the IgA dimer arrangement is that deduced from recent electron micrographic data (4), and the J-chain is assumed to be disulfide-linked (bonds not shown) in a conceiled and central position, as suggested by combined chemical and antigenic analysis. The SC chain is assumed to be coiled around the surface of the double-Fc

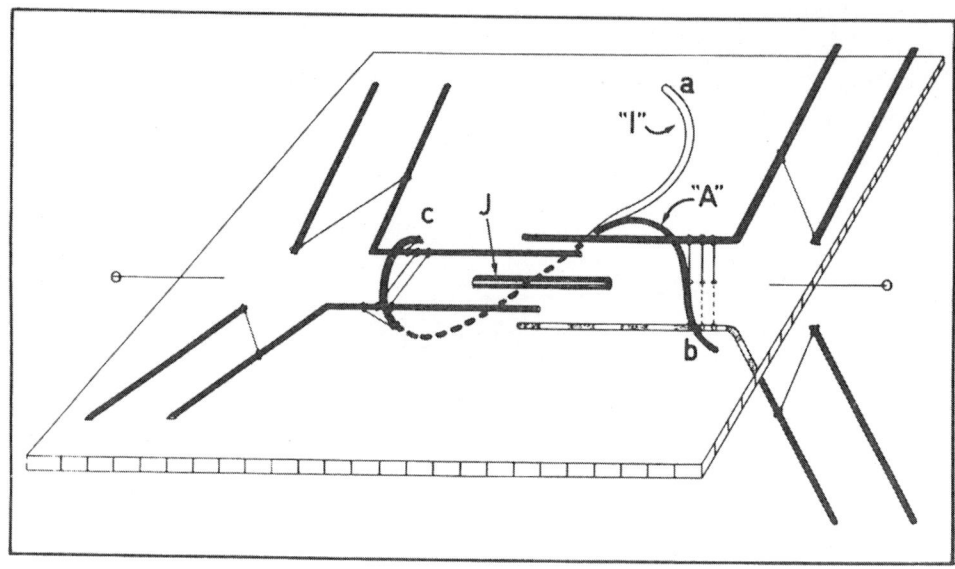

Figure 1.–Model proposed for the structure of Secretory IgA

cylinder, extending from the hinge region of one monomer to
the hinge region of the other monomer. The rationale for
this assumption is as follows. Firstly, the binding sites
for SC are known to be located in the Fc region, as shown
by α-chain disease proteins, and to include the hinge region,
as evident from combination studies with IgA_2 proteins (5).
The SC chain is long enough to span the hinge-to-hinge distance, but only when in the extended form. This configuration is also likely on account of the absence of any compact
SC "domains" in electron micrographs of S-IgA (4). The
strong reactions of S-IgA with antibodies to free SC suggests that much of the SC chain is exposed at the surface of
the complex. The SC coil around the Fc axis would nicely
account for the stabilization of S-IgA toward reductive dissociation. Intimate contact between SC and Fc over the
major part of their lengths is suggested by the finding that
both chains, taken separately, are very susceptible to proteolytic attack, yet efficiently protect one another when
present in the S-IgA complex (6). This concept of interaction over a wide area agrees with the finding that most of
the SC can be dissociated from human S-IgA after mere reduction in non-dispersing media, but only when a physical means
of separating the α and SC chains (e.g., gel-filtration) is
provided; in other words it appears that SC and Fc are bound
by a set of numerous yet weak non-covalent bonds. Combination and dissociation studies further suggest that disulfide

bonds are formed only secondarily, by SS interchange, and in some cases (e.g., the rabbit) may be lacking altogether.

The proposed structural model also provides some insight into the mode of formation of the S-IgA complex. $(IgA)_2$.J.dimers, provided by plasma cells, would be recognized via their Fc regions by free SC from epithelial cells (cf. below). The geometry of the IgA dimer would remain unaffected by this encounter, but the SC chain, by coiling around the double Fc axis, would change its configuration (from a to b in Fig. 1), thereby giving up some of its antigenic determinants ("I", ref. 7). The unusually high glycine content (10%) of the SC molecule (compared to 3% for α- or J-chains) would provide the flexibility required for this change. A system of multiple non-covalent linkages would form and subsequently become completed - though not in all cases - by disulfide bridges arising by SS interchange, notably in the hinge regions (as suggested for IgA_2 proteins).

2. ORIGIN OF SERUM IgA

In the human, serum IgA represents about 1/6 of the immunoglobulins (2.6 ± 1.1 mg/ml) and consists for about 85% (2.2-2.3 mg/ml) of monomer IgA, 10-15% (0.2-0.3 mg/ml) of $(IgA)_n$.J (chiefly dimers), and about 1% (0.004-0.05 mg/ml) of S-IgA. In most animals the concentrations of polymeric and secretory IgA in the serum are the same as in man, but monomeric IgA is greatly deficient or lacking, thus lowering the total serum IgA level to 0.03-0.8 mg/ml.

It is proposed (3) that these three forms of serum IgA each recognize a separate origin, as delineated in Fig. 2. This idea is supported by the already mentioned finding that the polymerization pattern of IgA is typical for the cell that produces it.

IgA monomers presumably originate mostly in the bone marrow, spleen and lymph nodes (other than the mesenteric nodes). This is suggested by the finding that IgA-cells in these sites are numerous in the human but rare in animals whose serum IgA is largely dimeric (e.g., the cat), whereas mucosal IgA-cells are equally numerous in all species. Also, extramucosal IgA-cells, in contrast to epithelium-associated IgA-cells, have been shown not to fix free SC in tissue sections, a property believed to indicate the monomeric nature of their product (8).

IgA polymers probably originate chiefly in mucosal and
glandular sites, particularly in the gut wall. That the IgA
produced by IgA-cells in these locations is largely dimeric
is attested by the fact that the two IgA halves of the S-IgA
molecule are identical with regard to L-chain type and H-
chain allotype, and hence cannot have been assembled at
random from serum IgA monomers; furthermore, in tissue sections, SC is fixed by subepithelial IgA-cells.

Anatomic considerations demand that IgA from mucosal
and glandular sites be drained off into the blood via the
lymphatics. This has been verified in the dog, by experiments showing that the IgA content of mesenteric lymph was
about 20 times higher than expected from the supply of IgA
from the circulation; also, the specific radioactivity of
mesenteric lymph IgA was much lower than that of serum IgA
after intravenous infusion of labeled IgA (9). Less complete but analogous demonstrations have been furnished in
rats and guinea-pigs. In mice a selective shut-down of the
supply of intestinal IgA to the blood can be produced by
mild irradiation of the gut which causes a rechannelling of
the IgA output of its mucosa in favor of secretion into the
lumen (10).

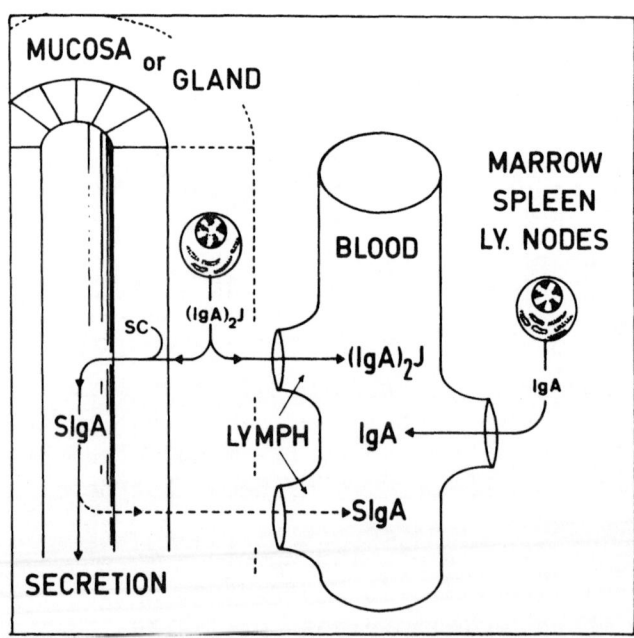

Figure 2.-Multiple origin of serum IgA (Proposed Model)

In man the contribution of intestinal IgA to serum IgA is probably as important as it is in animals, but this does not show up in the IgA content of thoracic duct lymph because of the presence of a 10-fold excess of monomeric IgA from extramucosal sources. Mucosal contribution to human serum IgA is nevertheless attested by perfusion studies on isolated bowel segments (11) and by the selective rise in serum IgA during mucosal infections.

The tiny S-IgA fraction probably represents S-IgA reabsorbed from secretions, since its concentration rises in inflammatory mucosal diseases and during lactation.

3. ORIGIN OF IgA IN SECRETIONS

The common statement that IgA is the predominant immunoglobulin in external secretions does not apply to all cases, when reference is made to absolute concentrations. It does seem of nearly universal application, however, when the secretion/serum ratios of the different immunoglobulin classes are considered. In most cases the S-IgA form represents the bulk of secreted IgA, except when the contribution from circulating IgA becomes important.

It is generally agreed now that the concept of secretory IgA largely, though not fully, coincides with that of "muco-antibodies", i.e., that most of the S-IgA is produced in situ by the mucosae and exocrine glands, following local antigenic stimulation. This concept is founded on the knowledge that (i) antigenically stimulated mucosae synthetize and assemble all the component polypeptide chains of S-IgA in vitro or during perfusion experiments; (ii) that fluorescent antisera reveal the presence in these tissues of large populations of plasma cells producing both IgA and J-chains, and of epithelial cells making the SC chain; (iii) that S-IgA antibodies are anatomically restricted to the very sites that have been stimulated by the corresponding antigen and (iv) are not assembled from serum IgA monomers (cf. above); and (v) that none of the forms of serum IgA is excreted by mucosal or glandular sites at a rate sufficient to account for the amounts of S-IgA found in secretions, as discussed in more detail below.

On the other hand it is equally clear that sizable amounts of plasma IgA may escape into secretions, together with other plasma proteins, whenever the capillaries of the

Table 1. Origin of IgA in canine secretions

	Saliva	Bile	Jejunal Fluid
Local synthesis	80%	40–45%	85%
Plasma origin Passive transfer	1%	2–3%	3%
Plasma origin Active transfer	19%	42–57%	12%

area involved are relatively permeable to macromolecules or
have been rendered so as a result of irritation or inflammation.

Recent excretion studies by our group (12), using dogs
intravenously infused with biosynthetically labeled plasma
proteins, have shown that the transfer of IgA from plasma
to secretions, as induced from specific radioactivity measurements, attains higher proportions in the dog than in the
human (Table 1). Furthermore the transfer process could be
resolved into a sum of three pathways whose relative importance could be established by comparing the clearance rates
of IgA as well as of proteins of exclusive plasma origin,
to their respective molecular radii. Pathway (i) consisted
of bulk transfer of unadulterated plasma, whereas pathway
(ii) involved molecular sieving through a membrane which,
in the case of the biliary tract, could be assigned to the
vascular walls rather than to the biliary epithelium, as
evidenced by studies on the composition of hepatic lymph.
Pathways (i) and (ii) together constitute "passive transfer".
In biliary, salivary and intestinal canine secretions it
turned out that only a small proportion of the plasma-derived
IgA could be accounted for by this process, the rest having
to be considered as representing "active transfer", selective
for IgA (Pathway iii), by the epithelial wall.

Anatomic reasons make it evident that both the IgA from
the plasma, to the extent that it is excreted, and the IgA
produced locally by mucosal or glandular plasma cells, must
join a common pre-excretory pool located in the interstitial
subepithelial fluid. It is therefore probable that the transfer of locally produced IgA through the epithelial barrier
proceeds through the same pathways, particularly the one involving active transport, that have been documented by the
above cited studies in the dog. Also, the discrepancy between the minimal excretion of human compared to canine plasma

IgA would vanish if it were supposed that the selective
transfer mechanism preferentially operated on dimeric rather
than on monomeric IgA.

A molecular model for the $(IgA)_2.J+SC = S-IgA$ reaction
has been proposed above. Marker proteins may infiltrate the
intercellular junctions but are not transferred; the absence
of excretion of preformed S-IgA indicates that the combination reaction does not take place in the intercellular space
but on or in the epithelial cell. The former hypothesis,
with SC cast in the role of a receptor for dimeric IgA located on the lateral cell membrane, is the more likely, i.e.,
because fluorescent antisera to SC stain the intercellular
contact region (probably the cell membrane). In this sense,
SC would truly be a "transport protein". One may further
speculate that it probably also serves to shield IgA from
cellular proteases during its transcellular (diacytotic ?)
passage, and in fact that SC is a homologue of the IgG-
specific conveyor-protector that has been assumed to ensure
the metabolic protection of IgG and its transfer through
fetal membranes (13). By extension one wonders whether the
antigen revealed by anti-SC reagents in tissues not involved
in the production or transfer of IgA represents genuine SC
or some related member from a whole family of immunoglobulin-
receptor proteins.

4. THE IgA ANTIBODY RESPONSE

Immunohistological studies in mice (14) disclosed that
parenteral administration of antigen (ferritin) prompted
intestinal plasma cells to an antibody response which,
though much weaker than that to orally given antigen, was
equally preferentially expressed by the IgA system. This
suggests that most of the mucosal lymphocytes are precom-
mitted to the production of IgA. Several authors have explained this by assuming that IgA-carrying circulating lymphocytes would be captured by IgA-receptors (SC ?) on epithelial cells; this concept would agree with the above proposed location of SC on the lateral walls of epithelial cells,
and with the known occurrence of "thelio"-lymphocytes in
the spaces separating these cells.

One may ask whether the frequent replacement of mucosal
IgA-cells by IgM-cells in subjects selectively lacking IgA
reflects a failure of a hypothetical IgM to IgA switch, or
the removal of a competition for SC binding by IgM- _versus_

IgA-cells, the latter normally dominating because of the higher affinity of SC for IgA than for IgM.

The local output of secretory antibody by an antigenically stimulated mucosa is frequently, though not always, associated with the more or less selective appearance of IgA antibodies in the blood. As explained in section 2.2, some of this IgA originates in the mucosal area involved, being drained into the blood via the lymphatics; but immunohistological data and Jerne plate assays concur in showing that part of it is produced by IgA-cells from distant, extramucosal lymphoid tissues. These cells, or their precursors, are probably emigrants from the antigenically stimulated, IgA-committed, mucosal immunocyte population.

Several reports indicate that the IgA system is endowed with only little, if any, immunological memory. What is more, a recent study by C. André and our own group (15) has shown that the primary splenic IgA response to sheep erythrocytes administered intragastrically to rats is followed by a refractory phase lasting several weeks, during which no significant recall of antibody formation can be elicited by renewed digestive administration of antigen.

5. POSSIBLE SIGNIFICANCE OF IgA ANTIBODIES

There is ample evidence that IgA, in the form of S-IgA, is indeed intrusted with an important role in the immunologic protection of mucosal surfaces, but that its absence causes no harm as long as IgA can be replaced by IgM. The complex of dimeric IgA with SC has probably been selected for this role because of its stability towards proteases. Extending the hypothesis (cf. 3) on the transport role of SC, one may surmise that SC, unlike the analogous receptor for IgG, has evolved so as not to dissociate from its substrate when the complex leaves the cell, because further protection is needed in the septic environment where IgA has to operate.

Whether IgA antibodies have effector functions mediated by ancillary systems such as complement, and leading to lysis or opsonization, remains controversial. Perhaps the reported absence of segmental flexibility in the hinge area (16), itself related to the lack of glycine residues in that region, may account for the poor performance of IgA antibodies in fixing C_1, since it would hinder the allosteric transition needed for that reaction.

In contrast, more direct effects of IgA antibodies, e.g., the neutralization of viruses, is better documented. The hypothesis that S-IgA may serve to keep harmful antigens out of the body, by forming non-absorbable complexes with them that would be carried away by the conveyor-belt action of the mucus coat, has been supported by the finding that oral immunization of rats with human serum albumin caused a subsequent 20-fold reduction in the absorptive capacity of the gut for the same antigen (C. Andre and J. F. Heremans, unpubl.). This, incidentally, might account for the "negative memory" effect mentioned above.

REFERENCES

1. Kobayashi, K., Vaerman, J.-P. and Heremans, J. F., Eur. J. Immunol. 3:185, 1973.
2. Raam, Sh.V. and Inman, F.P., J. Immunol. 110:1044, 1973.
3. Heremans, J.F., in The Antigens, Edited by M. Sela, Academic Press, Inc., in press.
4. Munn, E.A., Feinstein, A. and Munro, A.J., Nature 231: 527, 1971.
5. Jerry, L.M., Junkel, H.G. and Adams, L., J. Immunol. 109:275, 1972.
6. Kobayashi, K., Vaerman, J.-P. and Heremans, J.F., Immunochemistry 10:73, 1973.
7. Brandtzaeg, P., Immunology 21:323, 1971.
8. Brandtzaeg, P., Nature-New Biology 243:142, 1973.
9. Vaerman, J.-P., Studies on IgA Immunoglobulins in Man and Animals, Sintal, Louvain, 1970.
10. Bazin, H., Maldague, P., Schonne, E., Crabbé, P.A., Bauldon, H. and Heremans, J.F., Immunology 20:571, 1971.
11. Bull, D.M., Bienenstock, J. and Tomasi, T.B., Gastroenterology 60:370, 1971.
12. Dive, C., Nadalini, A.R. and Heremans, J.F., Eur. J. Clin. Invest., in press, 1973.
13. Brambell, F.W.R., Hemmings, W.A. and Morris, I.G., Nature 203:1352, 1964.
14. Crabbé, P.A., Nash, D.R., Bazin, H., Eyssen, H. and Heremans, J.F., J. Exp. Med. 130:723, 1969.
15. André, C., Bazin, H. and Heremans, J.F., Digestion, in press, 1973.
16. Weltman, J.K. and Davis, R.P., J. Mol. Biol. 54:177, 1970.

ORIGIN, DISTRIBUTION AND DIFFERENTIATION OF IgA-PRODUCING CELLS

Max D. Cooper, Paul W. Kincade, Dale E.
Bockman, and Alexander R. Lawton
Spain Research Laboratories, Depts. of
Pediatrics and Microbiology, University of
Alabama in Birmingham, Birmingham, Alabama and
Dept. of Anatomy, Medical College of Ohio,
Toledo, Ohio

A large body of experimental data relating to the on-togeny of cells capable of IgA synthesis has been obtained in diverse species over the past few years. In the aggregate, this information suggests that the initial development and distribution of IgA-bearing lymphocytes is relatively thymus- and antigen-independent, whereas normal maturation of B lymphocytes into IgA-secreting plasma cells depends both on antigen stimulation and T cell help. After examining some of the features of these distinct developmental stages of the IgA class of B cells, and their relationship to other classes of B cells, we will raise for discussion the theory that most IgA cells in the intestinal lamina propria are seeded from gut-associated lymphoepithelial tissues (GALT, i.e., Peyer's patches and the appendix) as a result of selection and stimulation by intestinal antigens which enter the lymphoid follicles via specialized follicle-associated epithelial cells.

STEM CELL ORIGIN

Cells of B and T lymphocyte lines, and other lines of cells in the blood, are derived from primitive multi-potential stem cells. The generation of cells capable of IgA synthesis from stem cells is particularly well illus-trated by our observations in an adenosine deaminase de-ficient infant whose lack of T and B cells was repaired by transplantation of fetal liver cells (Figure 1) (1).

13

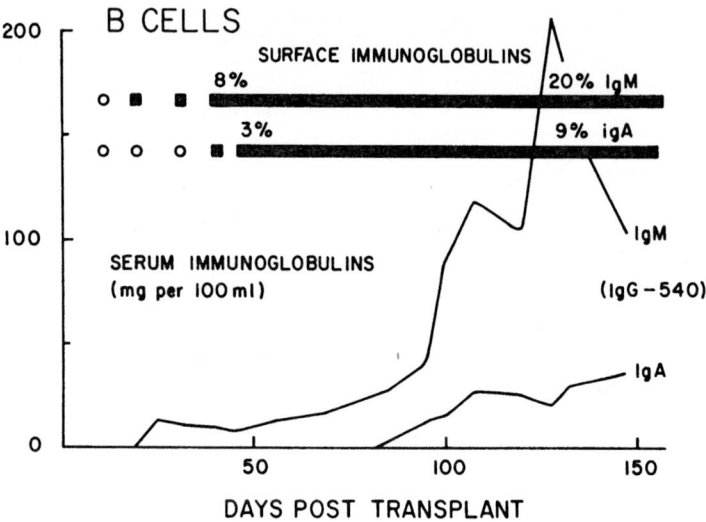

Fig. 1. Development of B-lymphocytes and immunoglobulins
in a patient with severe combined immunodeficiency following transplantation of fetal liver.

IgA-bearing lymphocytes appeared in the recipient's
blood around four weeks after transplantation, one week after
IgM-bearing cells were found. The emergence of IgG-bearing
lymphocytes was obscured by an abundance of IgG-coated mono-
cytic cells. The numbers of IgM- and IgA-bearing lymphocytes quickly increased, but almost three months elapsed
before IgA secreting cells had developed in sufficient numbers to produce detectable amounts of IgA in the serum. The
substantial time lag between the initial appearance of immunoglobulin-bearing B lymphocytes and the subsequent development of mature immunoglobulin-secreting plasma cells is a
feature of normal embryonic development in humans (2, 3);
here, too, the gap is greatest between IgA-bearing and IgA-
secreting cells. IgM-bearing lymphocytes are first found
around the ninth week of gestation. IgG- and IgA-bearing
cells follow in quick succession, and by 14 to 15 weeks all
three classes of B lymphocytes have reached adult proportions
in the circulating blood and spleen. In contrast to the
abundance of IgA-bearing lymphocytes in very young fetuses,
IgA-producing plasma cells have not been found before 31
weeks of fetal life, and serum IgA is usually not detectable
until around birth.
    Although the ontogeny of IgA-bearing cells has not been

so well studied in other species, IgM- and IgG-bearing B
lymphocytes have been shown to develop prior to birth in
pigs (4), guinea pigs (5) and chickens (6). In mice, guinea
pigs and chickens, IgM-bearing cells are the first class of
B lymphocytes to appear. Since immunoglobulin-bearing
lymphocytes, including those of the IgA class, make their
appearance and undergo expansion in an orderly pattern in
the antigen-sheltered intrauterine environment, we conclude
that exogenous antigens do not play a significant role in
their genesis. In support of this conclusion, B lymphocyte
development in the bursa could not be accelerated by de-
liberate antigenic stimulation of chick embryos (7), and
the proportion of splenic B lymphocytes and their class
distribution is similar in mice raised in germ-free and in
conventional environments (8). Development and distribution
of immunoglobulin-bearing B lymphocytes of all classes is
unimpaired in athymic mice (9) and humans (10), indicating
the thymus-independent nature of this stage of B lymphocyte
development.

INDUCTION SITE FOR B LYMPHOCYTES

In order to understand how B lymphocytes are generated,
one needs first to know where they are spawned. In birds,
a dorsal evagination of the hindgut serves this function.
Stem cells of yolk sac origin migrate into the bursal epithelium and are induced shortly after their arrival to produce small amounts of IgM (7). Later, cells are found which
produce detectable amounts of IgG, and still later cells containing small amounts of IgA can be detected. Early embryonic removal of the bursa produces total agammaglobulinemia
for the life of the bird. Bursectomy a little later produces
animals capable of only IgM synthesis in adult life, regardless of the extent of antigenic stimulation. Selective deficiency of IgA can be produced by bursectomy at a critical
time, whereas selective deficiencies of only one of the other
two classes cannot (11). Thus, IgM deficiency is always
accompanied by diminished levels of IgG and IgA, and IgG
deficiency is invariably associated with low or undetectable
IgA levels. In each of these instances, matching deficiencies
in terms of the classes of B lymphocytes and plasma cells are
produced by bursectomy. The first clues as to the basis for
the sequential generation and seeding of the different classes
of bursal lymphocytes were provided by the observations that
(i) IgG-producing cells always appeared in the midst of IgM-

producers in bursal follicles and (ii) many of the bursal lymphocytes containing IgG also appeared to contain IgM whereas "double producers" in the spleen were rare (7).

These observations led to the intrabursal "switch" hypothesis, in the order of IgM→ IgG→ IgA, and to the experiments which confirmed it. Early embryonic injection of goat antibodies to chick u-chain determinants suppressed lymphoid development in the bursa and subsequent synthesis of all three immunoglobulin classes throughout the body; either removal of the bursa after hatching or continued injections of antibodies to u-chains resulted in persistence of the suppression (11, 12). It was also shown that once IgG-committed bursal cells had seeded into the blood stream their subsequent development could not be checked by anti-u. The latter results and the studies employing bursectomy at various times during embryonation revealed the switch in classes to be confined to the bursal stage of B lymphocyte development. In other words, outside of their inductive microenvironment bursal lymphocytes are irrevocably committed as to the class, and probably the specificity, of the antibodies which they and their plasma cell progeny can synthesize.

Experiments employing antibody-mediated suppression of immunoglobulin classes in mice provide data which strongly support our hypothesis that a similar developmental switch in classes of B lymphocytes occurs in mammals (13, 14). Treatment of mice with anti-u from birth to maturity suppresses IgM-, IgG$_1$-, IgG$_2$- and IgA-producing cells. Anti-u treated mice have particularly striking deficits in development of Peyer's patches and thymic independent follicles of spleen and lymph nodes. Immunoglobulin-bearing B lymphocytes are greatly reduced in numbers, and antibody responsiveness is lacking. A striking finding has been the virtual absence of IgA-producing cells in the intestinal lamina propria. T cell development and function in such mice has been extensively examined and found to be normal. Evidence favoring the IgG to IgA part of the switch hypothesis has also been obtained in the immunoglobulin class suppression studies in mice (15). These animals were given anti-u for a short interval after birth to allow time for catabolism of maternally-derived IgG; after 1 week, anti-u injections were stopped and they were given antibodies to IgG$_1$ and IgG$_2$. More than half of the mice so treated had suppressed development of IgG$_1$- and IgG$_2$-producing cells; these mice were also deficient in IgA producing cells and circulating IgA. IgM synthesis was not impaired in any of the mice so treated.

Studies of immunoglobulin structure in humans and mice have revealed that the same heavy chain variable region may be found in association with μ, γ, and α constant regions (16, 17). Our hypothesis and supporting data suggest an orderly mechanism by which this is accomplished during normal development, before the onslaught of environmental antigens. Where this developmental switch in gene expression occurs in mammals is unknown. We have reasoned, by analogy to the chicken, that it may be confined to the bursa-equivalent, but until the location of this site is certain this idea cannot be tested.

ROLE OF ANTIGEN AND T CELLS
IN MATURATION OF IgA B LYMPHOCYTES

In contrast to the antigen-independent development of all classes of immunoglobulin-bearing B lymphocytes, antigens are clearly the major stimulus for division and terminal plasma cell differentiation. Perhaps the best example of this is the relative hypogammaglobulinemia of germ-free rodents, and the rapid increase in levels of immunoglobulins of all classes which occurs with transfer to a conventional environment (18).

For most antigens, complete evolution of the humoral immune response requires interaction of B-cells with macrophages and T-lymphocytes. This concept has been particularly well illustrated in studies of athymic mice. Antigens may induce B-lymphocyte proliferation in these animals without accompanying terminal differentiation (19). The defect in antibody synthesis involves primarily the IgG and IgA response, and can be repaired by a thymus graft (20). The striking thymic dependency of IgA responses has also been demonstrated in rats (21), rabbits (22, 23), and chickens (24), and probably also exists in man.

The precise mechanism of T cell helper activity is still debated but it appears to be mediated in part via macrophages (25). According to our model of B cell differentiation (Figure 2, ref. 26), the hierarchy which exists in the requirement for T cell help in triggering responses in different classes of antibodies is related to the function of the different immunoglobulin classes as B lymphocyte receptors. IgM receptors appear to be more efficient generators of signals to initiate antibody synthesis than IgG or IgA receptors. The reasons for this are unknown. The intensity of fluorescence is notably less for IgA-bearing

lymphocytes than for IgM B lymphocytes when the two are
assessed by fluorchrome-labeled antibodies. Although this
could be explained in several ways, it may be that IgA receptors are less dense than IgM on the surface of B lymphocytes, thus reducing the relative frequency of antigen-
binding to lymphocytes bearing IgA.

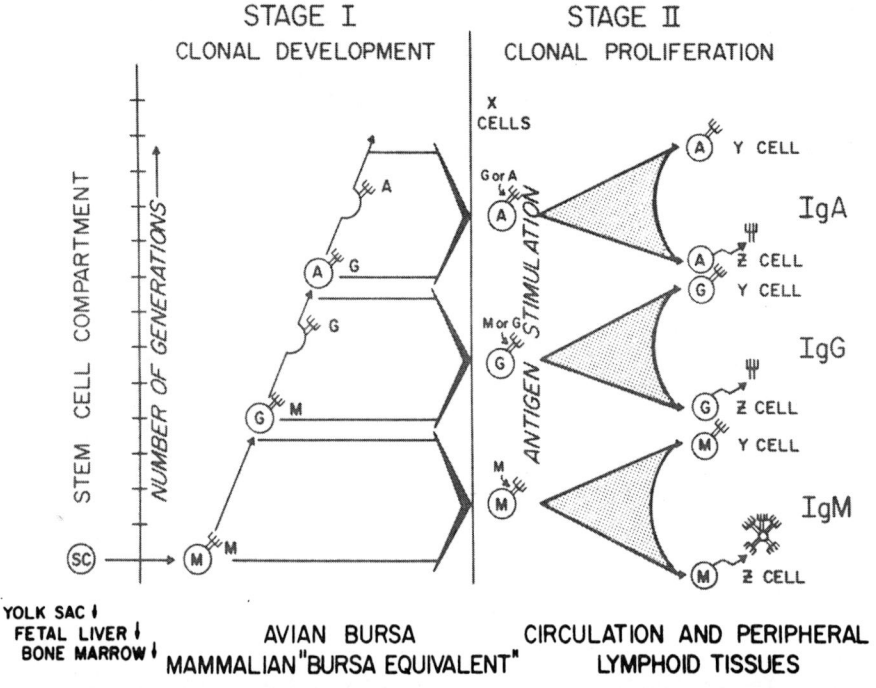

Fig. 2. A model for B-cell differentiation. Reproduced
from Cooper, M. D., Lawton, A. R., and Kincade, P. W.,
Clin. Exp. Immunol. 11:143, 1972 with kind permission of
Blackwell Scientific Publications Ltd.

ROLE OF GALT IN SEEDING IgA CELLS

Both T and B lymphocytes are found in gut-associated
lymphoepithelial tissues (27-29). Development of follicles
of B lymphocytes beneath the dome-shaped epithelium in
Peyer's patches and in the appendix begins during intrauterine life in most if not all mammals, whereas population
of thymus-dependent areas between the follicles does not
generally occur until after birth (30, our unpublished

observations). In porcine fetuses, which are sheltered from
exogenous antigens by a six-layered chorio-epithelial placenta, lymphoid follicles of Peyer's patches make their
appearance by 50 days of gestation (out of a total of about
114 days) (30); this is before significant development of B
cells can be found elsewhere (31). Follicular lymphoid
development in the human appendix also begins early in
fetal life. In the uninflamed appendixes of young children
B cells may predominate over T cells by as much as an eight
to one ratio (our unpublished observations).

In addition to the influx of T cells into GALT, striking
changes in the follicles of B lymphocytes are also seen
following birth (See ref. 32). There is a marked increase
in size of the follicles, whose base expands and comes to
lie against the muscle layer of the intestinal wall. In
addition, GALT follicles become compartmentalized into a
cortex, containing rapidly dividing medium-sized to large
lymphoblasts, and a less densely populated medulla, containing smaller and less active lymphoid cells. Intestinal antigens, including bacteria, are clearly involved in stimulating
these changes; cortico-medullary division of Peyer's patch
follicles may be totally undeveloped in germ-free mice unless
they are fed microorganisms (33).

An efficient epithelial channel by which intralumenal
antigens are transported into the follicular areas of GALT
has been found in chickens (bursa), rabbits, mice and man
(34). After the lymphoid follicles have begun their embryonic development, epithelial cells overlying them begin a
specialized pattern of cytodifferentiation. These follicle-
associated cells are characterized by sparse irregular micro-
villae and a dense apical cytoplasm containing numerous
micropinocytotic vesicles and vacuoles. Particulate substances placed in the lumen are rapidly transported to sub-
epithelial lymphoid areas through these specialized cells.

Not only do antigens induce proliferation and blast
transformation of B cells in GALT follicles of rats and
rabbits, but whether injected directly into the follicle or
placed in the intestinal lumen, antigens induce an exodus of
B cells to other sites where they may undergo plasma cell
differentiation (35, 36). The fate of the antigen-mobilized
B lymphocytes can be inferred by consideration of the
following related observations. Large lymphoblasts in
thoracic duct lymph of rats show a strong preference for
homing to the intestine (37, also see the paper by Guy-Grand,
et al., in this volume). When injected intravenously, they
they make their way to the intestinal lamina propria where

they become mature plasma cells, but they do not migrate
in significant numbers into Peyer's patches. Finally, it
has been shown that Peyer's patches of mature rabbits are
an enriched source of precursors of IgA-producing cells,
and when injected intravenously most of these migrate to the
intestinal lamina propria (38, see article by Cebra, et al.
in this volume).

The following hypothetical framework is offered for
discussion and should be easily testable. GALT are sites
of early antigen-independent development of B lymphocyte
clones. Subsequent specialized differentiation of highly
pinocytotic epithelial cells overlying the follicles provide
an efficient pathway for entry of intestinal antigens, including Gram negative bacteria. The intestinal antigens
select appropriate B lymphocytes, and, aided by lipopolysaccharide B cell mitogens, they expand their numbers by
inducing proliferation, trigger terminal differentiation,
and induce an exodus of stimulated B lymphoblasts into the
draining lymphatics. The latter make their way into the
bloodstream from whence they home to the intestinal lamina
propria and mature into antibody-secreting plasma cells.
In normal mature animals a majority of these cells produce
IgA antibodies, which in turn regulate the flow of ingested
antigens across the intestinal epithelium. Thus, an
efficient way is provided for the selection and distribution
of sentinel cells to patrol the vast border of the intestinal
absorptive surface, and perhaps other mucous surfaces as
well.

REFERENCES

1. Keightley, R.G., Lawton, A.R., Wu, L.Y.F., and Cooper,
      M.D., Exp. Hematol. In press.
2. Lawton, A.R., Self, K.S., Royal, S.A., and Cooper, M.D.,
      Clin. Immunol. Immunopath. 1:104-121, 1972.
3. Van Furth, R., Schuit, H.R.E., and Hijmans, W., J. Exp.
      Med. 122:1173-1188, 1965.
4. Binns, R.M., Feinstein, A., Gurner, B.W., and Coombs,
      R.R.A., Nature New Biol. 239:114-116, 1972.
5. Davie, J.M., and Paul, W.E. in Contemporary Topics in
      Immunobiology, Vol. 3, M.D. Cooper and N.L. Warner, eds.,
      Plenum Press, N. Y., 1973. In press.
6. Kincade, P.W., Lawton, A.R., and Cooper, M.D., J. Immunol.
      106:1421-1423, 1971.

7. Kincade, P.W., and Cooper, M.D., J. Immunol. 106:371-382, 1971.
8. Lawton, A.R., and Asofsky, R., Unpublished observations.
9. Bankhurst, A.D., and Warner, N.L., Aust. J. Exp. Biol. Med. Sci. 50:661, 1972.
10. Gajl-Peczalska, K.J., Park, B.H., Biggar, W.D. and Good, R.A., J. Clin. Invest. 52:919.
11. Kincade, P.W., and Cooper, M.D., Science 179:398-400, 1973.
12. Kincade, P.W., Lawton, A.R., Bockman, D.E., and Cooper, M.D., Proc. Nat. Acad. Sci. 67:1918-1925, 1970.
13. Lawton, A.R., Asofsky, R., Hylton, M.B., and Cooper, M.D., J. Exp. Med. 135:277-297, 1972.
14. Manning, D.D., and Jutila, J.W., J. Exp. Med. 135:1316-1333, 1972.
15. Lawton, A.R., Asofsky, R.M., Davie, J.M., and Hylton, M.B., Fed. Proc. 32:1012, 1973.
16. Wang, A.C., Wilson, S.K., Hopper, J.E., Fudenberg, H.H., and Nisonoff, A., PNAS 66:337-343, 1970.
17. Scornik, J., Kluskens, L., and Kohler, H., Fed. Proc. 32:989 Abs, 1973.
18. Fahey, J.L., and Sell, S., J. Exp. Med. 122:41, 1965.
19. Roelants, G.E., and Askonas, B.A., Nature New Biol. 239:63, 1972.
20. Pritchard, H., Riddaway, J., and Micklem, H.S., Clin. Exp. Immunol. 13:125, 1973.
21. Buckton, K.E., and Pike, M.C., Nature 202:714-715, 1964.
22. Perey, D.Y.E., Frommel, D., Hong, R., and Good, R.A., Lab. Invest. 22:212-227, 1970.
23. Clough, J.D., Mims, L.H., and Strober, W., J. Immunol. 106:1624-1629, 1971.
24. Perey, D.Y.E., and Bienenstock, J., J. Immunol. 111:633, 1973.
25. Feldman, M., J. Exp. Med., 135:1049, 1972.
26. Cooper, M.D., Lawton, A.R., and Kincade, P.W., Clin. Exp. Immunol. 11:143-149, 1972.
27. DeSousa, M.A.B., Parrott, D.M.V., and Pantelouris, E.M., Clin. Exp. Immunol. 4:637, 1969.
28. Raff, M.C., and Owen, J.J.T., Eur. J. Immunol. 1:27, 1971.
29. Levin, D.M., Rosenstreich, D.L., and Reynolds, H.Y., J. Immunol. III:980-983, 1973.
30. Chapman, H.A., Johnson, J.S., and Cooper, M.D., J. Immunol. In press.
31. Symons, D.B.A., and Binns, R.M., Int. Res. Commun. Sept. 1973.

32. Waksman, B.H., Ozer, H., and Blythman, H.E., Lab. Invest. 28:614, 1973.
33. Pollard, M., and Sharon, N., Inf. and Immunity 2:96, 1970.
34. Bockman, D.E., and Cooper, M.D., Am. J. Anat. 136:455-478, 1973.
35. Cooper, G.N., and Turner, K., Aust. J. Exp. Biol. Med. Sci. 45:363, 1967.
36. Hanaoka, M., and Waksman, B.H., Cellular Immunol. 1:316, 1970.
37. Hall, J.G., Parry, D.M., and Smith, M.E., Cell Tissue Kinetics 5:269, 1972.
38. Craig, S.W., and Cebra, J.J., J. Exp. Med. 134:188, 1971.

CELL TYPES CONTRIBUTING TO THE BIOSYNTHESIS OF sIgA

John J. Cebra, Susan W. Craig and Patricia
P. Jones
Department of Biology
The Johns Hopkins University
Baltimore, Maryland

INTRODUCTION

Almost a decade ago different isotypes of immunoglobulin were found, by immunohistochemical analysis, to be localized in different plasma cells and it was inferred that circulating IgA was synthesized by the unique class of plasma cells which contained this protein (1,2). Thus it seemed particularly encouraging to efforts to locate the sites of synthesis of secretory IgA (sIgA) when Tomasi and his colleagues found many IgA containing lymphoid cells in the interstitial tissue between acini of human salivary glands (3) and Heremans and coworkers found copious numbers of IgA immunocytes (400,000/mm³) in the lamina propria of human intestine (4). Our analysis of the rabbit ileum by double fluorescent antibody staining confirmed the abundance of IgA lymphoid cells in the lamina propria and revealed the skewed distribution of IgA containing lymphoid cells in favor of intestinal mucosa compared with spleen and peripheral lymph nodes (5). The IgA immunocytes comprise 80-90% of the total population of plasma cells in the rabbit intestinal mucosa but they only make up about 5% of the total in spleen and peripheral lymph nodes. A possible explanation for the preponderance of IgA containing cells in secretory tissue in contrast to their relative scarcity elsewhere is that there are "central" lymphoid tissues which give rise to IgA plasma cell precursors uniquely able to selectively populate gut lamina propria and the interstitia of exocrine glands. Alternatively, each locale may contain a mixed population of lymphocytes which include some that are pre-

23

committed to give rise to IgA-producing daughters and that
are selectively stimulated. If, however, lymphocytes are
not necessarily committed to the synthesis of a particular
Ig class before antigenic stimulation, it may be that the
secretory tissue environment can somehow influence plasma
cell precursors to generate cells producing IgA.

A few years ago we sought to assess the potential of
lymphoid cells taken from different sources to generate IgA
plasma cells and to re-populate intestinal lamina propria
by transferring allogeneic lymphoid cells from rabbits of
one Ig allotype (b5, kappa chain marker) into lethally-
irradiated recipients of another allotype (b4)(6-8). We
found that when equal numbers of cells from the peripheral
blood, popliteal lymph nodes and Peyer's patches from the
same donor rabbit were transferred separately into groups
of recipients, only cells from the Peyer's patches generated
plasma cells in the intestinal lamina propria (6). Extensive repopulation occurred with inocula of as few as 5 x
10^5 lymphocytes and almost all of the plasma cells bearing
the donor's allotype marker contained IgA. This finding
has prompted us to undertake an extensive analysis of Peyer's
patch lymphocytes with respect to their membrane immunoglobulin components, their proliferative and differentia-
tive potential, and their synthetic abilities. Further, we
have fractionated this heterogeneous population of cells
and have identified an immediate IgA plasma cell precursor
which has unique characteristics.

RESULTS

Potential of Peyer's Patch Lymphocytes to Generate
Plasma Cells in Vivo and in Vitro.

One method for assessing the proliferation and differ-
entiative potential of lymphocytes is by the allogeneic
transfer of cells from different tissues from rabbits of
one allotype into lethally irradiated (900R) recipients of
a different allotype. The spleens of the recipients, by 6
days after transfer, contain large clusters of plasma cells
that usually surround blood vessels in the red pulp of the
spleen (9) and most of the component cells contain the
donor's allotype marker. These re-populated spleens may be
rendered into single cell suspensions and the proportions of
total donor plasma cells containing each of three major isotypes of Ig can be determined by double fluorescent staining
of different samples for donor b marker and a particular
class of heavy chain. By this technique we have shown that

equal inocula of Peyer's patch and popliteal lymphocytes result in about equal numbers of donor plasma cells in recipients' spleens, although the Peyer's patch lymphocytes
yield predominantly IgA plasma cells while those lymphocytes
from popliteal nodes generate mostly IgG cells (6). Table I
shows the results from the assay of spleen cell suspensions
from eleven b^4/b^4 recipient rabbits which each received
5×10^6 Peyer's patch lymphocytes from one of two donor
rabbits (b^5/b^5 or b^9/b^9, respectively). The spleens examined six days after transfer, show a preponderance of
IgA cells and only about 1% of IgM cells. Thus, if there
are large numbers of IgM precursors cells in Peyer's patches,
they are not stimulated to divide and differentiate in the
allogeneic transfer system. Since few donor plasma cells
are found in recipient spleens before day 6 after transfer,
the possibility that a "switch" occurs from IgM producing
plasma cells to IgA cells seems unlikely. The fact that
popliteal lymph node cells generate very few IgA plasma cells

TABLE I

Frequency of Donor (b5 or b9) IgA, IgG and IgM Plasma Cells
in Spleens of b^4/b^4 Recipients of Peyer's Patch Cells Six
Days after Cell Transfer[1]

Recipient[2]	% Donor Cells Containing[3]:		
	IgA	IgM	IgG
1	98.5	0.3	6.0
2	89.0	0.6	7.5
3	81.5	0.8	12.5
4	77.0	0	14.0
5	77.0	0	10.5
6	76.0	0.4	13.0
7	75.0	0	7.0
8	79.0	0.1	10.0
9	98.7	1.3	0.3
10	99.0	1.2	0.3
11	100	0.5	0

1 Adapted from (7,8)
2 Recipients 1-8 received b5 cells, recipients 9-11 received b9 cells
3 Percentages calculated for each class of Ig separately
  taking the number of cells stained for donor b marker as
  100%.

in spleens of irradiated recipients (6) seems to rule out
the influence of the tissue milieu in distorting the proportion of IgA plasma cells generated by a given sample of precursor lymphocytes.

In the spleens alone from irradiated recipients repopu-
lated with Peyer's patch lymphocytes the yield of different
classes of donor plasma cells was 300-1,200 IgM cells/10^6
splenic white cells, 10,000-30,000 IgG cells/10^6 and 35,000-
100,000 IgA cells/10^6 at 6 days after transfer. Considering
that extensive re-population of the gut lamina propria with
donor IgA plasma cells also occurs, this in vivo assay would
appear to measure and weight particularly those precursor
cells capable of considerable proliferation and differentiation.

An alternative way to assess the potential of lymphocytes is to culture them in vitro in the presence or absence
of pokeweed mitogen. Micro-cultures, initially containing
2.5 x 10^5 lymphocytes, are incubated for 4 days (10); the
cells are then stained with fluorescent-antibody reagents
after fixation and the absolute numbers of cytoplasmic immu-
noglobulin-stained cells (CSC) and the relative numbers containing each isotype can be determined. Table II shows that
the proportion of plasma cells in fresh Peyer's patch cell
suspensions is extremely low - 0.6 to 1.2% - as has been re-

TABLE II

Plasma Cells Containing Different Classes of Ig Present before and after Culture of Peyer's Patch Lymphocytes [1]

Cells	% membrane stained for μ	% CSC[2]	% (of total CSC)		
			IgA	IgG	IgM
Before culture	34	1.0	43	0	55
" "	38	0.6	51	0	52
" "	35	1.0	42	3	53
" "	52	1.2	41	0	58
After culture	-	11	11	0	82
" "	-	6.5	14	0	83
" "	-	9.3	22	0	73
After culture(+PWM)[3]	-	18	60	0	41
" "	-	11	64	0	37
" "	-	20	67	0	30

1 Adapted from (12)
2 Cytoplasmic stained cells
3 Pokeweed mitogen

ported by others (11). Those CSC that are present seem
evenly divided between IgM and IgA cells. After culture for
four days, the proportion of surviving cells that are CSC
increases to 6.5-11%, and if pokeweed mitogen is present,
the percentage of CSC reaches 11-20. About 80% of the CSC
in unstimulated cultures are IgM cells. In contrast, 63%
of the CSC are IgA cells after Peyer's patch cells are cultured in the presence of the mitogen, a percentage of such
cells slightly higher than observed in the original inoculum.
Most cultures show an absolute increase of 2-5 fold with
respect to their original content of CSC. Since the number
of CSC usually drops in the first few days of culture and
then increases by day 4 or 5 it is likely that most of the
plasma cells in the four day cultures have come from differ-
entiating and/or dividing lymphocytes. Thus this in vitro
assay supports the observations with allogeneic transfers
indicating that precursors for IgA plasma cells occur in the
Peyer's patches, and it also shows, perhaps more clearly,
the potential of some lymphocytes from this source to generate IgM plasma cells.

The Membrane Immunoglobulin of Peyer's Patch
Lymphocytes and Its Replacement after Enzymic Removal

The B-lymphocyte precursors of plasma cells bear Ig
determinants on their plasma membranes, and these markers
may be visualized by either single-layer or double-layer
staining of the living cells with fluorescent anti-globulin
(13,14). We have analyzed populations of Peyer's patch
lymphocytes from many rabbits using goat anti-μ, anti-α,
anti-γ, anti-SC, and anti-b4 antibodies. All these reagents
were rendered specific by using a variety of appropriate
Sepharose-bound antigens to remove unwanted antibodies. In
addition, the anti-γ and anti-α were purified on columns of
Sepharose-IgG and Sepharose-IgA, respectively, to remove
naturally occurring goat anti-rabbit membrane antibodies.

The fluorescent anti-b4 and anti-μ were found to stain
directly a fraction of the cells. The indirect method,
using fluorescent rabbit anti-goat Ig, was obligatory for
visualization of SC, γ-chain and α-chain on the lymphocytes.
Table III tabulates the fraction of Peyer's patch lymphocytes bearing detectable amounts of each polypeptide on their
membranes. All the staining activity is removed if the
diagnostic anti-Ig used is first passed through a Sepharose-
Ig absorbant containing the homologous antigeneic determinants before it is applied to the cells. The data indicate that significant fractions of these lymphocytes bear

TABLE III

Percentage of Lymphocytes in Fresh Cell Suspensions from
Peyer's Patches Containing Various Ig Determinants on Their
Surface [1]

Rabbit #	b4 [2]	α [3]	γ [3]	μ [2]	SC [3]
1	30	43	7	28	41
2	29	44	8	26	43
3	23	-	7	30	-
4	36	43	9	-	40
5	36	61	7	-	32
6	29	44	-	-	39
7	27	52	-	-	46
8	36	43	-	-	40
Av. %	31	47	8	28	40

1 Adapted from (7).
2 Directly stained with labeled goat anti-Ig.
3 Indirectly stained with unlabeled goat anti-Ig followed
  by labeled rabbit anti-goat Ig.

b4, α, μ and SC determinants and that few cells carry detectable γ-chain determinants. The percentages given are not to
be taken as absolute or maximum figures since these values
vary with the instruments used for fluorescence microscopy,
the quality of the reagent antibodies and the method of
staining. For instance, use of another microscope or the
indirect method of staining often yields percentage of μ
and b4 stained cells 10-15% above those given in Table III.

In order to confirm the occurrence of polypeptide
chains containing b4, α, μ and SC determinants on the membranes of Peyer's patch lymphocytes we have used lactoperoxidase catalyzed, H_2O_2 driven radio-iodination to ex-
trinsically label these components on the surfaces of the
living cells (15,16). The characterization of polypeptide
chains labeled by this method is based not only on the use
of specific anti-globulin reagents to isolate and identify
labeled product but also on identification of the polypeptides by their electrophoretic mobility characteristics in
polyacrylamide gels (15,16). In this way the α-, μ-, SC-
and light (b4) polypeptides were isolated and clearly identified from NP-40 lysates of these lymphocytes.

The mere occurrence of any particular polypeptide on
the surface of a lymphocyte cannot be taken to signify synthesis of that component by the cell. For instance, we have

shown that a fraction of Peyer's patch lymphocytes from
$\underline{b}^4/\underline{b}^5$ or $\underline{b}^5/\underline{b}^9$ heterozygous rabbits bear both parental allotype markers on their surface (17). These cells may be
treated with pronase under conditions (0.25% pronase, 37°,
45 min.) that permit removal of all detectable membrane
light chain markers without affecting their viability. When
these cells are then cultured for 24 hours, they regenerate
one or the other parental allotype on their membrane, but
very few if any cells exhibit both allotypes (17). These
observations and others have led us to suggest that at least
some of the Ig determinants found on rabbit lymphocytes are
of exogenous origin, having been synthesized by cells
different from those to which they are found adhering. When
Peyer's patch lymphocytes were subjected to pronase digestion
under the above conditions most of the Ig determinants were
removed from the cells. During subsequent culture of the
cells for 24-48 hours, a progressive increase in the number
of cells with μ-chain and b4 markers occurred (see Fig. 1)
but no cells bearing SC, α- or γ-chain re-appeared. Usually
about 5-10% more of the cultured cells were positive for
light chain and μ-chain after this treatment than were
scored as positive in the original cell suspension. The
striking finding, however, was that the Peyer's patch lymphocytes did not appear to renew the elements of sIgA - α-chain
and SC-determinants - that were originally found on their
membranes. Since we have shown that Peyer's patches are a
rich source of precursors for IgA plasma cells, these observations raised the possibility that most or all IgA plasma
cells spring directly from B-lymphocytes bearing IgM receptors on their surfaces and we set about to test this notion.

Fluorescence-activated Cell Sorting of Peyer's Patch Lymphocytes Which Had Regenerated Surface Ig After Pronase Treat-
                ment and Subsequent Culture
        Herzenberg and his colleagues have developed an instru-
ment which sorts a cell population on the basis of the amount
of membrane-bound fluorochrome carried by individual cells
(18). The instrument imparts an electric charge to droplets
containing cells with a fluorescence emission above a pre-
determined level, and then pulls out these droplets in an
electric field without impairing the in vitro or in vivo
viability of the cells (18,19). We have collaborated with
the Herzenberg group to fractionate rabbit lymphocytes on
the basis of their surface content of two Ig polypeptides
of different allotypes (20) or different isotypes (12).
The living cells were membrane-stained consecutively with

antibodies of two different specificities labeled with contrasting fluorochromes using our standard procedures (21) and were then sorted out into different fractions on the basis of their membrane content of first one and then the other fluorochrome. In this way, by passing Peyer's patch lymphocytes twice through the cell sorter cells which were μ+b+, μ-b+, and μ-b- could be obtained.

The recovered fractions of the total lymphocyte population were tested for their ability to generate IgA plasma cells using the in vivo assay of allogeneic transfer and the in vitro assay of micro-culture with pokeweed mitogen. Table IV shows that only spleens from irradiated b4 recipients of 5 x 10^5 cells from the μ- or the μ-b5+ fractions contained significant numbers of donor CSC and these were almost all IgA plasma cells. Spleens from recipients of μ+b5+ or μ-b5- cells showed few, if any, donor plasma cells.

TABLE IV

Donor Plasma Cells in Spleens from Recipients of Fractionated Peyer's Patch Lymphocytes [1]

	Inoculum		No. b5 CSC/	% IgA
Recipient	Cells	No. x 10^5	10^6 total cells	(of total b5 CSC)
10	μ+	5.0	48	-
11	"	5.0	60	-
12	"	5.0	0	-
13	μ-	2.5	430	100
14	"	2.5	960	100
15	"	5.0	1030	99
16	μ-,b5+	2.5	6600	100
17	"	2.5	930	100
18	μ-,b5-	5.0	0	-
19	"	5.0	0	-

1 Adapted from (12).

In Table V, some representative data is given showing the striking difference in potential to generate particular classes of plasma cells between the μ+b5+ and μ-b5+ fractions in microculture. In the presence or absence of pokeweed mitogen, μ+ cells gave rise predominantly to IgM plasma cells while μ- cells generated mainly IgA CSC. Of the further fractions of μ- cells, the μ-b5+ cells clearly included the precursors for the IgA plasma cells while the μ-b5- cells yielded few CSC. In all cases most CSC have arisen by division and/or differentiation of cells in the inoculum since in positive cultures their absolute numbers exceeded

TABLE V
Recovery of Total Cells and of Plasma Cells after Culture
of Fractionated Peyer's Patch Lymphocytes [1]

Cells	PWM	No. viable cells/culture x 10^3	% CSC	% (of total CSC) IgA	IgG	IgM
μ+	-	21	22	2.7	0	98
"	-	27	7.5	3.5	0	98
"	+	28	28	3.0	0	96
"	+	45	9.0	5.0	0	96
μ-	-	51	1.1	88	0	8.0
"	-	88	18	98	0	2.0
"	+	54	18	99	0	0.7
"	+	146	30	95	0	3.0
μ-,b5+	+	84	12	97	0.7	0.7
"	+	75	11	100	0	0
μ-,b5-	+	22	0	-	-	-
"	+	40	0.1	-	-	-

1 Adapted from (12).

the CSC originally present by about 2-10X. Thus the immediate precursor of IgA plasma cells in the Peyer's patches
appears to occur in a sub-population of lymphocytes which
has no detectable membrane μ-chain and which comprises about
20% of the total population of cells which bear light chain
markers on their surface and about 8% of total lymphocytes.

DISCUSSION
        It is not known whether the μ-b+ cells among Peyer's
patch lymphocytes bear a class of heavy chain other than μ
on their surface. If these cells, which contain almost all
of the immediate precursors for IgA plasma cells as measured
by both in vitro and in vivo assays, do have elements of
α-chain on their membrane, its Fc portion must be cryptic,
i.e., inaccessible to our anti-α reagents. Perhaps this
presumptive heavy chain may be available for radioiodina-
tion by lactoperoxidase and hence eventually be identified.
At any rate, the μ-b+ cells make up, at most, only 10% of
the total lymphocyte population, so we do not think that
the 47% and 40% of cells in freshly prepared Peyer's patch
cell suspension which contain surface α-chain or SC respectively are necessarily related to the IgA plasma cell precursors or represent cells with self-made IgA receptors.
Thus our suggestion that local SC in lamina propria or

secretory tissue interstitia may affect the selective lodg-
ing of IgA precursors (6) must be held in reserve until
further surface properties and tissue distribution of the
µ-b+ population of lymphocytes can be evaluated.

     In vitro, almost no IgG plasma cells are generated by
any of the fractions of cultured Peyer's patch lymphocytes. Further, despite the abundance of IgA plasma cells
in the spleens of recipients of allogeneic Peyer's patch
cells, only a small fraction of the CSC are IgG plasma cells
and these do not appear earlier than IgA cells. These observations lead us to doubt the validity of a proposal by
Cooper and his colleagues that plasma cell precursors pass
through a sequence depicted as IgM → IgG → IgA cells (22).
We feel our data indicate that the immediate precursor
lymphocytes for clones of IgA plasma cells are distinct
from those bearing membrane IgM. However, the sum of our
observations is consistent with these precursors being
generated directly from lymphocytes bearing IgM without any
intervening synthesis of IgG.

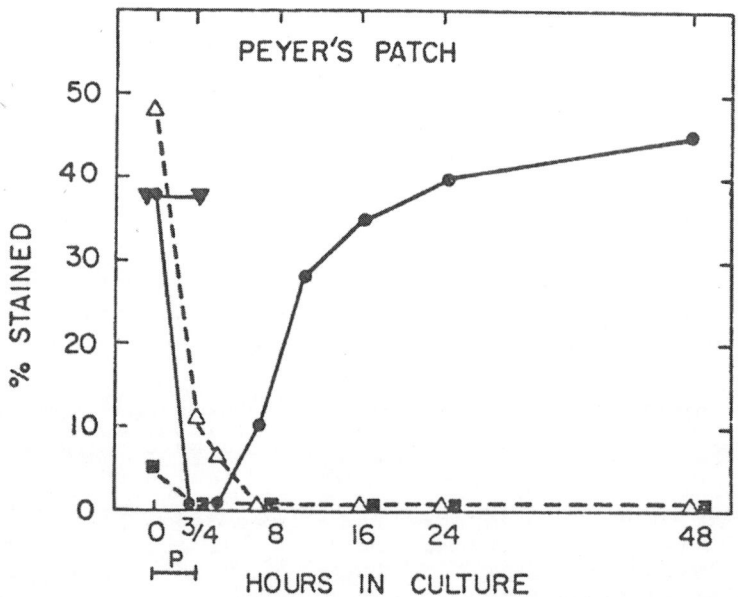

Figure 1. In vitro regeneration of membrane Ig after removal
with pronase.   ⊢P⊣ , duration of enzyme treatment; ● —— ●,
cells stained with anti-µ; Δ --- Δ, cells stained with
anti-α; ■---■, cells stained with anti-γ; ▼ —— ▼, not
pronase treated but stained with anti-µ.

REFERENCES

1. Mellors, R.C. and Korngold, L., J. Exp. Med. 118:387, 1963.
2. Bernier, G.M. and Cebra, J.J., J. Immunol. 95:246, 1965.
3. Tomasi, T.B., Jr., Tan, E.M., Solomon, A. and Prendergast, R.A., J. Exp. Med. 121:101, 1965.
4. Crabbe, P.A., Carbonara, A.O. and Heremans, J.F., Lab. Invest. 14:235, 1965.
5. Crandall, R.B., Cebra, J.J. and Crandall, C.A., Immunology, 12:147, 1967.
6. Craig, S.W. and Cebra, J.J., J. Exp. Med. 134:188, 1971.
7. Craig, S.W., Rabbit Secretory Immunoglobulin A: Cellular Studies, Dissertation, Johns Hopkins University, 1973.
8. Craig, S.W. and Cebra, J.J. in New Approaches for Inducing Natural Immunity to Pyogenic Organisms. Edited by R.M. Krause, J.B. Robbins and R.E. Horton. Govt. Printing Press (in press).
9. Frensdorff, A., Jones, P.P., Berwald-Netter, Y., Cebra, J.J. and Mage, R.G., Science 171:391, 1971.
10. E. Lennox, personal communication.
11. Faulk, W.P., McCormick, J.N., Goodman, J.R., Yoffey, J.M. and Fudenberg, H.H., Cell Immunol. 1:500, 1971.
12. Jones, P.P., Craig, S.W. and Cebra, J.J. (in preparation).
13. Raff, M.C., Steinberg, M. and Taylor, R.B., Nature 225:553, 1970.
14. Pernis, B., Forni, L. and Amanti, L., J. Exp. Med. 132:1001, 1970.
15. Marchalonis, J.J., Cone, R.E. and Atwell, J.L., J. Exp. Med. 135:956, 1972.
16. Vitetta, E.S., Baur, S. and Uhr, J.W., J. Exp. Med. 134:242, 1971.
17. Jones, P.P., Cebra, J.J. and Herzenberg, L.A., J. Immunol. 1973 (in press)
18. Bonner, W.A., Hulett, H.R., Sweet, R.G. and Herzenberg, L.A., Rev. Sci. Instrum. 43:404, 1972.
19. Lulius, M.H., Masuda, T. and Herzenberg, L.A., Proc. Nat. Acad. Sci. 69:1934, 1972.
20. Jones, P.P., Cebra, J.J. and Herzenberg, L.A. (in preparation).
21. Cebra, J.J. and Goldstein, G., J. Immunol. 95:230, 1965.
22. Cooper, M.D., Lawton, A.R. and Kincard, P.W., Clin. Exp. Immunol. 11:143, 1972.

DISCUSSION

Dr. Good - I have a question for Dr. Cebra. Have you looked for any other B-cell markers on these cells that do not seem to have surface immunoglobulins but that can act as precursors to IgA. For instance, do they have the C3 receptor or the Fc receptor for IgG?

Dr. Cebra - No we have not. Of course they have one very characteristic B-cell marker which is the light chain (the κ chain) on their plasma membrane. We have not looked for any of the other B-cell markers that you have mentioned.

Dr. Good - The reason for raising this question is the possibility that the precursors may not be determined with respect to immunoglobulin class until after stimulation. That is somewhat different from the way we have ordinarily thought about it. These cells that are preliminary or precursor to the B-cells might not have light or heavy chains until after this step in differentiation.

Dr. Cebra - I would like to ask Dr. Cooper whether, in any of his suppression experiments done in mice, he used anti-allotype reagents raised in mice to the IgG_{2a} or IgG_{2b} allotypes so that he could be quite sure that he was ablating their IgG response with antibodies directed against the γ chain?

Dr. Cooper - No, allotype markers were not used in the IgG suppression studies of Lawton and Asofsky, but the anti-antibodies were isolated from IgG affinity columns after several passes over affinity columns bearing IgM or IgA.

It is surprising to me, Dr. Cebra, that you view your results as not being predicted by our model. As a matter of fact, our switch model is the only one stating that outside of the induction microenvironment B-cells are committed to the immunoglobulin class that they and their progeny can make. Others have viewed the switch in classes as a later event which is triggered by antigens. Your results in rabbits showing class commitment closely parallel our data obtained in chickens indicating that B-lymphocytes

outside of the bursa are irrevocably committed as to the
class of immunoglobulins which they and their progeny can
make.

The failure of resynthesis of surface immunoglobulins of non-IgM classes following pronase stripping is
most intriguing, but may not disprove the notion that the
immunoglobulin found on the cells before pronase treatment
was made by the cells bearing it. One possibility is that
you are facing difficulties based on different thresholds
of detection of the various immunoglobulin classes on the
surface of B-lymphocytes. In the first place, fluorescence
of IgM positive cells is always far brighter than that of
IgG- and IgA-bearing cells, as indicated in your experiments
by the need to use a double antibody technique to detect
the latter two classes on the surfaces of cells. This
suggests that the density of surface immunoglobulins detectable by your fluoresceinated antisera is less for IgG- and
IgA-bearing cells than for IgM-bearing cells. This would
favor detection of IgM synthesis over surface IgG and IgA
replacement, particularly if less than optimum conditions
for cell culture were used. For example, Dr. Frank Wu in
our laboratory could show, under conditions that were
probably suboptimum for culturing human peripheral blood
lymphocytes, that by two days all of the B-lymphocytes in
culture had lost surface immunoglobulins in detectable
amounts. Even so, he could still add pokeweed mitogen at
that point and induce perfectly normal generation of
immunoglobulin producing and secreting cells of all classes
five days later.

There are certain circumstances in which B-
lymphocytes bearing M, G and A can be demonstrated in the
total absence of plasma cells making and secreting those
classes of antibodies, as for example in agammaglobulinemic
patients with B-lymphocytes and under normal conditions early
in fetal life. In each of these circumstances exogenous
sources are lacking for the immunoglobulins which the B-
lymphocytes bear; it would be interesting to see if resynthesis of surface IgG and IgA could be demonstrated under
your culture conditions.

Dr. Cebra - I would go along with your interpretation that
our results could be considered as complementary to your
own. We can begin to detect IgM or the b-locus markers of
light chain within 4 hours after pronase stripping and by
12 hours the intensity of staining is about the same as at
48 hours. I believe that if there are alpha chain markers

present, they are situated differently from those that we
see on fresh Peyer's patch cells. I also am quite convinced
(see J. Immunol. Nov., 1973) that there is a considerable
amount of adventitious immunoglobulin on lymphocytes and
that this accounts for some of the isotypic determinants
observed on fresh lymphocytes. In an effort to detect alpha
chain on stripped and cultured cells we have done biosynthesis studies and looked for incorporation of ^{3}H-leucine
into each isotype. I omitted the results of these studies
after having heard Dr. Melchers at the Physiology meetings
(Sept., 1973, Woods Hole). As little as one-half percent
of plasma cells in a suspension of lymphocytes can account
for most of the products synthesized. Our Peyer's patch
lymphocytes, which after Ig stripping do not contain
detectable membrane IgA, do synthesize and incorporate ^{3}H-
leucine into IgA but we can't rule out that it is a product
of a few percent or less of the cells. I do agree with your
general comment that we should look harder for heavy chain
markers on the μ-b+ cells - for instance for variable region
markers (a markers) and the f and g allotypic markers of
alpha chain.

Dr. Leslie - We have been doing some work on immunoglobulin
class suppression in the chicken and have results that are
very comparable to what Dr. Cebra suggested and not entirely
inconsistent with Max's work. We have been trying to do
selective IgA suppression using anti-alpha and have been only
partially successful in doing this even in conjunction with
neonatal bursectomy. We found using specifically purified
anti-μ, anti-α and combinations thereof, that anti-α
produces significant suppression of both IgA and IgM. If
we give anti-μ about the time of hatch we still get suppression of M and A and no suppression of what Max calls
IgG in the chicken and what we call IgY. The combined
administration of anti-μ and anti-α had greater suppressive
effects on IgM and IgA than either antibody alone and had
no suppressive effect on IgY production. So we feel that
this differentiation process appears to involve an M to A
switch with very few cells going through the postulated
intermediate pathway of M to G or G to A.

Dr. Bienenstock - Dr. Perey, Rudzik, and myself have carried
out some of the experiments that were so elegantly described
by John Cebra. Craig and Cebra's model used allogeneic
transfer from one rabbit into another. We in fact have used
transfer from one rabbit into the same rabbit, an isogeneic

system. We take out the Peyer's patches, irradiate the
animal, and then transfer the Peyer's patch cells back into
the same individual. The results are rather strikingly
different from those reported and shown today. They suggest
that the turning on of these cells to IgA production which
occurs in the spleen is not found in the syngeneic system.
We find no increase in IgA cells over the normal background
in the spleen; however, when we look at the gut, we find
large numbers of IgA producing cells just as reported with
the allogeneic Peyer's patch cell transfer. Maybe this
brings a little confusion into the sort of data reported
before because we are not dealing with an entirely physiological situation. It does suggest that the allogeneic
mechanism may be one of several for switching on the
potential precursor cells into IgA production.

Dr. Cebra - I just wanted to comment that I feel your autologous transfer system gives results very complementary to
our own obtained with an allogeneic transfer system. Presumably what you observe is gut-stimulated IgA-cell maturation. That you are not getting this maturation in the
spleen probably indicates that allogeneic differences are
playing a role in the allogenic system in inducing proliferation of lymphocytes. I would further like to comment
that the two kinds of assays (in vivo and in vitro assays)
we are using are quite different but that they lead to
similar conclusions. One assay - allogenic transfer - measures cells capable of extensive proliferation to yield a
lot of daughters making IgA. The in vitro assay probably
measures cells that either don't divide but go directly to
plasma cells or divide once or twice and then mature to
plasma cells. Thus we are measuring the potential for
synthesis of isotype in higher proportions of the population
in the in vitro assay. The in vivo transfer system probably
measures a lower proportion of the population - only that
fraction with considerable proliferation potential prior to
maturation.

Dr. Lehner - I was very pleased to hear Dr. Cooper mention
that IgA differentiation may be thymus dependent, as I am
sure he knows Arnason has shown the same in thymectomized
rats. The problem there was that Arnason wasn't quite sure
whether it was IgA that was depressed in thymectomized
animals. Unfortunately, Humphrey and Askonas were unable to
confirm this. It was later that Robert Good and others
pointed out a relationship between thymus function and IgA

in clinical situations. Now on analysis of oral diseases
there seems to be a very interesting association between
cell mediated immunity and IgA. I wonder if I could ask Dr.
Cooper to clarify this point - whether he has found following thymectomy that the proportion of IgA staining B-
lymphocytes and plasma cells, as well as serum and salivary
IgA, were in fact decreased?

Dr. Cooper - It is unfortunate that Dr. Warner is not here
today since he was to present his data on this issue. In
the congenitally athymic "nude" strain of mice, the development of all classes of immunoglobulin-bearing B-lymphocytes
appears to proceed normally. If anything, the number of
IgA-bearing cells are increased in proportion to IgG- and
IgM-bearing cells, at least in thoracic duct lymph, although
the mice showed marked deficiencies in serum immunoglobulins,
particularly IgA. In athymic humans also, the distribution
of IgM, IgG and IgA bearing cells does not seem to be
significantly distorted despite the lack of T cells. The
studies of Pritchard and colleagues in "nude" mice have
further shown that the serum deficiencies of IgG and IgA
can be repaired by a thymus graft. Having said that, I
cannot give a precise answer to your question about the
levels of IgA in secretions of athymic individuals. My
colleague Sandy Lawton tells me that the numbers of IgA
containing cells in the intestinal lamina propria of the
congenitally athymic mouse are reduced in comparison to
littermate controls, but they are not lacking entirely.
          In response to the comments by Drs. Tomasi and
Leslie, I would like to emphasize that we do not consider
that the G to A switch in our model is established conclusively. There are two special problems in approaching this
question using antibody-mediated suppression of various
immunoglobulin classes. The first is that the switch we are
discussing is primarily an embryonic event in most mammalian
species. The other very practical problem in the class
suppression approach to this question is the umbrella of
circulating IgG provided by the mother. In essence this
throws up a curtain which prevents efficient homing of anti-
IgG antibodies to the target IgG-bearing cells. In order to
try to circumvent these problems, Dr. Lawton and Dr. Asofsky
first gave newborn mice antibodies to IgM in order to hold
B cell development in abeyance while maternal IgG was cata-
bolized. After a week they stopped the anti-μ injections
and proceeded then to give antibodies to IgG_1 and IgG_2.
More than half of the animals so treated later showed

significant suppression of cells capable of IgG_1 or IgG_2
synthesis. In these same animals they found a corresponding
deficiency of IgA; IgA producing cells along the gut were
almost totally absent in some instances. On the other hand,
IgM producing cells were normally developed in the treated
mice. It is difficult to envision a basis on which to
explain these results other than our idea that IgA-producing
cells derive from cells formerly capable of making IgG_1 and
IgG_2. Nevertheless, this is a question that demands much
more work, and it would be helpful to have other experimental approaches to supplement the information that can
be gained from antibody-mediated class suppression.

GUT-ASSOCIATED LYMPHOBLASTS AND INTESTINAL IgA PLASMA CELLS

Delphine Guy-Grand, Claude Griscelli, and
Pierre Vassalli
Laboratory of Immunology, Hôpital Necker-
Enfants Malades, Paris, and
Department of Pathology, University of Geneva
Faculty of Medicine, Geneva

The term "gut-associated lymphoid system" (GALS) can be applied, in the mouse and in the rat, to the lymphoid cells present in 1) the Peyers' patches (PP); 2) the intestinal mucosa, where these cells consist of disseminated lympho-cytes and IgA secreting plasma cells; 3) the mesenteric lymph nodes (MLN), into which the lymphatic system of the gut drains, and 4) the thoracic duct lymph (TDL), which receives the efferent MLN lymph. It has been shown in the rat that the TDL and MLN "lymphoblasts" (i.e. large dividing cells which are labeled after in vitro incubation with ^{3}H thymidine) display, after transfer into syngeneic recipients, a strong tendency to migrate to the intestinal mucosa (1,2,3), the PP, and to some extent the MLN (2). This migration pattern is not observed with the blasts obtained from immunized peri-pheral lymph nodes (PLN); these blasts do not migrate to the gut and home more in the PLN than in the MLN (2). Preferen-tial migration is characteristic of only the GALS blasts, since it is not found in transfer experiments when the total lymphoid population from TDL or MLN is labeled (2). Since these observations indicate that some of the GALS blasts have special properties, it was decided to investigate further the nature and properties of the various GALS cells in the mouse and in the rat.

The lymphoid cells from PP, TDL, MLN and immunized PLN (obtained 3 days after the last of 3 daily foot pad injec-tions of sheep red blood cells) were stained with T and B-specific antisera (rabbit anti MSLA and anti MBLA (4) and

antisera directed against $\mu, \gamma, \alpha,$ and κ chains (4)). The blasts
were labeled by one hour of _in vitro_ incubation with ^{3}H thymidine (2) and at once characterized by a combination of
immunofluorescence and radioautography (4). After transfer
experiments (2) the nature of the labeled cells was determined by immunofluorescence studies of cell suspensions of
various organs, or of tissue sections, in which the intracellular Ig chains, or the T nature of the cells (5) can be
easily detected.

Table I.A shows in a summarized form the nature of the
mouse GALS and PLN blasts, as judged by their cell surface
antigenic determinants. An important point is that IgA is
the predominant surface immunoglobulin among GALS blasts,
while it is predominant neither among the PLN blasts, nor
among the total lymphoid cells of GALS or PLN. The predominance of cells bearing surface IgA among the B cells is
therefore a characteristic of the GALS blasts.

Table I.B shows the results observed when blasts from
the same sources are studied for their intracellular Ig
content. While there are few blasts containing Ig chains
among PP blasts, and still fewer containing IgA, a high
percentage of IgA containing blasts is found in MLN and TDL.
Thus, in TDL, 75% of the blasts bearing surface IgA (which
represent themselves the vast majority of the TDL B blasts)
also contain intracellular IgA; this has been ascertained by
double immunofluorescence staining with rhodamine anti-α antiserum for surface staining and fluorescein anti-α antiserum
for cytoplasmic staining. This observation indicates the
existence, among the blasts bearing surface IgA, of a maturation process which leads to the progressive accumulation of
intracellular IgA, this process being almost completed when
these blasts reach the thoracic duct.

Table I. Nature of Blasts from Mouse GALS and Peripheral Lymph Nodes

A. Cell Surface

	$\%\dfrac{\text{blasts}}{\text{total cells}}$	% T/B blasts	$\%\dfrac{\text{sIgA}}{\text{sk}}$ blasts*	$\%\dfrac{\text{sIgA}}{\text{sk}}$ total cells**
1)Periph.LN (immunized)	∿2	∿60 B, 40 T	5	10
2)PP	>4	∿80 or more B	50	20
3)Mesent.LN	∿2	∿50 B, 50 T	50	20
4)TD lymph	∿0.5	∿67 T, 33B	85	25

B. Intracellular Ig Chains

	% Ig containing blasts	% IgA	$\%\dfrac{\text{intracell.}\alpha\text{***}}{\text{intracell. Ig}}$	$\%\dfrac{\text{intracell.}\alpha\text{****}}{\text{surface }\alpha}$
1)Periph.LN (immunized)	∿7	∿0.4	6	0
2)PP	∿2	∿0.7	35	2
3)Mesent.LN	∿8	∿6.5	85	50
4)TD lymph	∿16–20	∿16–20 (up to 40 in the rat)	100	75

*   Percentage of blasts (or total cells**) bearing surface α chains among blasts (or total cells**) bearing surface k chains.

*** Percentage of blasts containing α chains among all blasts containing Ig chains.

**** Percentage of blasts containing α chains among blasts bearing surface α chains.

The homing properties of these various blasts after transfer into syngeneic recipients have been determined by radioautography of the recipient mouse tissues, comparing the density of labeled cells per field in different organs and in the spleen, 1 day after transfer. The results confirm and extend those found in the rat (2): 1) PLN blasts do not home in the gut and home more to the PLN than to the GALS (if the density of labeled cells/field in the spleen is taken as 100%,

that in PLN is 64%, MLN 25%, PP 7% and gut mucosa 0%; 2) PP
blasts home in the gut and more in the GALS than in the PLN
(PLN : 34, MLN : 90, PP : 62, gut : 40%); 4) TD blasts home
massively in the gut, and much more in the GALS than in the
PLN (PLN : 8, MLN : 43, gut : 63%). It must be stressed
again that this peculiar migration pattern of some of the
GALS blasts is in total contrast with that of the whole
lymphoid population of these sources, which has completely
different homing properties.

   Various types of experiments were performed to explore
the possible role of gut antigens in the gut homing properties of some of the GALS blasts. All led to the conclusion
that this migration is not antigen driven, the most definitive of these experiments being performed with transfer of
PLN, MLN and TDL blasts in mice and rats bearing a graft of
foetal intestine placed under the kidney capsule. The degree
of homing in the graft was found to exactly parallel that
observed in the recipient's own gut: absent with PLN blast,
conspicuous with MLN and still more striking with TDL blasts.
Since these grafts were never exposed to intestinal antigen,
it is clear that the GALS blasts gut homing is not antigen
driven.

   To explore the nature and ultimate fate of these gut
homing blasts, combined immunofluorescence and radioautography were performed on sections of the recipient's own gut
and of the grafted gut, using antisera against different Ig
chains, and also the rabbit anti T ('anti MSLA") antiserum
(4), which recognizes very easily the T lymphocytes on tissue
sections (5). The labeled cells homing in the gut wall were
found to be of two sorts only: IgA plasma cells, present in
the lamina propria, and T lymphocytes, present both in the
lamina propria and the intestinal mucosa. When the nature of
the labeled transfered blasts was compared to the nature and
density of cells which had, after transfer, homed in the gut,
it became apparent that the amount of labeled IgA plasma cells
found in the gut is related to the number of blasts having both
surface and intracellular IgA present in the transferred cells.
Blasts having only surface but not intracellular IgA, such as
the PP blasts, do not home to the gut, at least within 1 day
after transfer.

   In the interpretation of these various observations, the
problems of the gut homing tendency of the IgA containing
blasts and of the T blasts should be considered separately.

There is indeed evidence that the gut homing of the T blasts
is unrelated to that of the IgA blasts, since it appears
that all the T blasts spontaneously released in the circulation, probably whatever the stimulating antigen, and
possibly whatever the stimulated lymphoid organ, do home in
the gut mucosa and epithelium (6). Thus, only the problem of
the generation of the intestinal mucosa IgA plasma cells will
be discussed here. The likeliest interpretation of the observations made with the IgA blasts is that the gut IgA plasma
cells are the progeny of the proliferating germinal center
cells of the PP. The patches might be considered as the
equivalent of the superficial cortex of LN, with follicles
separated by interfollicular areas of T lymphocytes; these
interfollicular areas are indeed brightly stained when the
rabbit MSLA (T) antiserum is applied on tissue sections of
the gut. In the absence of antigen, as in germ free mice (7),
or of T cells, as in nude mice (8), there is no germinal
center formation. In normal conditions, in contrast, germinal
centers develop, which explains the high proportion of blasts
found among the PP cells. Since the majority of these blasts
bear surface IgA, their migration to the MLN through the
existing lymphatic channels, accompanied by some degree of
maturation, would explain the high percentage of blasts not
only bearing but also containing IgA which is found in the
MLN, and finally in the thoracic duct. In order to explain
why the acquisition of intracellular IgA develops in parallel
to the acquisition of the gut homing capacity, one should
explore the possibility that the accumulation of intracellular IgA coincides with a shift from the synthesis of monomeric
to that of polymeric IgA. Such a shift might be related to the
gut homing mechanism, since the presence of polymeric IgA on
the cell surface of the more "mature" blasts might explain,
in view of the known affinity of polymeric IgA with the
secretory component (SC) (9) why these last blasts migrate
to places where SC is present, as in the gut. If proliferating
and migrating IgA bearing blasts from the PP germinal centers
are really the progenitors of most of the intestinal wall IgA
plasma cells, the failure of development of the patches'germinal centers, because of the lack of T cells, should result
in a lack of gut IgA plasma cells. This is in fact what is
observed in the nude mice: their PP have no germinal centers,
and the content of the gut in IgA plasma cells is 10 to 15
times below normal. This is not due to the lack of lymphocytes
bearing surface IgA since such lymphocytes are found among
the non-proliferating patches' lymphocytes (6). It appears
that, in the absence of T cells, these IgA bearing lympho-

cytes cannot be stimulated: thus their proliferation, migration and seeding to the gut to become IgA plasma cells cannot take place.

Acknowledgments: This work was supported by grants from INSERM (ATP 2 and 16) and from the Fonds National Suisse de la Recherche Scientifique (no 3.408.70).

REFERENCES

1. Gowans, J.L. and Knight, E.J. Proc. Roy. Soc. Ser. B. Biol. Sci. 159:257, 1964.
2. Griscelli, C., Vassalli, P. and McCluskey, R.T. J. Exp. Med. 130:1427, 1969.
3. Hall, J.G., Parry, D.M. and Smith, M.E. Cell Tissue Kinet. 5:269, 1972.
4. Lamelin, J.P., Lisowska-Bernstein, B., Matter, A., Ryser, J.E. and Vassalli, P. J. Exp. Med. 136:984, 1972.
5. Gutman, G.A. and Weissman, I.L. Immunology 23:465, 1972.
6. Guy-Grand, D., Griscelli, C. and Vassalli, P. (in preparation).
7. Crabbé, P.A., Nash, D.R., Bazin, H., Eyssen, H. and Heremans, J.F. Lab. Invest. 22:448, 1970.
8. Mitchell, J., Pye, J., Holmes, M.C. and Nossal, G.J.V. Austr. J. Exp. Biol. and Med. Sc. 50:637, 1972.
9. Mach, J.P. Nature (Lond.) 228:1278, 1970.

BRONCHIAL LYMPHOID TISSUE

Bienenstock, J., Rudzik, O., Clancy, R.L. and
Perey, D.Y.E.

McMaster University
Hamilton, Ontario, Canada

The role of the respiratory tract in the defense
against potential pathogens has been a subject of interest
to microbiologists, virologists and immunologists for many
years. The description of the secretory IgA system,
common to mucosal surfaces throughout the body, has
extended the interests of immunologists in the mechanisms
of mucosal resistance (1). Like the gastrointestinal
tract, the respiratory tract is characterized by the
predominance of IgA containing cells in the lamina propria,
by the presence of secretory IgA in bronchial and nasal
secretions, and the demonstration of secretory component
in the glandular epithelia. Further, the demonstration of
local antibody, mainly of the IgA class, following
immunization by nose drops or aerosol with a variety of
antigens has shown that this system must play a major role
in immunological responses to local antigen (2,3).
Resistance to infection by certain organisms has been
correlated with the presence of some local antibody and a
lack of correlation exists between resistance and serum
antibody. That immunity to infection in the respiratory
tract is not only mediated by humoral antibody responses
has been clearly shown in experiments of local
immunization in animals and man in which specific release
of migration inhibition factor has been found in lymphocytes from bronchial washings (4,5).

It is the purpose of this paper to discuss the
possible role of the bronchus associated lymphoid tissue

(BALT) which we have recently described and its potential relationship to mucosal immunity (6,7).

BALT may have been first described by Burdon-Sanderson in 1868 (8), however in 1875 Klein (9) wrote "lymphoid follicles in the bronchial walls are therefore in every respect analogous to the lymph follicles found in other mucous membranes, e.g. tonsils and in the intestine." Recent awareness of the BALT appears to be limited as judged by our search of the literature. Because of the resemblance of the BALT to gut associated lymphoid tissue we have compared studies of one with the other.

We first became aware of organized sub-epithelial lymphoid aggregates in the bronchial tract of rabbits while studying the response of rabbits to immune complexes instilled into their respiratory tract. This BALT bears a striking morphologic similarity to intestinal Peyer's patches (Fig. 1).

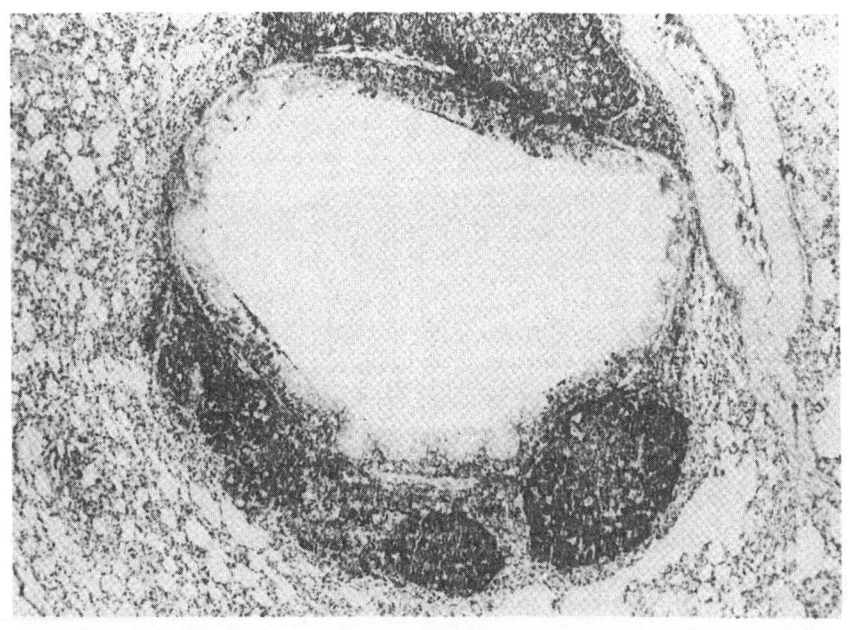

Fig. 1. Cross section of rabbit bronchus showing BALT follicles with overlying lymphoepithelium.

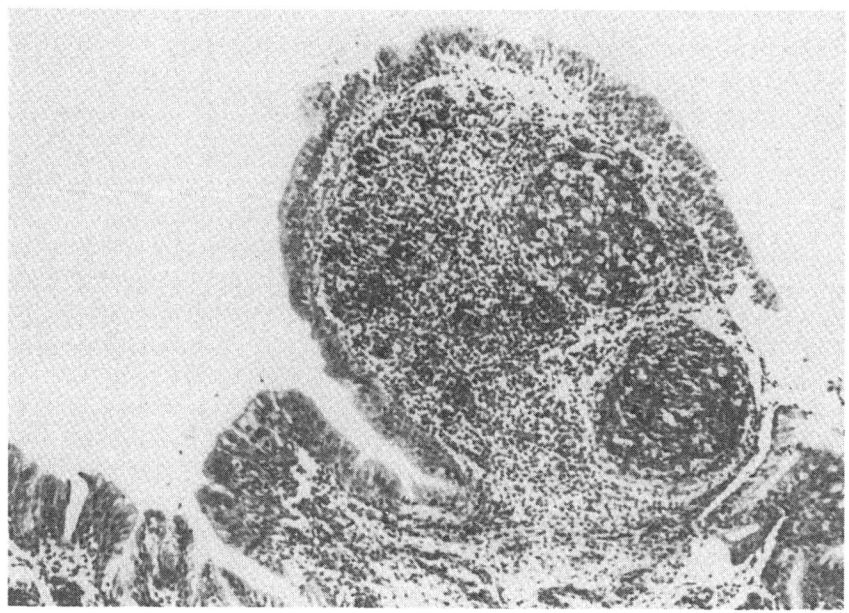

Fig. 2. Chicken BALT showing two distinct germinal centres.

The lymphoid tissue is made up of one or two
follicles containing loosely organized sheets of lymphocytes, with a clear epithelial relationship. It often
lies between plates of cartilage with the major mass of
the BALT below the cartilage and a minor sub-epithelial
mass connected to it by a stalk.   The BALT is present in
rabbits, dogs, mice, rats, pigs, guinea pigs, chickens and
man.

The epithelium overlying the BALT is flattened,
heavily infiltrated with lymphocytes and, in contrast with
the surrounding epithelium, does not stain with periodic
acid–Schiff or Alcian Blue. This lymphoepithelium is not
ciliated.

We have been unable to demonstrate plasma cells on
the basis of histochemistry, ultrastructure, and immunofluorescence with anti α, μ or γ heavy chains inside the
BALT of rabbits and chickens. Chicken BALT however
contains germinal centres characteristic of that species
(Fig. 2).

The BALT is present in germ free rats although less well developed than amongst conventionally raised animals. Similarly primitive BALT follicles developed in mouse fetal lungs transplanted subcutaneously into syngeneic recipients.

In cytokinetic studies using a single pulse of intravenously injected ^{3}H–thymidine the following results were obtained (7). In animals killed 1 hr after injection two labelling patterns were seen in BALT. In some instances randomly scattered heavily labelled cells were seen throughout the BALT follicles, while in others, sometimes superimposed upon this pattern, were localized areas of highly labelled cells frequently at the periphery of follicles. Only very rare labelled cells were seen in the lymphoepithelium. In animals killed at 24 hr one could still identify heavily labelled cells randomly scattered throughout lymphoid follicles, but approximately one half of BALT follicles also contained crescent shaped areas of densely packed less heavily labelled cells. Such areas did not bear any obvious relationship to the overlying bronchial epithelium.

We have recently performed experiments in which we studied the fate of thoracic duct lymphocytes labelled _in vitro_ with either ^{3}H–uridine or ^{3}H–thymidine and subsequently reinfused intravenously in autologous recipients. Animals were killed at 24 hr and autoradiography performed on tissue sections. Following prolonged exposure, autoradiographs in recipients of uridine labelled lymphocytes revealed evenly distributed lightly labelled cells throughout the loose lymphocyte sheet of BALT and outlined crescent shaped areas devoid of radioactivity which we interpreted as corresponding to those areas labelled following intravenous injection of ^{3}H–thymidine. In recipients of ^{3}H–thymidine labelled thoracic duct lymphocytes only rare randomly scattered heavily labelled cells could be seen in BALT and bronchial lamina propria. This suggests that BALT is made up in part of recirculating lymphocytes as well as rapidly dividing locally derived cells (Fig.3).

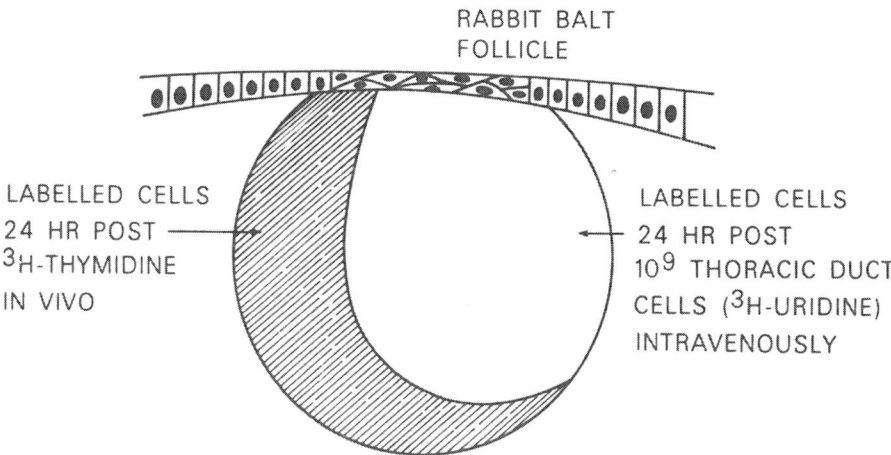

Fig. 3. Schematic drawing of results of cytokinetic studies
in rabbit BALT.

The distribution of a rabbit thymus lymphocyte
antigen (RTLA) as originally described by Frandezi et al
(10) was studied in cell suspensions prepared from various
rabbit lymphoid organs using the standard complement
dependent cytotoxicity test. As seen in Table 1 the
distribution of this antigen corresponds to various
reported values obtained with anti- antisera in the mouse.
The percentage cytotoxicity of lymphocytes in both BALT
and Peyer's patches were similar (18% and 17% respectively).

In order to assess the presence of B cell markers in
the same cell populations we performed membrane immunofluorescence with specific conjugated heavy chain antisera
with an F/P ratio greater than 2.5/1 (11). The results are
seen in Table 1 expressed as percentages. The ratios of
distribution of μ and α were remarkably similar within
each cell population for BALT, Peyer's patches and
thoracic duct lymphocytes although the absolute values
differed. Absorption of anti-μ antiserum with IgA did not
appreciably alter the results. Similar conclusions were
obtained for absorption experiments of anti-α with IgM.
Controls included anti-μ and anti-α absorbed with IgM and

TABLE 1

Distribution of surface markers on rabbit lymphocytes

Cells	RTLA* % ± S.E.	Membrane Fluorescence % ± S.E.		
		IgG	IgA	IgM
Thymus	95.0+2.9	<1	<1	<1
Thoracic duct	72.0+5.0	6.7+0.8	10.5+1.1	11.3+1.6
Blood	43.9+7.9	nd	nd	nd
BALT	18.4+3.9	8.1+1.0	18.8+2.7	19.0+3.3
Peyer's patches	16.6+4.0	16.8+1.5	30.0+4.5	32.0+4.8

* As % cytotoxicity with anti RTLA (10)

IgA respectively. Attempts to demonstrate the presence of μ and α on the same cells with double labelling techniques have so far been unsuccessful. The percentage of BALT cells staining for any cytoplasmic immunoglobulin was under 1%.

The effect of isolated or combined extirpation of central lymphoid organs in the chicken at hatching were studied in white leghorn chickens (12). Serum immuno-globulin levels were determined. Simple surgical bursectomy at hatching led to moderate reduction of serum IgA levels but in only 1 of 12 birds did we fail to detect serum IgA at 5 months of age. Simple thymectomy at hatching also led to a slight reduction of serum IgA although it was not detectable in 3 or 18 birds at 5 months of age. Combined surgical bursectomy-thymectomy at hatching led to a total absence of both serum and secretory IgA in 6 out of 6 birds at 5 months of age. In none of 41 sham operated birds did we fail to detect serum IgA. The absence of IgA in bursectomized-thymectomized birds was further documented by immuno-fluorescence and organ culture studies with radiolabelled amino acids.

Bursectomy or thymectomy alone produced no recognizable

changes in the BALT of the respective birds. However combined
surgical bursectomy-thymectomy led to a marked depletion of
lymphoid elements of BALT which were grossly disorganized
and lacking in germinal centres as well (Fig. 4). Germinal
centres in cecal tonsils from the same birds were quite
prominent (Fig. 5).

From the above observations, BALT can be described as
subepithelial collections of organized lymphoid tissue made
up of follicular or crescent shaped areas of rapidly
replicating cells surrounded by a sheet of more loosely packed
lymphocytes which appear to consist in large part of
recirculating lymphocytes. The latter are lightly labelled
with 3H-uridine and are devoid of cells taking up 3H-
thymidine. BALT is always closely associated with the
bronchial epithelium which forms a distinct lympho-epithelium
resembling that associated with the lymphoid submucosal
aggregates of other surfaces. Studies aimed at detecting
T cell markers reveal that in rabbit BALT cell suspensions,
some 20% of the cells are lysed in the presence of RTLA
antibody and complement. The presence of recirculating,
non dividing lymphocytes and cells possessing RTLA within
BALT strongly suggests that T cells make up part of these
lymphoid aggregates. Conversely, nearly 20% of BALT cells

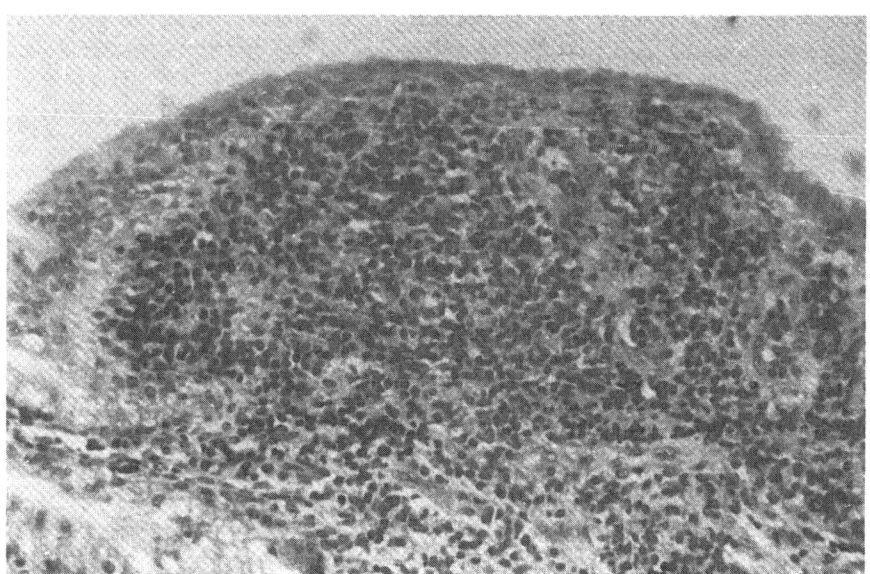

Fig. 4. Depleted BALT follicle in 5 month old chicken after
surgical bursectomy-thymectomy at hatching.

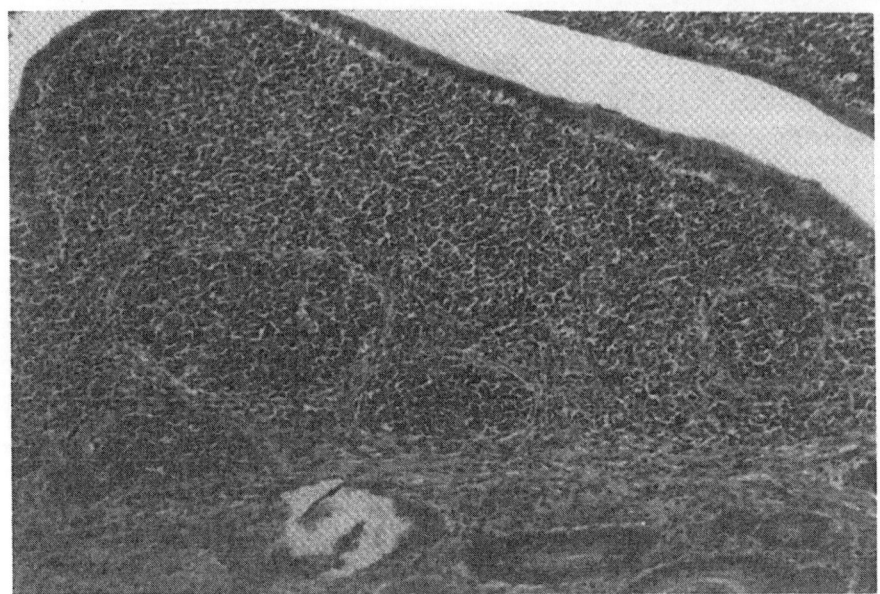

Fig. 5. Prominent germinal centres in cecal tonsil of same
bird as seen in Fig. 4.

in suspension possess either μ or α chain determinants on
their surface as detected by membrane immunofluorescence
although no cytoplasmic fluorescence can be demonstrated with
anti-heavy chain monospecific antibodies in frozen sections
or BALT cell suspensions. This suggests that B cells
precursors, if not mature B cells, make up at least a part
of BALT.

     In an attempt to assess the thymus- or bursa- dependence
of cells within BALT, we performed extirpative studies in
newly hatched chicks and observed partial depletion of cells
within the lymphocyte sheets of BALT following thymectomy and
sublethal total body x-irridiation.

     Germinal centres normally seen in BALT were absent in
agammaglobulinemic chickens following bursectomy and sublethal
total body x-irridiation. The BALT of birds undergoing combined
bursectomy-thymectomy at hatching (without subsequent x-
irridiation) lacked germinal centres completely and were made
up of grossly depleted and disorganized lymphoid accumulations;
this was associated with total absence of both serum and
secretory IgA, nevertheless, germinal centres were clearly

seen in the spleen and cecal tonsils of these IgA deficient birds. It is important to note that the cecal tonsil synthesizes predominantly IgG as judged by immunofluorescence and radio-labelled amino acid incorporation in organ culture (13). Despite this apparent influence of both thymus and bursa upon the development of chicken BALT, in preliminary studies we have been unable to demonstrate a proliferative response by rabbit BALT cell suspensions in the presence of phytohemagglutinin or pokeweed mitogen. This may reflect the relative immaturity of BALT cells.

Several lines of indirect evidence suggest that the thymus may be involved in the differention of IgA-producing cells. Serum IgA levels in nude mice are extremely low (14) and neonatal thymectomy in rabbits leads to low levels of serum IgA and markedly reduced serum IgA antibody responses to arsenyl-azo-bovine albumin (15). Similarly, adult thymectomy combined with lethal total body x-irradiation and reconstitution with allogeneic rabbit fetal liver cells resulted in decreased serum IgA (16).

The origin of IgA-producing cells is not known, however Craig and Cebra (17) have shown that rabbit Peyer's patch cells unlike peripheral blood and lymph node lymphocytes, when transferred into lethally irradiated allogeneic recipients, predominantly synthesize IgA. We have described striking similarities between BALT and Peyer's patches (6,7). The present report further underlines these similarities and suggests that BALT may be another source of cells with IgA-producing potential. Although Peyer's patches of mice (18) and rabbits possess cells with T cell surface markers they do not appear to contain effector T cells capable of mediating a graft versus host reaction (19,20) or an allogeneic effect (21). However, helper T cell function has been demonstrated in mouse Peyer's patches (21).

Our current working hypothesis is that BALT and Peyer's patches are the sites of differentiation of IgA-producing cells. This differentiation requires interaction between immature B cells and T cells to allow phenotypic expression, and may occur within the submucosal lymphoid aggregates themselves.

REFERENCES

1. Tomasi, T.B. and Bienenstock, J., Advances in
    Immunology, Edited by F.J. Dixon, Jr., and H.G. Kunkel,
    vol. 9., p.1. Academic Press, N.Y., 1968.
2. Rossen, R.D., Kasel, J.A. and Couch, R.B., Porgress in
    Medical Virology 13:195, 1971.
3. Fazekas De St. Groth, S. and Donnelley, M., Austr. J.
    Exp. Biol. Med. Sci. 28:45, 1950.
4. Henney, C.S. and Waldman, R.H., Science 169:696, 1970.
5. Waldman, R.H., Spencer, C.S. and Johnson, J.E. III.,
    Cell Immunol. 3:294, 1972.
6. Bienenstock, J., Johnson, N. and Perey, D.Y.E., Lab
    Invest. 28:686, 1973.
7. Bienenstock, J., Johnson, N. and Perey, D.Y.E. Lab
    Invest. 28:693, 1973.
8. Burdon-Sanderson: Eleventh report of the medical office
    of the Privy Council, 1868, p.101, 102 (sic) quoted in
    ref. 9 below.
9. Klein, E.E., The Anatomy of the Lymphatic System, Vol.
    II, Smith, Elder and Co., London, 1875.
10. Fradelizi, D.P., Chou, C.T., Cinader, B. and Dubiski, S.
    Cell.Immunology 7:484, 1973.
11. Lawton, A.R., Asofsky, R., Hylton, M.B. and Cooper, M.D.
    J. Exp. Med. 135:277, 1972.
12. Perey, D.Y.E. and Bienenstock, J., J. Immunol. 111:
    633, 1973.
13. Bienenstock, J., Gauldie, J. and Perey, D.Y.E., J.
    Immunol. 111, In press.
14. Luzzati, A.L. and Jacobson, E.B., Eur. J. Immunol. 2:
    473, 1972.
15. Clough, J.D., Mims, L.H. and Strober, W., J. Immunol.
    106:1624, 1971.
16. Perey, D.Y.E., Frommel, D., Hong, R. and Good, R.A.,
    Lab. Invest. 22:212, 1970.
17. Craig, S.W. and Cebra, J.J., J. Exp. Med. 134:188,
    1971.
18. Raff, M.C. and Owen, J.T.T., Eur. J. Immunol. 1:27,
    1971.
19. Perey, D.Y.E. and Guttmann, R.D., Lab. Invest. 27:427,
    1972.
20. Heim, L.R., McGarry, M.P., Montgomery, J.R., Trentin,
    J.J. and South, M.A., Transplant 14:418, 1972.
21. Katz, D.H. and Perey, D.Y.E., J. Immunol. In press.

THE ORIGIN OF MONOMERIC AND POLYMERIC FORMS OF IgA IN MAN

J. Radl, Henrica R.E. Schuit, J. Mestecky* and
W. Hijmans
Institute for Experimental Gerontology, T.N.O.,
Rijswijk (Z-H), The Netherlands, and* the
Department of Microbiology, University of
Alabama in Birmingham, U.S.A.

INTRODUCTION

A distinctive feature of immunoglobulin A is its
tendency to occur in different molecular forms. In contrast
to that in most mammalian species, the majority (85 to 90%)
of the serum IgA in man occurs in a monomeric form. This
prompts a question as to where the monomeric and the polymeric serum IgA is formed and by which cells. Peripheral
lymph nodes, spleen, and intestinal lymphoid tissue have long
been considered the main sources of circulating IgA (1).
However, Hijmans et al. (2) have shown that human bone
marrow, because it carries such a large number of cells that
contain IgA, can be regarded as a major source of the circulating IgA. Test systems at the cellular level which specifically distinguish between the different molecular forms of
IgA may help to clarify this problem.

In the present study we used 3 such systems in an
investigation of bone marrow cells and sera from patients
with and without an IgA paraproteinemia and from normal
individuals. For these tests, 3 markers that specifically
recognize polymeric IgA were used: an antiserum that recognizes only the dimeric (polymeric) determinants of IgA, an
antiserum against J chain, and the ability of polymeric
IgA1 to bind the secretory component (SC) in vitro.

MATERIAL AND METHODS

Analyses were made of bone marrow cells and serum from 17 patients with an IgA1 paraproteinemia (16 myelomas and 1 idiopathic paraproteinemia; 7 paraproteins were of the κ and 10 of the λ type), from 7 patients with various diseases but without a paraproteinemia, and from 5 healthy adults. In the myeloma group, the proteinemia was determined by the biuret technique, and the approximate paraprotein concentration in the serum was calculated from agar electrophoretic slides by scanning in a densitometer (Vernon Phi 5, Paris). The sub-class specificity and the light chain type were analyzed by immunodiffusion techniques, and the form of the paraproteins was estimated by analytical ultracentrifugation as described previously (3). Antisera against the individual class and the light chain immunoglobulin determinants were produced in rabbits or sheep. All adsorptions of the antisera, as well as the isolation of specific antibodies, were done on solid immunoadsorbents as described previously (4). Globulin fractions or isolated specific antibodies were conjugated with FITC or TRITC. The speicificity was tested by the immunodiffusion techniques and by performance tests on monoclonal bone marrow cells (5).

Test systems for polymeric IgA:

1) Antiserum that recognized only the dimeric (polymeric) determinants of IgA (DiA). A detailed description of this antiserum will be published elsewhere. In principle, 2 antisera (made available by Nordic Immunological Laboratories, Tilburg, The Netherlands) produced in 2 sheep by hyperimmunization with isolated human secretory IgA (S-IgA) contained antibodies to α class specific determinants, to Ig light chains, and to SC. After adsorption with normal human serum and with SC, the antisera still gave precipitin lines in immunodiffusion systems with S-IgA and with dimeric and other polymeric forms of IgA, but not with the monomer. In some instances, there was an indication that precipitation was inhibited by 7S IgA. No reaction was obtained when the antisera and conjugates were tested against free SC from human milk, against J chain isolated from 10S IgA paraprotein, and against free α chains from sera of patients with α chain disease. In immunofluorescence (IF), the isolated and labeled anti-DiA antibodies did not react with monoclonal bone marrow cells from IgG, IgM, IgD, κ and λ myeloma, or with lymphocytes that contained α common class determinants intracellularly or had α receptors on the membrane.

2) Antiserum against J chain. J chain from a polymeric IgA paraprotein was isolated as described previously (6). Conjugates were prepared from rabbit and guinea pig antisera by labeling the globulin fraction or specific antibodies that were isolated on a cross-linked, reduced, and alkylated polymeric IgA paraprotein. When tested in immunoelectrophoresis and by double diffusion, the antisera reacted only with isolated J chain. No precipitation was obtained with any Ig of the 5 classes, including native polymeric IgA and S-IgA. No staining was obtained in IF on monoclonal bone marrow preparations when the cells contained IgG or IgD of any light chain type. The Bence Jones myeloma cells of both the κ and the λ types were also negative. However, in 3 cases (2 λ and 1 κ) a positive reaction was observed in the myeloma cells that showed a different pattern in the double staining with anti-light chain conjugates. In a number of cases of Waldenstrom's macroglobulinemia some of the cells that contained IgM showed a positive staining for J chain. J chain in serum samples was revealed by immunoelectrophoresis after 2 hours incubation of 5 λ of serum combined with 45 λ 9M urea and 0.2M mercaptoethanol (pH=8.6). Normal human serum exhibited no reaction in dilutions above 1:5 to 1:8. Some bone marrow preparations were examined after being treated with mercaptoethanol (30 min.) and iodoacetamine (10 min.).

3) Binding of SC in vitro. Analysis of the binding of SC by the paraproteins in sera is described elsewhere (3). The test system for bone marrow cells was as follows: in a simple 2 step procedure, free SC was isolated from milk of a mother who had agammaglobulinemia. The defatted milk was first passed over an adsorbent of insolubilized anti-lactoferrin antibodies. Then the milk samples without lactoferrin were applied on an adsorbent column consisting of a cross-linked polymeric IgA paraprotein that was capable of specific retention of all the free SC from the milk on the column. By using a 0.1M glycine-HCl buffer, pH=2.4, about 80% of the SC was then eluted from the adsorbent in a pure state.

The cell suspension on the slide was reacted with the pure, free SC at a 60 µg/ml concentration for 30 min. After washing the cells in phosphate buffered saline for 10 min., a monospecific anti-SC conjugate was applied.

Slides were viewed under the fluoresence microscope by the 2 wavelength method (2,7) and the 3 markers were

TABLE I

Demonstration of polymeric IgA by three immunochemical markers specific for the polymeric form in serum and bone marrow cells of patients with IgA1 myeloma.

Pati-ent	Serum					Bone marrow			
	Para-protein in gr %	Polymeric form % of total	SCB	DiA	J	SCB	DiA	J	J-ME
1.	5.6	± 100	+	+	+	+	+	-	±/+
2.	5.6	± 90	+	+	+	+	+	+	
3.	6.0	70	+	+	+	+	±	+	
4.	5.3	47	+	+	+	+	+	-	±
5.	4.3	46	+	+	+	+	+	+	
6.	2.8	43	+	+	+	+	+	+	
7.	4.0	30	+	+	+	±	+	-	± G
8.	4.3	28	+	+	+	-	±	-	+
9.	5.3	25	+	+	+	+	+	+	+
10.	5.1	12	u	u	u	-	±	-	±/+
11.	5.6	10	u	u	u	±/+	+	+	
12.	4.3	6	u	u	u	G	G	G	
13.	5.2	6	-	u	-	G	G	G	
14.	2.0	2	-	u	-	-	+	±	-
15.	2.8	<1	-	-	-	-	-	-	-
16.	3.1	<1	-	-	-	-	-	-	-
17.	3.7	<1	-	-	-	-	-	-	-

SCB   = secretory component binding in vitro
DiA   = antiserum against dimeric determinant of IgA
J   = antiserum against the J chain
J-ME = antiserum against the J chain after treatment of the cells with mercaptoethanol and iodoacetamide
+   = positive test, many cells with brilliant fluorescence
-     = negative test, no positive cells in fluorescence
±   = few cells and weak fluorescence
G   = fluorescence restricted only to the Golgi zone
u   = positive only in undiluted sera or low diluted sera, in dilutions above 1:10 negative

evaluated in correlation with the staining by an antiserum
against common α class specific determinants.

RESULTS

Tests with the myeloma sera (Table 1) gave consistent
reactions to the 3 markers for polymeric IgA. Paraproteins
that had a polymer concentration of more than 25% of the
total paraprotein level were precipitated by the anti-DiA
serum, contained J chain, and were able to bind the SC
in vitro, even when test sera were diluted 1:80. On the
other hand, paraproteins with polymer levels of less than
1% of the total paraprotein content gave completely negative reactions to all 3 markers. In samples which had polymeric fractions that varied from 2% to 12%, the test systems
were usually positive only with undiluted sera. Some of the
sera gave positive tests in dilution, but never in titer
exceeding 1:10.

In the majority of the bone marrow preparations, the
presence of J chain in IgA-containing cells usually paral-
leled the positive tests for the DiA conjugate and the SC
binding (Table 1). However, exceptions were also noted. In
the cases in which the serum contained almost pure 7S IgA
paraprotein, either no positive bone marrow cells were evidenced by a reaction to the 3 markers, or the fluorescence
was restricted to the Golgi zone of the cell. The numerical
relationship between the polymer positive and alpha positive
cells varied considerably among the cases with a polymeric
IgA paraprotein, occasionally reaching nearly 100%. The
intensity and the localization of the fluorescence within
the cells also varied in different patients.

The serum of normal persons and that of patients without
paraproteinemia showed no appreciable reaction in any of the
systems. The number of bone marrow cells exhibiting a positive reaction with the 3 markers was generally low. The
mean percentages with the standard deviation for SC-binding,
anti-DiA and J chain, before and after mercaptoethanol treatment, were as follows: 7.3 ± 5.1, 21.6 ± 16.0, 0.5 ± 1.2 and
4.7 ± 5.2, respectively. There was no substantial difference
between the patients and the normal persons.

The pattern of fluorescence differed somewhat in the
myeloma and nonmyeloma groups. In myeloma cells, the
fluorescence in positive cases was often diffuse with maxima,

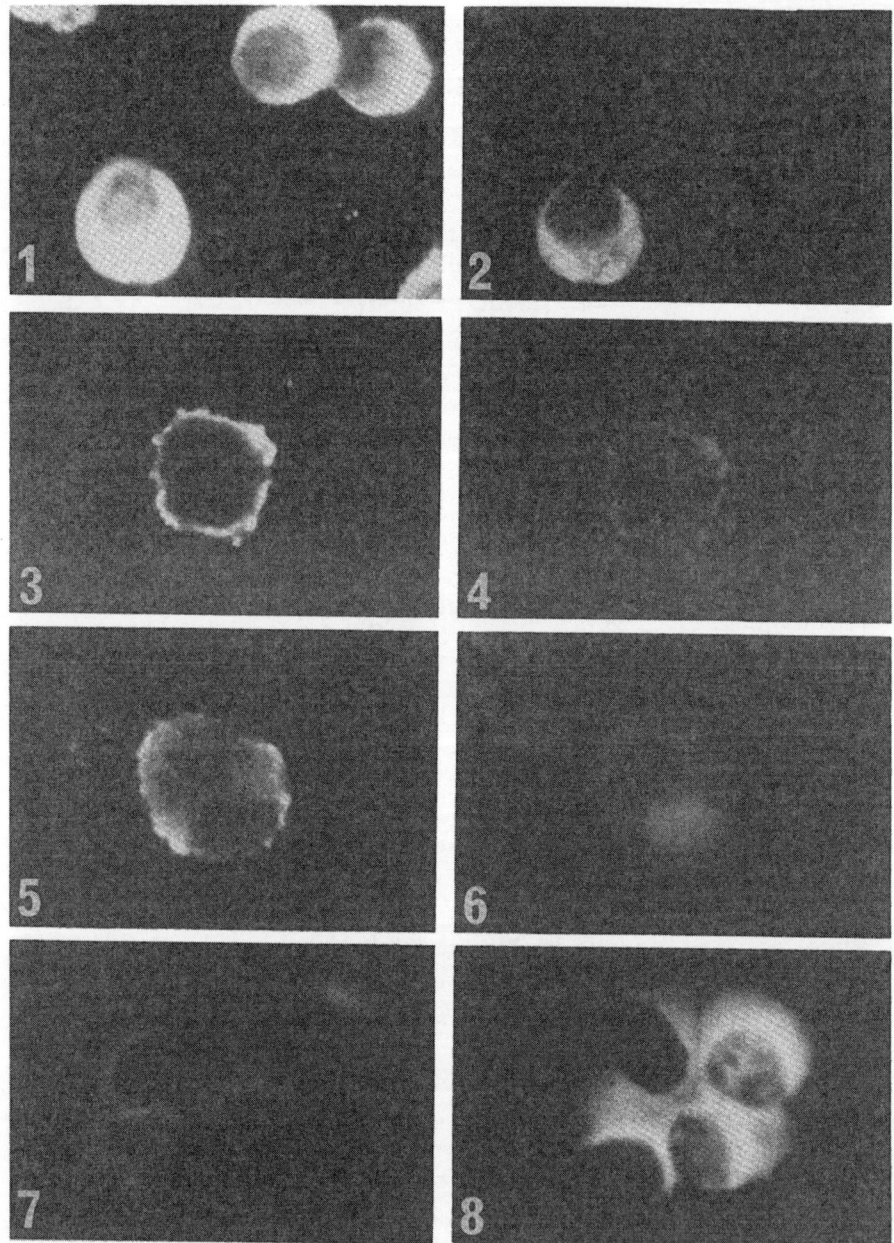

Fig. 1. Immunofluorescent pattern in myeloma (1.2.5.6.7.8) and normal bone marrow (3.4). Examples of different localization: diffuse SC binding (2), DiA at the rim (4), SC binding in the Golgi zone (6); α common staining of the same cells (1.3.5). Effect of mercaptoethanol on J chain staining (8), no treatment (7).

sometimes at the rim of the cells or in the Golgi zone; in
normal bone marrow, the IF was mainly situated at the rim
of the cells (Fig. 1). This was most pronounced with the
antiserum against DiA.

DISCUSSION

At the serum level, the results of our study correspond
with the data in the literature (3,8-12). New findings were
projected as a result of the IF investigations at the cellular level. It is noteworthy that the antiserum against DiA
and the SC showed the presence of corresponding determinants
already within the cell. Parkhouse reported (13) that, in
mouse plasma-cell tumors which produced dimeric IgA, the
intracellular IgA was most prevalent in its monomeric form.
Grey et al. (14), who used a similar technique, reported a
definite predominance of monomeric forms in mouse IgA myeloma
cells, but approximately 20% of the intracellular IgA was in
the polymeric form. In contrast to these reports, the fluorescence staining for markers of the polymeric IgA in human
myeloma cells showed rather frequently a brilliant fluorescence throughout the cytoplasm, in some cases, with a maximum at the rim of the cell and in the area corresponding to
the Golgi zone. The same holds for cells that contain IgM
(15), wherein we found numerous cases of intracellular
binding of free SC. This suggests that the IgM in the cell
contains some complete pentamers of higher polymers as well.
Here too, however, positive reactions were restricted to the
plasma cells, especially to those containing Russell bodies.

The restriction of the fluorescence to the Golgi zone,
with all 3 marker systems, in 2 cases of myeloma in which
the production of 10S IgA was very low may deserve special
attention. According to the suggestion of Sherr et al. (16),
the assembly of the Ig molecules is completed in the Golgi
apparatus where the molecules are incorporated into membrane-
bound vesicles before being secreted, by reverse pinocytosis,
into extracellular space. It may be possible that the Golgi
apparatus is also the place where the J chain is added and
mediates the polymer formation or stabilization.

The demonstration of the J chain in cells of 3 Bence-
Jones myelomas might indicate that these malignant clones
originally produced IgA or IgM. Such a conjecture prompts
the idea that it would be of value also to test the J chain
production in malignant cells from cases of so called
"empty myeloma".

Our results can be discussed from the point of view of
the extent of the potential contribution of bone marrow to
circulating IgA. The investigation of the myeloma group
indicates that the number of cells in the bone marrow that
were positive for polymeric IgA appropriately reflects the
level of polymeric IgA paraprotein in serum. Similarly, in
normal individuals and nonmyelomatous patients, the bone
marrow contained cells, positive for markers of polymeric IgA
in numbers that were proportionate to the reported amount of
polymeric IgA in serum. This supports findings of Hijmans
et al. (2) and extends the suggestion that, in man, the bone
marrow is a major contributor of both the mono- and polymeric
IgA that occurs in the circulation.

SUMMARY

Sera and bone marrow cells from patients with IgA1
myeloma and from those with other diseases as well as from
normal individuals were tested by immunodiffusion and
fluorescence techniques with specific antisera for the
presence of α dimeric (polymeric) determinants and J chain,
and for their ability to bind SC in vitro. Polymeric IgA in
all sera and in the majority of bone marrow cells reacted with
the 3 markers, whereas these containing monomeric IgA did not.
As demonstrated by immunofluorescence, the determinants
specific for polymeric IgA are already detectable within the
cells that are producing polymeric IgA. Human bone marrow
can be regarded as a major source of both monomeric and
polymeric serum IgA in myeloma patients as well as in normal
individuals.

Acknowledgements: The authors are grateful to Miss P.v.d.Berg,
Mrs. P.C. Moree-v.d.Linde, and Miss A.M.G. Aijer for their
skillful technical assistance. Supported in part by research
grant USPHS AI 10854 (J.M.).

REFERENCES

1. Tomasi, T.B., N. Engl. J. Med. 287:500, 1972.
2. Hijmans, W., Schuit, H.R.E. and Hulsing-Hesselink, E.
    Ann. N.Y. Acad. Sci. 177:290, 1971.
3. Radl, J., Klein, F., v.d. Berg. P., de Bruyn, A.M. and
    Hijmans, W., Immunology, 20:843, 1971.
4. Radl, J., v.d. Berg, P., Voormolen, M., Hendriks, W.D.H.
    and Schaefer, U.W., Clin, exp. Immunol. in press.
5. Hijmans, W., Schuit, H.R.E. and Klein, F., Clin. exp.
    Immunol. 4:457, 1969.

6. Mestecky, J., Zikan, J., Butler, W.T. and Kulhavy, R., Immunochem. 9:883, 1972.

7. Ploem, J.S., Leitz-Mitt. Wiss. u. Techn. 4:225, 1969.

8. Brandtzaeg, P., Human secretory Immunoglobulins, Universitetsforlaget, Oslo, 1970.

9. Mach, J-P., Nature, 228:1278, 1970.

10. Apicella, M.A. and Allen, J.C., J. Immunol. 104:455, 1970.

11. Halpern, M.S. and Koshland, M.E., Nature, 228:1276, 1970.

12. Mestecky, J., Hammack, W.J., Schrohenloher, R.E. and Bennett, J.C., in Protides of the Biological Fluids, Edited by H. Peeters, Pergamon Press, Oxford, p. 279, 1973.

13. Parkhouse, R.M.E., FEBS Lett. 16:71, 1971.

14. Grey, H.M., Abel, C.A. and Zimmerman, B., Ann. N.Y. Acad. Sci. 190:37, 1971.

15. Askonas, B.A. and Parkhouse, R.M.E., Biochem. J. 123:629, 1971.

16. Sherr, C.J., Schenkein, I. and Uhr, J.W., Ann. N.Y. Acad. Sci. 190:250, 1971.

CYTOPHILIC PROPERTIES OF IgA TO HUMAN NEUTROPHILS

Hans L. Spiegelberg, David A. Lawrence
and Peter Henson

Scripps Clinic and Research Foundation
Department of Experimental Pathology
La Jolla, Calif. 92037

INTRODUCTION

In 1961 Boyden and Sorkin demonstrated that antigens
can be bound to spleen cells which have previously been
incubated with specific antisera (1). The term "cytophilic"
immunoglobulins was coined for this type of antibody. Subsequently, it was shown that immunoglobulins attach via the
Fc fragment to receptors on phagocytic cells such as macrophages (2,3), monocytes (4) and neutrophils (5). The
biological importance of the cytophilic antibodies appears
to be promotion of phagocytosis (opsonization) of antigens.
Not all immunoglobulins are cytophilic. In rodents, IgG of
slow electrophoretic mobility, $\gamma 2G$, is cytophilic whereas
$\gamma 1G$, the anodally migrating IgG is not (3). In man, it has
been shown by inhibition studies that IgG1 and IgG3 are
cytophilic for monocytes (4) and neutrophils (5). Most of
these findings were made by studying "rosette" formation,
that is the adherence of antibody coated red cells to phagocytes (3,4,5). More recently, cytophilic properties have
also been studied by measuring the uptake of radiolabeled
immunoglobulins on macrophages (6) or by release of histamine
from basophils (7). Relatively little is known about cytophilic properties of IgA, probably because it is difficult
to obtain pure IgA antibodies suitable for cytophilic testing.
Since the cytophilic reaction depends on the Fc fragment,
immunoglobulins having no demonstrated antibody activity such
as myeloma proteins can also be used as a source of IgA.
Isolated IgA myeloma proteins were therefore used in this

study. First, the release of lysosomal enzymes from neutrophils following incubation with aggregated IgA was analyzed
(8) and second, the uptake of radiolabeled IgA onto neutrophils was measured and compared to that of other immunoglobulin classes (9).

METHODS

The procedures used to isolate myeloma proteins and to
determine release of β-glucuronidase from neutrophils have
recently been described (8). Five million neutrophils were
incubated for 60 min. at $37^{o}C$ in BTS in presence of 500 μg
of heat or bis-diazotized benzidine aggregated immunoglobulins. The release of β-glucuronidase into the supernatant
was determined and expressed as percent of total release
obtained with triton x-100. The detailed procedure employed
to study the uptake of radiolabeled immunoglobulins on cells
will be reported elsewhere (9). The myeloma proteins were
labeled with ^{125}I employing the chloramine T method (10) and
centrifuged at 100,000 g for 90 min. before use. In order to
determine the uptake of labeled immunoglobulins 40 ng of
labeled proteins were mixed with 5×10^{6} cells in BSS, incubated for 30 min. at $4^{o}C$ and washed twice through fetal calf
serum. EDTA in a concentration of 0.7 mM and 0.25% bovine
serum albumin was added to the BSS. The uptake of radiolabeled protein was expressed in $pg/10^{6}$ cells.

RESULTS

Release of enzymes from neutrophils

When antigen-antibody complexes are mixed with neutrophils, the complexes adhere to the cells and are phagocytosed.
During this reaction the neutrophils release lysomal enzymes
into the medium. Phagocytosis, however, does not appear to
be a prerequisite since enzymes are also released by exocy-
tosis when the complexes are bound to surfaces too large to
be phagocytosed such as microphore filters (11). The release
of enzymes can therefore be used as an indicator of a cytophilic reaction of neutrophils with immunoglobulins. As
shown in Fig. 1, insoluble aggregates of the four IgG and,
interestingly, the two IgA subclasses induced release of
β-glucuronidase from neutrophils, whereas IgD, IgE and IgM
did not. The release of β-glucuronidase was not the result
of cell lysis since no significant release of lactic dehydro-
genase occurred during incubation. Microscopically, the

neutrophils could be seen to adhere to large insoluble
complexes of IgA and IgG but not to complexes of the other
immunoglobulin classes. Examination of neutrophils by
electron microscopy showed that the insoluble IgA aggregates
had been phagocytosed. The amounts of insoluble aggregates
that caused release of β-glucuronidase were similar for both
IgA and IgG myeloma proteins. Nonaggregated or soluble
complexes of the myeloma proteins were inactive in this system.
However, when the soluble aggregates were adherend to micro-
pore filters again aggregated IgA as well as IgG proteins
caused release of enzyme whereas aggregated IgD, IgE and
IgM proteins and unaggregated IgA and IgG proteins did not.
As in all previously reported cytophilic reactions, complement did not appear to play a role in this system since
addition of 10% fresh serum did not significantly change the
release of β-glucuronidase. Not all the enzyme content could
be released and a considerable variation existed in the

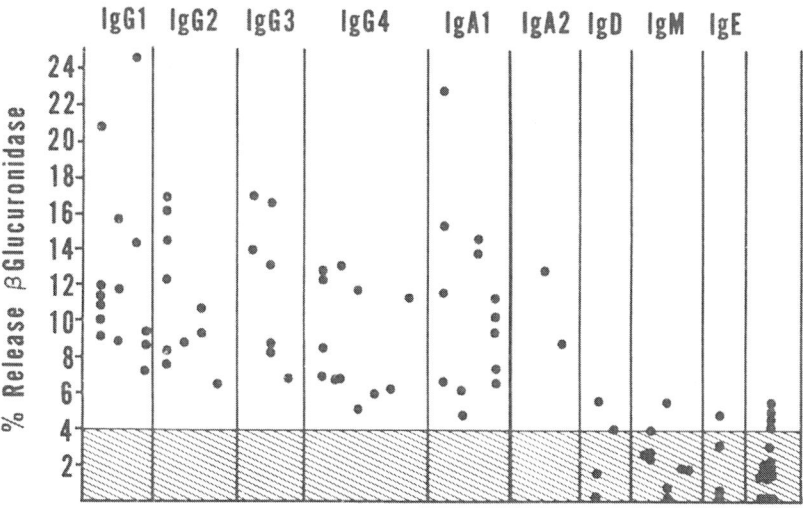

Fig. 1. Release of β-glucuronidase from human neutrophils.
Each column represents a myeloma protein and each point the
mean of a duplicate determination of an individual donor.

percent release from neutrophils of different donors. Furthermore, aggregates of certain myeloma proteins within a
subclass consistently caused better release independent of
the donor of the neutrophils. The reason for the variations
is not known. Despite the considerable variation, it did
not appear that significant quantitative differences existed
in activity between the different subclasses of IgG and IgA.
IgG tetanus-antitetanus complexes were about twice as active
on a mg basis, suggesting that a large proportion of the
artificial aggregates were biologically active. Mild reduction and alkylation of IgA and IgG reduced the release of
enzyme. Similarly, fragments of IgG were less active. Fc
fragments, however, were more active than F(ab')$_2$ fragments
and Fab fragments and light chains were inactive, suggesting
that the Fc portion of the heavy chain was mainly responsible
for the reaction. Attempts to inhibit the enzyme release by
addition of large excess of unaggregated IgA and IgG were
unsuccessful.

Binding of ^{125}I-labeled proteins to neutrophils

The binding of iodinated unaggregated myeloma proteins,
secretory IgA (kindly provided by Dr. Tomasi) and normal
IgG to neutrophils is shown in Fig. 2. Although there was
a considerable variation within a subclass, it was apparent
that IgG1 and IgG3 proteins bound best, followed by IgA1 and
IgA2 proteins. Somewhat more IgG4 was bound than IgG2, IgM,
IgD and IgE. The uptake of secretory IgA was similar to the
IgA myeloma proteins Ka and Wu, and normal IgG was bound to
a similar extent as most IgG1 and IgG3 proteins tested. The
uptake was also determined following incubation at 37°C.
More protein was bound under these conditions; however, the
relative binding of the different classes was not significantly changed. The ability to inhibit the binding of IgG1,
IgG3, IgA1 and IgA2 proteins was investigated by preincu-
bating the neutrophils with a 50–100 fold excess of unlabeled
intact proteins. Binding of IgG1 protein Ma and IgG3 protein
Ni was inhibited by 58 to 84% by both IgG1 and IgG3 proteins.
IgA immunoglobulins (Pu, Wu and S-IgA) inhibited the binding
of proteins Ma and Ni by 8 to 20%. Protein Ma inhibited the
binding of IgA1 protein Pu by 40% but did not significantly
affect the binding of proteins Wu and S-IgA. Protein Wu
inhibited the binding of protein Pu by 42%. Fc fragments of
IgG1 and IgG3 proteins equally inhibited the uptake of intact
IgG proteins, whereas Fab fragments were inactive in this
respect. F(ab')$_2$ fragments showed a slight but significant

inhibition of IgG1 and IgG3 proteins. One IgG1 (Ma) and one
IgA1 (Pu) protein bound much better than all other proteins
tested. In order to determine if the Fc fragment of protein
Ma was responsible for the better binding, its Fc fragment
was labeled and the uptake compared to the Fc fragment of
protein Ba (IgG1). Less of the fragments was bound to the
cells; however, the uptake of the two Fc fragments was
similar.

Since no significant difference was found in the release
of β-glucuronidase from neutrophils in comparing aggregated
IgG and IgA proteins, we attempted to determine the uptake
of the different proteins following aggregation with F(ab')$_2$
fragments of a rabbit antilight chain antiserum. The uptake
of all proteins increased after aggregation, however, the
uptake of IgG2, IgG4, IgA1 and IgA2 proteins increased as
much as 10 fold, whereas binding of IgG1, IgG3 and IgM
proteins increased by only 3 to 5 fold.

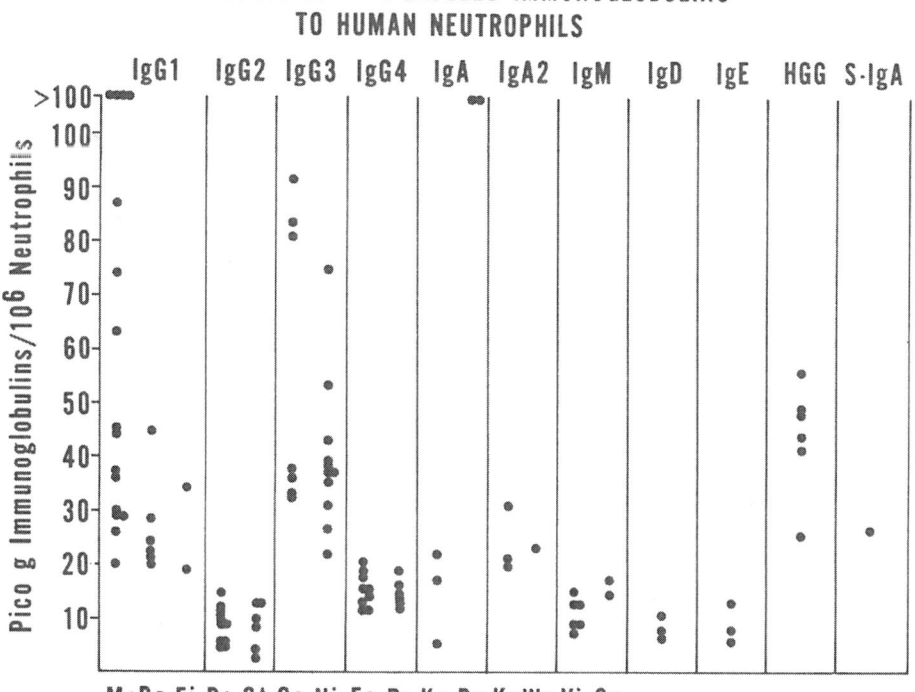

Fig. 2. Uptake of ^{125}I-labeled myeloma proteins, secretory
IgA (S-IgA) and normal IgG. Each point represents mean of
duplicate determinations.

DISCUSSION

The reported experiments demonstrate that both aggregated and unaggregated IgA immunoglobulins react with human neutrophils, suggesting that neutrophils have receptors specific for IgA. Aggregated IgA1 and IgA2 myeloma proteins caused release of lysosomal enzymes in quantities similar to IgG whereas IgM, IgD and IgE myeloma proteins did not. Unaggregated IgA1 and IgA2 myeloma proteins as well as secretory IgA bound to neutrophils, although less than IgG1 and IgG3 myeloma proteins which appear to have the strongest affinity to neutrophils. The receptors for IgA appear to be different from those of IgG since binding of the IgA proteins could not easily be inhibited with IgG myeloma proteins and vice versa. The presence of receptors on neutrophils for IgA suggests that IgA antibodies have an opsonic role and support previous data on bactericidal activity of IgA (12). Hitherto, no effector or secondary function of IgA after it had reacted with antigen had been known. Recently it has been shown, however, that IgA activates the alternate pathway of complement fixation (13,14). However, it appears unlikely that the opsonic role of neutrophils is related to the activation of the alternate complement pathway, since addition of normal serum to the neutrophil-IgA mixture did not change the release of lysosomal enzymes.

The affinity of unaggregated IgA to neutrophils appears to be low. The enzyme release of neutrophils could not be inhibited by unaggregated IgA proteins and less unaggregated IgA was bound to the cells than IgG1 and IgG3. The weak binding of unaggregated IgA is not unexpected since a similar phenomenon was previously shown for $\gamma 2G$ antibody to guinea pig macrophages (3). In these experiments, rosette formation was difficult to inhibit when the antibodies had reacted with the red cells but easily inhibited when the antibody was first added to the macrophages. The low affinity of unaggregated IgA suggests that the opsonic function of IgA antibodies manifests itself mainly following reaction with antigen. Whether allosteric changes after reaction with antigen or the formation of a complex of many IgA molecules causes the increased binding is not known; however, the fact that artificially aggregated myeloma proteins also show strong binding suggests that the latter possibility is more likely.

The reason why the IgG1 protein Ma and IgA1 protein Pu bound much better than the other myeloma proteins of the same subclass is unexplained. In the case of protein Ma, it does not appear to be the result of a different structure in the

Fc fragment since the Fc fragment of protein Ma did not bind
better than the Fc fragment of another low binding IgG
myeloma protein. It has been shown that some myeloma proteins have antiimmunoglobulin activity (15). If proteins
Ma and Pu would have such an activity, the high binding
could result from reaction with cytophilic IgG on the cells
which was not washed off during cell isolation. Alternatively, the Fab fragment may modulate the site on the Fc
fragment which is reacting with the cells. Such a modulation
has been postulated in order to explain the variation seen in
turnover rates of myeloma proteins with a given subclass (16).
In any event, since the normal secretory IgA and normal IgG
bound to an extent similar to the majority of the myeloma
proteins of the same class, it is most likely that the high
binding of proteins Ma and Pu does not reflect the cytophilic
property of most normal IgG and IgA antibodies.

SUMMARY

IgA has been shown to be cytophilic to human neutrophils.
Unaggregated IgA myeloma proteins and secretory IgA bind to
neutrophils, and aggregated IgA myeloma proteins adhere to
neutrophils, release lysosomal enzymes from these cells, and
become phagocytosed.
Publication No. 769 from the Department of Experimental
Pathology, Scripps Clinic and Research Foundation, La Jolla,
California.

REFERENCES

1. Boyden, S.V., and Sorkin, E., Immunology 4:244, 1961.
2. Boyden, S.V., Immunology 7:474, 1964.
3. Berken, A. and Benacerraf, B., J. Exp. Med. 123:119, 1966.
4. Huber, H. and Fudenberg, H.H., Int. Arch. Allergy and
   Applied Immunology 34:18, 1968.
5. Messner, R.P. and Jelinek, J., J. Clin. Invest. 49:2165,
   1970.
6. Inchley, C., Grey, H.M. and Uhr, J.W., J. Immunol. 105:
   362, 1970.
7. Ishizaka, K., Ann. Rev. Med. 21:187, 1970.
8. Henson, P.M., Johnson, H.B. and Spiegelberg, H.L., J.
   Immunol. 109:1182, 1972.
9. Lawrence, D.A. and Spiegelberg, H.L., in preparation.
10. Unanue, E.R., J. Immunol. 107:1168, 1971.
11. Henson, P.M., J. Exp. Med. 134:114s, 1971.

12. Adinolfi, M., Glynn, A.A., Lindsey, M. and Milner, L.M., Immunology <u>10</u>:517, 1966.
13. Spiegelberg, H.L., and Götze, O., Fed. Proc. <u>31</u>:655, 1972.
14. Tomasi, T.B., these meetings.
15. Grey, H.M., Kohler, P.F., Terry, W.D., and Franklin, E.C., J. Clin. Invest. <u>47</u>:1875, 1968.
16. Spiegelberg, H.L., Fishkin, B.G. and Grey, H.M., J. Clin. Invest. <u>47</u>:2323, 1968.

DISCUSSION

Dr. Pruitt - I have a question for Dr. Spiegelberg. I believe in your paper you showed that aggregated serum IgA interacted preferentially with the surface of the neutrophils when compared to the unaggregated serum IgA. I'd like to ask whether you made the same observation with secretory IgA?

Dr. Spiegelberg - Yes. Bis-diazoitized, benzene-aggregated secretory IgA reacted very similarly to the myeloma proteins.

Dr. Pruitt - That is very interesting; it parallels the work that Dr. Boackle and I have done with regard to the difference between the interaction of aggregated serum IgA and secretory IgA with the complement system. We found that unaggregated serum IgA or secretory IgA does not interact with complement but that aggregates of serum IgA or secretory IgA produced by a lyophilization, or simple drying, did interact with the complement system.

Dr. Spiegelberg - What kind of complement system?

Dr. Pruitt - I'll turn this over to Dr. Boackle at this time.

Dr. Boackle - Lyophilized or evaporated preparations of secretory and serum IgA were interacted with human serum as a source of complement and the complement profiles taken. We found that these interfacially aggregated preparations removed functional C3 through C9 activity, but not C1 activity.

Dr. Spiegelberg - What about C2?

Dr. Boackle - In studies with guinea pig complement, no C2 activity was removed.

Dr. Robert Waldman - I would like to ask Dr. Bienenstock whether, when he injected the BALT cells in the transfer experiments, he looked to see if they preferentially homed to secretory surfaces? Was there a difference between the respiratory surface and the gastrointestinal surface in this regard? In Dr. Cebra's experiments, did he ever look at the respiratory mucosa to see whether the cells that he transferred went there or only to the gastrointestinal tract?

Dr. Bienenstock - The answers to your questions are yes. The cells derived from the bronchial lymphoid tissue go to the gut. I showed you a photograph of that. As far as one can see, they also home to the bronchial lymphoid tissue area but not into the lymphoid follicle itself. The cells in gut and spleen are considerably greater in terms of numbers than they are in the bronchial lymphoid tissue. There are, in fact, very few plasma cells detected by immunofluorescence with anti-alpha chain or anti-any immunoglobulin serum in the lamina propria of normal animals' bronchial tracts. As regards the question of Peyer's patch cells going to these areas - Peyer's patch cells migrate to the bronchial areas in much the same way as cells from bronchus-associated lymphoid tissue. In contrast, lymph node cell transfer does not result in any immunoglobulin-producing cells of any type in these areas.

Dr. David Rowe - I'd like to address a question to Dr. Cooper, Dr. Bienenstock, Dr. Cebra or anybody who might like to answer. It's a paradox at the moment that the previous work on the secretory system has emphasized the local nature of the immune response. I would cite Dr. Waldman's work and Dr. Ogra's work, indicating that exposure to local antigen results in a local antibody response. Now we hear that the driving mechanism for the distribution of IgA cells from precursors in GALT and BALT is the arrival of antigen in these specialized lymphoid areas. This, then, implies that antigen may result in the distribution of antibody synthesizing cells very widely throughout the lamina propria of the gastrointestinal and respiratory tracts. Now the marker that's been used, of course, has been IgA. Would anybody like to comment on the antigenic specificity of the cell populations triggered in this way? In practical terms of immunizing people against infections that occur in particular places, this may be very important.

Dr. Bienenstock - I'll try and answer you, David, however, there is no direct answer that I could suggest. If we go back to the experiments of Ray Ogra showing local antibody production, I think it is fair to say that we are talking about low titers of antibody, of the order of 1:8 to 1:32. In other words, the difference between a local response and

no response is not very great. In view of the very large
numbers of antigens bathing these sites and presumably
triggering IgA production, it is perhaps not surprising that
the titer to a specific antigen might be low. I would suggest that one is going to have to go to the cells themselves,
to look at the frequency of cells producing antibody of a
given specificity, rather than simply look at the secretions
as the reflection of how much antibody is being produced.

Dr. Hanson - I would like to ask something that has been
puzzling me for some time. Where do the cells in the mammary gland come from and how do the proper antigens reach
those cells - that is, the antigens that should cause
formation of the antibodies that the neonate needs to
protect its gastrointestinal tract. Can anybody answer that?

Dr. Cebra - A lot of us would like to be able to use antigen
binding as a marker for plasma cells that are making antibody of a given specificity and to follow the route of
precursors of such cells to the tissue location where they
may be expanded out. The precursors for particular IgA
antibody forming cells may initially be expanded out in the
Peyer's patches. There already is a paper published suggesting antigen priming in the gut by Dr. Bazin. He and
his colleagues fed sheep red blood cells to the mouse and
then assayed for indirect IgA plaque forming cells by
facilitation. They found them to occur and increase in
number first in mesenteric lymph nodes. Later on such PFC
peaked in the spleen. It remains an open question whether
PFC with the same specificity would also be found elsewhere
in secretory tissue. Now, to talk to the point concerning
what stimulates the cells in mammary tissue. One might
imagine that antigen driven proliferation by the antigens
passing through the dome epithelium in the Peyer's patches
results in the expansion of clones of B-cells with specificity for environmental antigens, followed by emigration
of these cells to other secretory tissues. We now know that
many of these B-cells can be turned on with pokeweed mitogen,
with lipopolysaccharide, and with a hose of other nonspecific
agents unrelated to the original priming antigen. It is
possible that a second antigen encounter by these immediate
precursors of IgA is not necessary for their maturation in
exocrine tissue and lamina propria to plasma cells.
           I have a question for Dr. Vassalli. He stressed
his interest in the blast cells from the gut associate
lymphoid tissue. I wonder if he ever observed, coexisting

on the plasma membrane of these cells, both IgA markers and
Thy-1 or TL markers.   I would be interested in knowing
whether or not there is any feedback of IgA onto T-
lymphocytes and thus whether or not there might be adherent
IgA on the surfaces of T-lymphocytes from the gut associated
lymphoid tissues.

Dr. Vassalli - No.   You mean whether blast cells from GALS
show at the same time a T-cell marker and IgA?   No, certainly
not.

Dr. Good - I was very much interested in Dr. Bienenstock's
observations, particularly the lympho-epithelial relationships in the respiratory apparatus.   In looking over a wide
range of separate phylogenetic divisions, we have found all
sorts of different apparent associations of this lympho-
epithelial type.   I think that this may be a very common
concomitant of antigen associated stimulation at these sites.
I know that the theme this morning has been that the
development of these sites is independent of antigenic
stimulation but I am not sure that we should close the book
on this.   Dr. Kim working with us has been studying what are
truly antigen free animals, the piglets of pathogen-free
sows that have an extremely impermeable placenta.   These
piglets do not develop these sites in the lung nor in the
gastrointestinal tract until after they are exposed to
antigen.   Now barnyard pigs are quite unacceptable for this
kind of investigation.   I was encouraged to find that the
Czech investigators, using models that we would think are
satisfactory, find neither B cells in the circulation (except
for a very, very few IgM producing cells), nor these lympho-
epithelial sites that we have all been so attracted to as
candidates for development of the B-lymphocytes.   I think it
may very well be that an early stage of B-cell differentiation
may require antigen drive just as well as the later stage
requires it, although perhaps at a lower level of antigen
exposure.

Dr. Montgomery - Mr. Chairman, I have a few comments in reply
to your question concerning the mechanism of localized antibody production and the arrival of IgA producing cells in a
secretory site.   We have evidence in the rabbit system -
after oral stimulation with dinitrophenylated pneumococcus -
that no serum antibodies are induced while these animals are
producing secretory IgA antibodies at a remote secretory
site - the mammary gland.   We shall elaborate on the details

of these studies Thursday morning. Although we did not
directly look at antibody producing cells, we feel that our
observations on antibody production suggest that IgA precursor cells may be migrating out from the intestinal area
(assuming that oral immunization stimulates the gastrointestinal mucosa) and seeding a remote secretory site.

Dr. Cooper - I just want to answer my mentor, Bob Good. I
agree that it is an unsettled issue whether development of
B-lymphocytes require no exogenous antigen or just tiny
amounts of antigens relative to that required to trigger
B-lymphocytes to become mature plasma cells. However, the
studies in fetal pigs published by Binns and colleagues
gave very different results than the ones you mention. Now
his pregnant sows may have a different microbial flora,
but they were from specific pathogen free herds. At any
rate, these investigators find significant numbers of B-
lymphocytes in the pig fetus beginning after the 50th
gestational day (out of a 114-day total gestation), and
there is a regular and rapid increase in numbers beginning
around 65 days. These results fit well with the onset of
antibody responsiveness at about 70 days of gestation as
demonstrated in studies by English and Czech workers.

Dr. Parkhouse - I wish to make a comment on Dr. Radl's paper.
It is perfectly true that we have shown for both IgM and IgA
in the mouse that the intracellular species present is the
7S monomeric form. Now Buxbaum, Zolla, and Scharff have
examined human bone marrow samples taken from cases of IgM
myeloma. They showed that there are two patterns of intracellular assembly: one which looks very much like the mouse
and another in which there is a gradual build-up within the
cell of the polymeric form of the IgM. The latter situation
may be similar to what Dr. Radl reports for human IgA.
Alternatively, although the evidence looks convincing, it has
to be remembered that in our studies, and in the studies of
Scharff's group as well, the material is always examined
eventually under dissociating conditions, whereas, in these
fluorescent studies the conditions obviously are not dissociating. The key experiment to do here, I would imagine,
is a biosynthetic experiment; to analyze radiolabeled intracellular IgA on a dissociating gel and to determine that
there really are disulfide-bonded polymeric forms in the
cells.

Dr. Reynolds - I have a question that I would like to direct
to Dr. Radl or perhaps to Dr. Heremans. This question
regards the origin of 7S monomeric IgA in the lungs of
humans. In an analysis of about 35 specimens of bronchial
washings obtained from a subsegmental lung lobe of humans
through a transnasal fiber-optic bronchoscope, we have
been surprised to find, in addition to typical 11S secretory IgA, a substantial amount of 7S monomeric IgA. This
7S IgA does not have identifiable secretory component and
apparently lacks J chain as well. It seems to be the same
IgA species that is found in predominance in the serum. I
might add that the bronchial fluids have not been frozen
but have been separated by chromatography or on sucrose
density gradients. Should we interpret from the discussion
this morning that this 7S monomeric IgA has passively dif-
fused from the serum into the lungs or is it conceivable
that it is formed by a local synthetic process? I might
say that this finding of 7S IgA in humans is in contra-
distinction to findings in the dog and rabbit, where
washings of the lungs contain primarily 11S IgA.

Dr. Heremans - I think the best way to answer your question
is experimental. What you have to do is compare the excretion rate of the 7S IgA you are interested in with the
excretion rate of proteins which you are quite certain are
not synthesized locally, such as albumin, transferrin, alpha
2 macroglobulin, etc. If in that case there is an excess of
the 7S IgA form you know that it must either have been
transferred selectively or that it is formed locally. Specific activity measurements will help decide between these
two possibilities.

Dr. Fudenberg - I would like to comment if I may on Dr.
Reynolds' question. Do I understand that these washings
from humans were obtained from normal lung, and if so, how
do you get this by a human experimentation committee? We
have been unable to obtain such permission at our institution.
I think that using the dog as a model to see if this is
secreted or synthesized or merely passive diffusion is not
valid because in the dog about 85 percent, as I recall, of
the IgA is in dimer form in the serum. I would, if these
are diseased lungs, assume that the 7S IgA represents leak-
age from the serum through diseased capillaries or something
of that nature. The dog is not a suitable control.

Dr. Plaut - I also want to respond to Dr. Reynolds and point
out that the presence of low molecular weight or 7S "IgA"
in secretions may actually be Fc fragments of IgA and not
whole IgA itself. We are going to discuss this evening
bacterial enzymes present at mucosal sites which split IgA
proteins to yield Fc fragments. While one usually looks at
secretions with class specific antisera, I think that it is
now incumbent to insure that light chains are present on
these smaller substances which seem to be IgA.

Dr. Reynolds - Could I respond? Dr. Fudenberg, these bronchial washings were from, let's say, "normal patients,"
that is, people who had an indication for the procedure.
However, we have also been using normal volunteers. I think
normal volunteers are being used extensively around the
United States to obtain bronchial washings for experimental
purposes. With the fiber-optic bronchoscope, this is a very
nonhazardous procedure. To respond to Dr. Plaut's question,
that is why I indicated the special care taken in handling
of these bronchial secretions. Obviously you can introduce
all sorts of artifacts with careless handling. These seem
to be intact 7S molecules.

Dr. Tomasi - There is another possible source for 7S IgA
in secretions. There are higher polymers of IgA which are
present in many of these secretions and these are extremely
sensitive to reducing conditions, so that concentrations as
low as .01 molar mercaptoethanolamine, which are very weak,
will reduce them. I would suggest that you might try adding
iodoacetamide to see whether this has any effect.

Dr. Hanson - I would just like to come back to a point that
Dr. Heremans made this morning. He suggested that there was
no secondary response in the secretory IgA system since the
antibodies themselves would prevent the antigenic stimulus.
Now if that is true it would mean that breast-fed neonates,
having the maternal secretory IgA antibodies in their gut,
would also be prevented from receiving many antigenic
stimuli, resulting in a lower immune response at the local
level as compared to nonbreast-fed infants. As a matter of
fact there are reports of lower immunoglobulin levels in
breast-fed infants. This has been suggested to be due to
more infections in the nonbreast-fed ones, but may have this
additional cause. Would you agree to such an idea, that the
milk antibodies would prevent antigenic contact, Dr.
Heremans?

Dr. Heremans - Your point is that the higher antibody level to certain infectious agents in newborns that are fed cow's milk does not necessarily indicate that they have a higher infection rate but may indicate that they are easily immunized because they are not prevented from recognizing the antigen. However, the difficulty is that pediatricians would probably not agree, because the rate of clinical infections is higher in formulae-fed infants than it is in breast-fed infants. At least that is what I have been told - I am not a pediatrician myself.

Dr. Hanson - This is only partly true. It can be proven in some groups (i.e. from developing countries) but not among children living under rather good hygienic and public health circumstances. For example, in Sweden, a significant difference has not been shown in frequency of infection between breast-fed and formulae-fed infants.

Dr. Bockman - I would like to ask Dr. Heremans if I understood correctly that he was indicating a molecular sieving effect of the blood vessels both in the small intestine and the liver, and I would indicate that perhaps in the liver fenestrae, or holes, in the vascular walls are much too large to sieve any of the molecules that were shown. Perhaps this would be a good comparison for showing the effects of epithelial cells with or without the molecular sieving of the endothelial cells proper.

Dr. Cooper - In considering the local immune response along mucous surfaces of the body, it seems to me that there is an important issue that we have been dancing around. In order to elicit a local antibody response by any one of perhaps a million different clones of B cells, it is necessary to have an effective mechanism to bring the antigen into contact with members of the proper clone. In lymph nodes this mechanism seems to be provided by the antigen trapping capabilities of dendritic histiocytes and the continuous flow of B-lymphocytes through the lymph nodes, thus acting in a way analogous to a solid immunoadsorbent column. In most areas underlying mucous surfaces, however, there does not seem to be a steady stream of B-lymphocytes passing by nor has an efficient means for trapping antigen yet been demonstrated. In considering this problem, I find the Peyer's patches and the appendix theoretically attractive as sites where these requirements could be fulfilled. Regardless of whether or not one accepts the hypothesis that

these are the mammalian bursa-equivalent, it is established
that follicles of B-lymphocytes are generated in these
locations very early in life. Thus, if one were looking for
a place where antigens might enter and select the proper
clones of B-lymphocytes, what better place to go than where
clonal diversity is being generated? We suggest that antigen
crosses from the lumen via the pinocytotic follicle-
associated-epithelial cells, selects the proper B-lymphocyte
clone, induces expansion, stimulates emigration to lamina
propria of mucous surfaces elsewhere, and results in antibody production in these secondary locations. As was
elaborated in Dr. Vassalli's paper, there is a large amount
of data regarding homing of such cells from the lymph to the
small intestine. Whether or not this seeding occurs along
the lamina propria of other internal body surfaces needs
further exploration. The role of B cell mitogens, such as
lipopolysaccharides of gram-negative bacteria, in augmenting
antigen responsiveness of B-lymphocytes in GALT follicles
also deserves further study.

SESSION B

STRUCTURE, BIOSYNTHESIS AND GENETICS

CHAIRMAN: J. CLAUDE BENNETT

CHARACTERISTICS OF SC-Ig COMPLEXES FORMED IN VITRO

Per Brandtzaeg

Institute of Pathology, Rikshospitalet
Oslo, Norway

INTRODUCTION

A stabilized dimeric IgA is the predominant immunoglobulin of most human exocrine secretions. During its passage
through glandular cells the dimer becomes conjugated with an
epithelial glycoprotein called "secretory component" (SC).
IgM is also selectively transmitted through glandular epithelium (1). It has recently been proposed that SC may act
as a specific epithelial Ig receptor and hence determine the
selective external transfer of dimeric IgA and 19S IgM (2,3).
Mach (4) first demonstrated that when dimeric IgA is mixed
with free SC a spontaneous complexing occurs. He also mentioned that IgM is able to bind SC. This was independently
observed by Rádl et al. (5), who claimed that only the higher
polymers (25-30S) exhibit affinity for SC.

Here I report that free SC combines as readily with 19S
IgM as with dimeric IgA, and that the structural characteristic determining the molecular affinity is introduced at the
intracellular stage of Ig formation. The forces involved in
the SC-Ig interactions are defined, and the quaternary structure of SC-Ig complexes produced in vitro is partially characterized.

MATERIALS AND METHODS

Free SC of at least 98% purity was isolated from pooled
human colostrum by gel filtration and anionic-exchange
chromatography (6) combined with immunological removal of

contaminants. Monoclonal monomeric, dimeric and polymeric
IgA preparations were purified from sera of patients with
myelomatosis by anionic-exchange chromatography followed by
Sephadex G-200 filtration. Polyclonal monomeric and dimeric
IgA samples were similarly isolated from the serum of a
patient (K.M.) with an undefined intestinal disorder. Human
albumin, lactoferrin, colostral IgA (col.IgA), IgG and monoclonal IgM were obtained as reported elsewhere (7-9). Purified samples were labelled electrochemically with ^{125}I (10).
Dissociation and denaturation of Igs (8), electrophoretic
demonstration of J chain (9), immunochemical analyses (7,8),
production of rabbit antisera (7,8), preparation and characterization of fluorescent conjugates (11,12), processing of
biopsy specimens for immunohistochemistry (3), and microscopy with conditions for selective demonstration of green or
red immunofluorescence (12) have been described before.

SC affinity of Ig molecules in solutions of various
ionic strengths was analyzed by ultracentrifugation. After
incubation for 1 hr at $37^{\circ}C$ and overnight at $4^{\circ}C$, the samples
were centrifuged at 42,000 rev/min (rotor: Beckman SW 56 Ti)
and $4^{\circ}C$ for 20 hr on a 10-35% sucrose gradient made in the
pertinent buffer solution. The percentage of radioactive SC
contained in the Ig fractions served as a measure of binding
capacity. SC affinity of intracellular Ig components (3) was
tested on intestinal tissue from a patient with Crohn's disease. Serial sections were first incubated with unlabelled
SC at 7-15 µg/ml in a 0.3-0.5% (w/v) solution of rabbit IgG
for 1 hr at room temperature. Control sections were incubated with rabbit IgG alone. After a 20 min saline wash, all
sections were treated with a MRITC-labelled ("red") anti-SC
conjugate combined with a FITC-labelled ("green") anti-Ig
conjugate (Table I).

Table I. Conjugates used in the SC affinity test

Specificity	Label	Conc.(mg/ml)	Ppt.units	OD ratios
Anti-human SC	MRITC*	1.9	1/3	5.7
Anti-human α-chain	FITC*	1.2	1/5	1.7
Anti-human µ-chain	FITC	1.0	3/4	2.2
Anti-human γ-chain	FITC	0.3	2/3	1.8

* Rhodamine (MRITC) and fluorescein (FITC) isothiocyanates.

RESULTS

All of eight dimeric or polymeric IgA preparations, containing readily detectable J chain, bound SC when tested in
PBS (0.15M NaCl, 0.01M phosphate buffer, pH 7.5) or in 0.1M
Tris-HCl buffer, pH 8. When 2.5 µg SC was mixed with 100 µg
IgA the binding capacity was 60-75%, but it decreased dras-
tically with increase in the salt concentration. This held
true both for a monoclonal (not shown) and for a polyclonal
preparation (Fig. 1). The binding capacity of six IgM preparations containing readily detectable J chain was 65-74% and

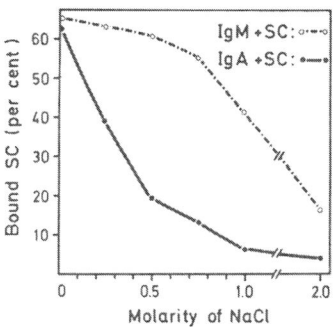

Figure 1. Binding capacity of 19S IgM (J.N.) and dimeric
IgA (K.M.) after incubation with 2.5 µg SC/100 µg in 0.1M
Tris-HCl buffer, pH 8, containing various molarities of NaCl.
Bound SC was determined by centrifugation on sucrose gradi-
ents made in corresponding buffer solutions.

only slightly affected by salt concentrations below 0.7M NaCl
(Fig. 1). Density gradient ultracentrifugation demonstrated
that 19S IgM as well as larger polymers bound SC (Fig. 2).
Based on the assumption that there was homogeneous labelling
of polypeptide chains, the fractions of larger polymers were
calculated to be 15.3-24.4% for three preparations of radioactive IgM. For the corresponding unlabelled proteins, the
binding capacity per µg could then be estimated to be about
45% higher for the 19S than for the larger polymer fractions
(Table II). Pooled IgG and eleven monomeric IgA samples did
not bind SC. Furthermore, IgM and dimeric IgA had no detectable affinity for radioactive IgG, albumin or lactoferrin.

Immunochemical and physico-chemical analyses were performed on SC-Ig complexes isolated by filtration through
Sephadex G-200 (Fig. 3). Before chromatography the immunoglobulins were incubated with about 10µg unlabelled plus
2 µg radioactive SC/100 µg in PBS. The final molar SC:Ig

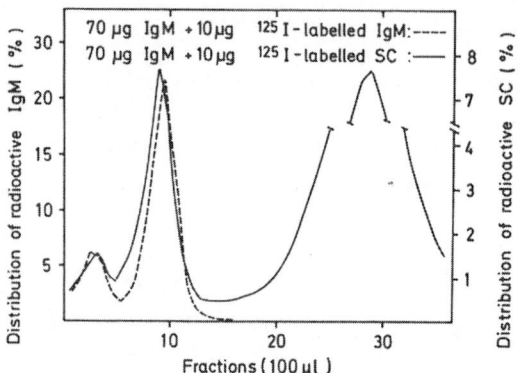

Figure 2. IgM (Karl.A), and complexes of IgM (Karl.A) and
SC, analyzed by density-gradient ultracentrifugation in 0.1M
Tris-HCl buffer, pH 8, containing 1M NaCl. Bottom of gradi-
ents to the left.

ratio averaged 1:7.5 for the IgA fraction and 1:2.5 for the
IgM fraction. The complexes had a relatively "loose" quaternary structure since they produced distinct precipitin rings
with anti-I (Fig. 4). With anti-SC, active against both A
and I determinants (8), double rings were formed by the SC-
IgA complexes demonstrating the presence of two molecular
species, one with accessible and another with inaccessible
I determinants. (A similar pattern is obtained for col.IgA
preparations when SC is partially released by reduction.)
Dialysis against 0.1M Tris-HCl buffer, pH 8, for at least 20
hr at 4°C, or bubbling of O_2 through the sample for 6 hr,
resulted in a "packing" of the SC-IgA complexes as revealed
by disappearance of the I determinant (Fig. 4). Similar
treatment did not decrease the I reactivity of the SC-IgM
complexes. When the samples had been stored at 4°C for 4
months most of the I reactivity was lost in the SC-IgA complexes, and it was moreover distinctly decreased in the SC-
IgM complexes. In the latter, two molecular species were now
distinguished by anti-SC reacting with both A and I determinants (Fig. 4).

Table II. Binding of SC to 19S and larger IgM polymers

| IgM pre-paration | Distribution of radioactive IgM and SC* | | | | | |
| | 19S fraction | | | Larger polymer fraction | | |
	IgM%	SC%	SC%:IgM%	IgM%	SC%	SC%:IgM%
Karl.A	75.6	81.7	1.08	24.4	18.3	0.75
Karl.B	84.7	88.9	1.05	15.3	11.1	0.73
L.H.	76.4	83.3	1.09	23.6	16.7	0.71

* Determined by density-gradient ultracentrifugation (Fig. 2).

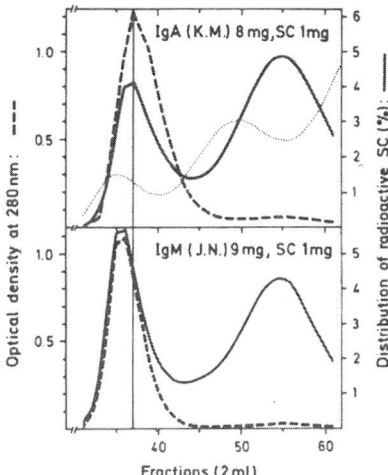

Figure 3. Chromatography of SC-IgA (top) and SC-IgM (bottom) complexes on a column (2.5 x 40 cm) of Sephadex G-200 equilibrated with 0.1M Tris-HCl buffer, pH 8, containing 1M NaCl. Flow rate (upward): 2.3 ml cm^{-2} hr^{-1}; sample volumes: 1 ml. Vertical line indicates fractions of equal SC content. For reference, part of the OD pattern of 1.5 ml lipid-free normal human serum filtered through the same column is indicated by a dotted line (top).

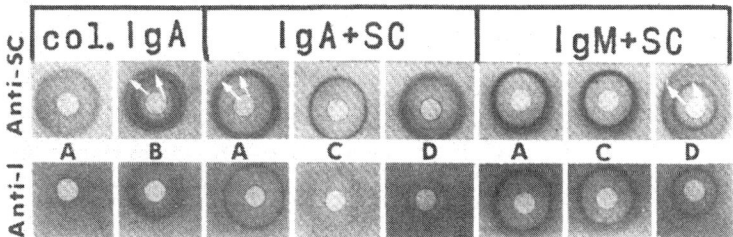

Figure 4. Single radial immunodiffusion with an antiserum to SC (top) and with an antiserum monospecific for the I determinant of SC (bottom). Complexes of IgA+SC and IgM+SC were isolated by gel filtration and subjected to the following treatments: storage at $-20°C$ for less than four months (A); dialysis against 0.1M Tris-HCl buffer, pH 8, for 35 hr at $4°C$ (C); or storage for 4 months at $4°C$ (D). Reference samples were col.IgA in its native state (A) and after reduction with 0.05M βME (B). In some preparations two molecular species (arrows) were revealed by anti-SC.

The "packing" of SC-IgA complexes after dialysis or O_2 bubbling was parallelled by a highly significant ($p<0.001$; Student's $\underline{t}$ test) stabilization as demonstrated by density

containing 1M NaCl (Table III). A less pronounced effect
($p<0.05$) was obtained for the SC-IgM complexes, although
these initially were significantly ($p<0.001$) more stable than
those of SC-IgA (Table III). The latter were, on the contrary, more resistart to denaturation by acid urea (Table
III); but both types of complexes were less resistant to such
treatment than col.IgA (Fig. 5). ("Resistant" refers to
dissociation and not to aggregation which was pronounced for
IgA after denaturation.) Assuming a homogeneous labelling
of all polypeptide chains, it was calculated that no more
than 25% of the bound SC was released from radioactive col.
IgA by acid urea, whereas 57-67% was released from the SC-Ig
complexes. However, the percentage of bound SC increased
upon prolonged storage before the treatment, especially for
the SC-IgA complexes (Table III). The above results show
that complexes formed spontaneously in vitro are less covalently stabilized than native col.IgA. The SC-IgA complexes
were slightly less resistant to β-mercaptoethanol (βME) than
those of SC-IgM (Table III); but the indirect effect of reduction on non-covalent interactions can hardly be evaluated
since the quaternary structures of dimeric IgA and 19S IgM
are highly sensitive to βME. Very low concentrations of βME
increased the stability of SC-IgM complexes (Table III),
probably by enhancing disulfide interchange. While 60% of
col.IgA remained polymerized after reduction with 0.05M βME,
only 30% of dimeric IgA (K.M.) was intact following such
treatment (Fig. 5). This superior stability of col.IgA can
most likely be ascribed to incorporation of SC. Thus, despite the pronounced sensitivity of dimeric IgA (K.M.) to

Table III.   Stability of SC-Ig complexes isolated by
             gel filtration

Sample treatment	Percentage ($\pm$ S.D.) of bound SC*	
	SC-IgA	SC-IgM
Storage at -20°C	59.2 $\pm$ 2.5 (n=8)	66.6 $\pm$ 1.0 (n=3)
Dialysis at 4°C	81.0 $\pm$ 2.3 (n=12)	72.9 $\pm$ 2.9 (n=3)
Urea, 6M, pH 3.3	42.3 (56.0)**	33.2 (40.8)**
βME, 0.002M	77.6	80.3
βME, 0.005M	77.9	77.7
βME, 0.010M	65.6	72.8
βME, 0.050M	45.1	50.9
βME, 0.075M	28.2	34.6

*   Determined by density-gradient ultracentrifugation.
** Samples stored at -20°C for 40 additional days.

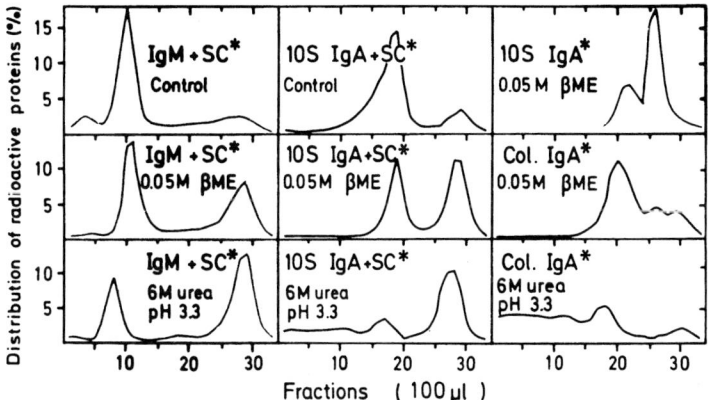

Figure 5. Isolated complexes of IgM+SC and IgA+SC, serum-type dimeric (10S) IgA, and secretory (col.) IgA analyzed by density-gradient ultracentrifugation in 0.1M Tris-HCl buffer, pH 8, containing 1M NaCl. Before the analyses the samples were dialyzed against 0.1M Tris-HCl buffer, pH 8, for 20 hr (Controls), or subjected to reduction or denaturation as indicated. The radioactive components are labelled with asterisks. Bottom of gradients to the left.

reduction, it was sufficiently stabilized by combination with SC to retain 45% of the bound component after treatment with 0.05M βME (Fig. 5).

As reported before (3) most IgA and IgM immunocytes adjacent to glandular epithelium bound SC in vitro. In test sections positive immunocytes were identified by red fluorescence (Fig. 6). Control sections incubated without SC showed immunocytes with pure green colour signifying their Ig content, whereas red fluorescence was confined to glandular cells producing SC. The specificity of the SC affinity was confirmed by testing the blocking effect of various proteins (Table IV). Lysozyme, neurophysin (gift from Dr. O.Trygstad) and albumin were selected because of their high content of half cystine, but they did not interfere with the SC binding. Neither did IgG, monomeric IgA or IgE (gift from Dr. T. Michaelsen) exhibit any inhibiting effect, whereas dimeric IgA and expecially 19S IgM efficiently blocked the reaction. Non-covalent forces were responsible for the affinity between SC and cytoplasmic Ig components since it was inhibited by dissociating reagents and NaCl (Table V; Fig. 6). These forces were clearly stronger for IgM cells than for IgA cells. The inhibiting effect of the alkylating reagents, revealed at relatively high molarities, should most likely be ascribed mainly to an ionic effect rather than to blocking of

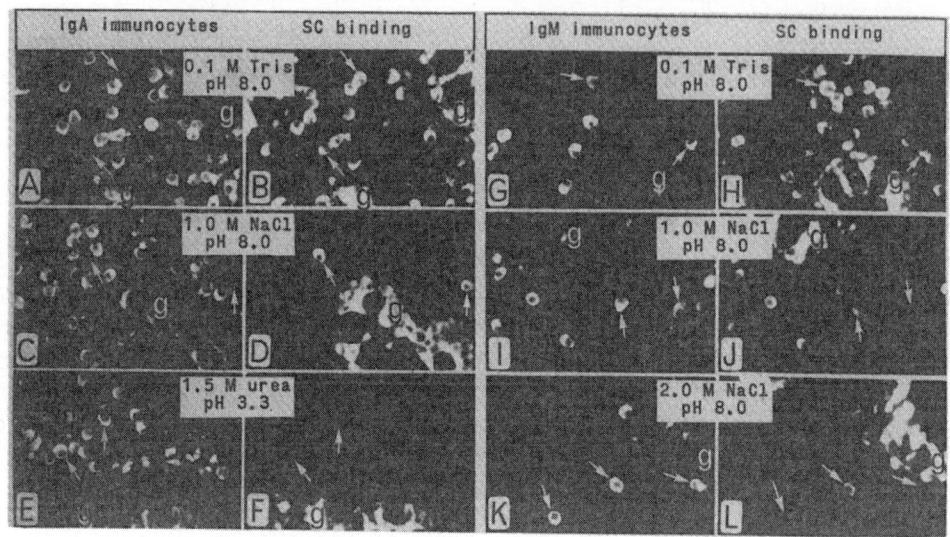

Figure 6. Immunohistochemical SC affinity tests performed
on IgA and IgM immunocytes in sections of human intestinal
mucosa. A pair of letters (e.g. A-B) refers to the same
field photographed through a green filter to reveal the Ig
class (A etc.) and through a red filter to reveal SC (B etc.).
Red fluorescence of immunocytes, after incubation with SC in
various reagents as indicated, demonstrates a positive affinity test, whereas red fluorescence related to the crypts
represents innate SC in glandular cells (g), which also contain some IgA and occasional traces of IgM. Examples of
identical positions in pictures of the same field are indicated by arrows. Original magnification: 180x.

Table IV. Specificity of the binding of SC to
immunocytes

Type	Blocking protein		Cytoplasmic fluorescence*	
	Conc. (mg/ml)	Addition (µg/µg SC)	IgA cells	IgM cells
Rabbit IgG	5.0	360	++	++
Egg-white lysozyme	5.0	360	++	++
Human neurophysin	2.0	150	++	++
Human albumin	5.0	360	++	++
Human 7S IgA	2.7	200	++	++
Human IgE	0.5	70	++	++
Human dimeric IgA	0.5	70	-	±
Human 19S IgM	0.5	70	-	-

* Graded on the average (duplicate sections) from negative
(-) through negligible (±) and faint (+) to intense (++).

Table V. Effect of various alkylating and dissociating
          reagents on the binding of SC to immunocytes

Reagent			Cytoplasmic fluorescence*	
Type	Molarity	pH	IgA cells	IgM cells
IAAM**	0.25	8.0	+	++
IAMM	0.50	8.0	±	+
IAMM	1.00	8.0	-	±
IAAC**	0.10	8.0	+	+
IAAC	0.20	8.0	-	+
IAAC	0.40	8.0	-	±
CH₃COOH	1.00	2.7	-	-
Urea	0.75	5.8	+	+
Urea	1.50	3.3	-	-
NaCl	1.00	8.0	±	++
NaCl	2.00	8.0	-	±

* Graded as in Table IV.
** Iodoacetamide and iodoacetic acid

SH groups. The difference between iodoacetamide and iodoacetic acid might be explained by the fact that while the
former was dissolved in 0.1M Tris-HCl buffer, the latter
needed a considerable addition of NaOH for adjustment to pH 8,
which is necessary to ensure selective reactivity with SH
groups. Pre-incubation of the sections for 1 hr and of the
SC for 10 hr with these reagents had no additional effect.

DISCUSSION

This investigation has demonstrated that SC exhibits
specific non-covalent affinity for 19S IgM and dimeric or
polymeric IgA. The affinity seems to be determined by the
presence of J chain in the polymer structure as indicated by
recent experiments on IgM (9); our subsequent studies of IgA
have supported this view (unpublished data). Dose-response
curves based on interactions in PBS have revealed a relatively high affinity and a limited capacity with a maximum molar
SC:Ig ratio of 1:1.5-1:2.5 for isolated complexes (unpublished data). This ratio drops markedly for the SC-IgA complexes when they are exposed to higher salt concentrations
(cf. Fig. 3); the non-covalent forces are not so strong between SC and IgA as between SC and IgM. Subsequent covalent
stabilization, on the other hand, takes place more readily
for the SC-IgA complexes, as demonstrated by lowered I determinant reactivity and decreased dissociation of bound SC.

These observations are in agreement with the fact that while
virtually all native secretory IgA polymers are conjugated
with SC, only 60-70% of 19S IgM purified from external
secretions contains bound SC; secretory IgM moreover exhibits
a distinct I determinant reactivity indicating a relatively
"loose" quaternary structure (unpublished data).

The binding of SC to immunocytes is also due to non-
covalent interactions. The inhibiting effect of salt on the
SC affinity of IgA and IgM cells parallelled the observations
made with dimeric IgA and 19S IgM. These findings strongly
support the idea that the cytoplasmic SC affinity is mediated
by completed IgA dimers and IgM polymers containing J chain.
This would be in agreement with recent studies indicating
that cells from most IgM-producing human tumors accumulate
fully assembled 19S molecules intracellularly (13).

The concept that SC may function as an epithelial Ig
receptor (2,3) is supported by the following observations.
1. Spontaneous interaction of SC with dimeric IgA and 19S
IgM depends on non-covalent binding sites of relatively high
affinity and limited capacity; 2. Immunofluorescence has indicated the presence of SC in glandular cell membranes, and
IgA is apparently bound in the same locations (14); 3. While
the I determinant of SC present in the Golgi region of secretory cells is fully exposed, it becomes increasingly inaccessible in their membranes and apical cytoplasm (14). It seems
likely, therefore, that SC mediates the selective epithelial
reception of dimeric IgA and 19S IgM, and that the SC-Ig complexes formed in the cell membranes are externally transmitted due to pinocytosis and subsequent secretion. Their
intracellular stabilization by disulfide bonds may be enzymatically catalyzed. Since most gland-associated immunocytes
synthesize dimeric IgA or 19S IgM, their products would be
readily available for external transfer by the proposed
mechanism.

Acknowledgments. Supported by the Norwegian Cancer Society
and the Norwegian Research Council for Science and the
Humanities.

REFERENCES

1. Brandtzaeg, P., Clin. Exp. Immunol. 8:69, 1971.
2. Brandtzaeg, P., in Host Resistance to Commensal Bacteria,
    Edited by T. MacPhee, p. 116, Churchill-Livingstone,
    1972.

3. Brandtzaeg, P., Nature New Biology 243:142, 1973.
4. Mach, J.-P., Nature 228:1278, 1970.
5. Rádl, J., Klein, F., van den Berg, P., de Bruyn, A.M. and Hijmans, W., Immunology 20:843, 1971.
6. Brandtzaeg, P., Acta Path. Microbiol. Scand., Section B, 79:189, 1971.
7. Brandtzaeg, P., Fjellanger, I. and Gjeruldsen, S.T., Scand. J. Haematol. Suppl. 12, 1970.
8. Brandtzaeg, P., Acta Path. Microbiol. Scand., Section B, 79:165, 1971.
9. Eskeland, T. and Brandtzaeg, P., Immunochemistry, In press.
10. Solheim, B.G., Harboe, M. and Deverill, J., Immunochemistry 8:939, 1971.
11. Brandtzaeg, P., Scand. J. Immunol. 2:273, 1973.
12. Brandtzaeg, P., Scand. J. Immunol. 2:333, 1973.
13. Buxbaum, J., Zolla, S., Scharff, M.D. and Franklin, E.C., J. Exp. Med. 133:1118, 1971.
14. Brandtzaeg, P., J. Immunol (In press).

ASSOCIATION OF S-IgA SUBUNITS

Jiri Mestecky, Ralph E. Schrohenloher, Rose
Kulhavy, Genesis P. Wright and Milan Tomana
Institute of Dental Research, Department of
Microbiology, Cancer Research and Training
Center, and Division of Clinical Immunology
and Rheumatology, University of Alabama in
Birmingham, Birmingham, Alabama 35294

INTRODUCTION

The differentiation of secretory component (SC) and J
chain as two separate polypeptides (1,2) raised questions
concerning the role played by these two subunits in the
stabilization of secretory IgA (S-IgA) molecules. Of special
interest is the clarification of the relationship between the
presence of J chain and the binding of SC. When added to
serum or to fixed cells, SC was selectively bound to free or
intracellular polymeric immunoglobulins of the IgA and IgM
classes (3-6). Since all polymeric immunoglobulins that bind
SC contain J chain, it was suggested that this subunit might,
in a way as yet undefined, mediate the binding of SC (3,5).
Both polypeptides have been found to be linked to the Fc
region of the α chain (7-10). The enzymatic and disulfide
bond cleavages did not, however, permit a clear distinction
between the possibilities that SC is attached either to Fc
through J chain or it is attached directly to the α chain,
even though the process might be mediated by J chain.

Amino acid analyses of isolated SC and J chain revealed
the absence of methionine from SC and the presence of one
residue in J chain (11-15), whereas α chains contained 3-6
residues (16). Therefore, cyanogen bromide (CNBr) cleavage
of the polypeptide chains at the methionine residues should
yield fragments of S-IgA that are composed of entire SC, with
parts of J chain in the first case, or alternatively with
fragments of α chain.

99

MATERIALS AND METHODS

Purification and Characteristics of S-IgA and Myeloma
IgA. S-IgA was obtained from human colostrum and myeloma
IgA from blood plasma of a patient with IgA myelomatosis
(Fel) after the removal of fibrinogen by recalcification.
Crude gamma globulin fractions from both sources were
obtained by ammonium sulfate precipitation to 50% saturation.
Details of subsequent gel-filtrations through Sephadex G-200
and Sepharose 6B, and ion-exchange chromatography on DEAE
Sephadex have been described (17). Final purity was tested
by immunoelectrophoresis with polyvalent antisera to normal
serum and colostrum. The IgA myeloma protein belonged to
the IgA2 subclass, with λ chains covalently attached to α
chains. The S_{20w} of 9.5 was determined (18).

Preparation of Polypeptide Chains and CNBr Fragments.
To obtain α and L chains, S-IgA or myeloma IgA proteins were
totally reduced and alkylated or S-sulfonated, then gel-
filtered through Sephadex G-200 column (2.6 x 100 cm) in
5M guanidine·HCl (17). J chain that was present in the L
chain fraction was separated by DEAE-Sephadex chromatography
under conditions used in previous experiments (2). Sephadex
G-10 in 1% ammonium bicarbonate was used for desalting.

Purified intact S-IgA and myeloma IgA and totally
reduced and alkylated α and J chains were dissolved in 70%
formic acid at 2% protein concentration and subjected to
CNBr cleavage. A twofold amount of CNBr was added, and the
reaction was allowed to proceed at room temperature for 4
hours. Samples were then diluted with 10 volumes of dis-
tilled water and lyophilized.

Analytical Procedures. Disc electrophoresis in polyacrylamide gel containing sodium dodecyl sulfate (SDS) was
performed under conditions and with standards described
previously (17). For J chain detection, alkaline urea gels
at pH 9.4 (19), and immunoelectrophoresis with anti-J chain
serum were used (2).

Techniques employed for amino acid (2) and carbohydrate
analyses (18) and for peptide mapping (2) were reported
earlier. Molecular weights of peptides were determined by
sedimentation equilibrium ultracentrifugation (20).

RESULTS

After cleavage of disulfide bonds, J chain was released from both secretory-and myeloma IgA proteins and was detectable by disc electrophoresis and by immunoelectrophoresis. When examined by ultracentrifugation (Fig. 1), myeloma IgA

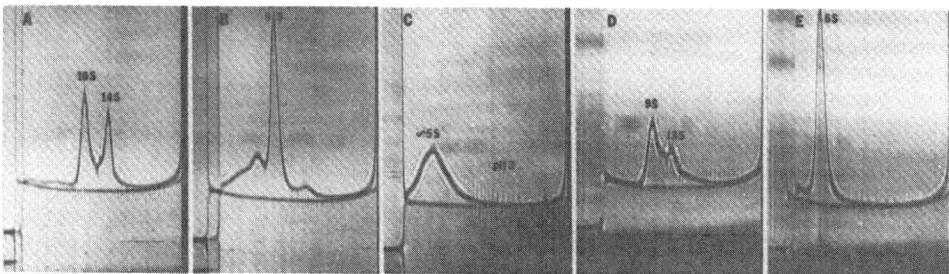

Figure 1. Ultracentrifugation patterns of (A) untreated secretory IgA, (B) and (C) reduced and alkylated secretory IgA, (D) untreated myeloma IgA and (E) reduced and alkylated myeloma IgA. Samples (A), (B), (D) and (E) were analyzed in pH 7.5 sodium phosphate buffer (0.076M). Sample C was analyzed in pH 3 glycine buffer (0.1M). Patterns (A),(B) and (C) were recorded after 32 min. at 56,100 rpm. Patterns (D) and (E) were recorded after 24 min. at the same speed. Sedimentation rates of major components are indicated.

dissociated into a monomeric form (6.5S) as a consequence of reduction; to achieve the dissociation of S-IgA, a decrease in pH was required after reduction. At pH 3, components in the mixture had approximate sedimentation rates of 4-, 5-, and 6S. This indicated that the association with SC was involved in stabilizing S-IgA, in concert with J chain that was present in both proteins. Had SC been attached exclusively to J chain so that no interaction with H chains would occur, then no difference would have been expected.

An improved insight into structures of S-IgA and myeloma IgA was afforded by analyzing fragments derived from these proteins by CNBr cleavage and separated by Sephadex G-200 filtration in 5M guanidine·HCl (Fig. 2). Most of the material was eluted early and had a high molecular weight. Fragments with a low molecular weight were examined by disc

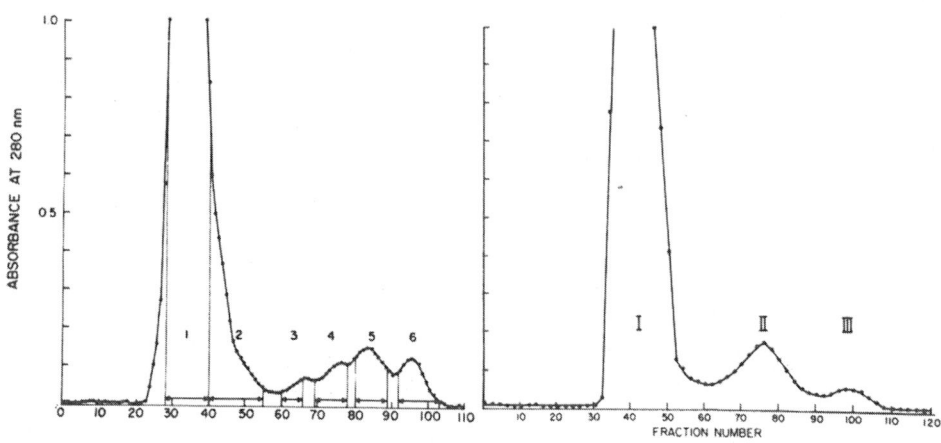

Figure 2. Gel filtration of CNBr-cleaved S-IgA (left) and
myeloma IgA (right) through Sephadex G-200 (column 2.6 x
100 cm) in 5M guanidine·HCl.

electrophoresis at pH 9.4 and by immunoelectrophoresis with
an anti-J chain serum (Fig. 3). Protein with the antigenic
determinants and electrophoretic mobility of J chain was
present mainly in fraction 4 of S-IgA and fraction II of
myeloma IgA. Comparative analyses showed that peptide maps
and amino acid compositions were highly similar in fraction
4 and J chain purified from S-IgA.

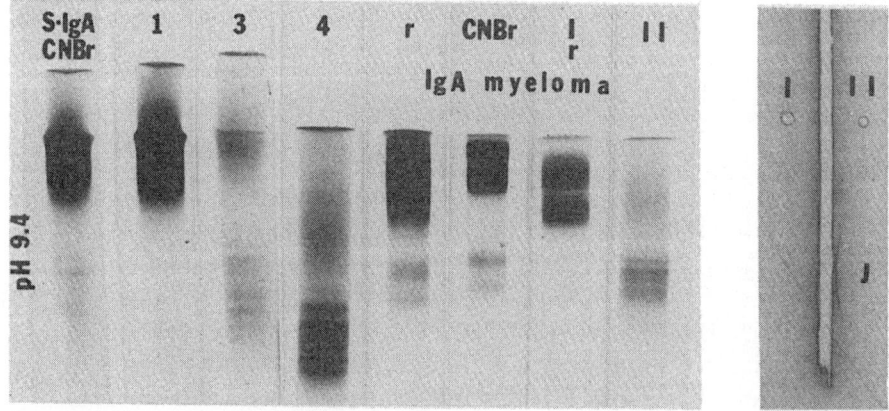

Figure 3. Disc electrophoresis at pH 9.4 and immunoelectrophoresis of CNBr-cleaved S-IgA and myeloma IgA and their
fractions (Fig. 2). (r) indicates reduced.

The proteins with high molecular weights (fraction 1
and I) contained no J chain, whether untreated or reduced
and alkylated. By SDS disc electrophoresis, the molecular

weights of proteins present in fraction 1, before disulfide
bond cleavage, were estimated to fall in the range of
170,000-320,000. After cleavage (by oxidative sulfitolysis)
of the disulfide bonds in fraction 1 from S-IgA, the resulting polypeptides were separated by gel-filtration through
Sephadex G-200 in 5M guanidine·HCl (Fig. 4). These polypeptides were identified on the basis of their apparent
molecular weights on SDS disc electrophoresis, and by their
amino acid and carbohydrate compositions. The first fraction
contained aggregated and/or unsplit material; the second
fraction was identified as SC on the basis of its position
on SDS gel and the composition of amino acids and
carbohydrates which are characteristic of SC (11-13, 21),
specifically, in this case, the absence of homoserine residues
and a large amount of fucose. An antiserum to SC was produced
by immunization with the protein in fraction 2. A large
fragment of the α chain, which was found in the third
fraction, had a molecular weight that was 25-30% less than
that of the original α chain; and thus allowed a good
separation from SC. Galactosamine that is restricted to α
chain (21) was found in this fraction. The fourth fraction
was identified as L chains because of the molecular weight,
banding pattern at pH 9.4, antigenic determinants, and the
absence of carbohydrates. The J chain which would have been
eluted with L chains under these conditions was missing.

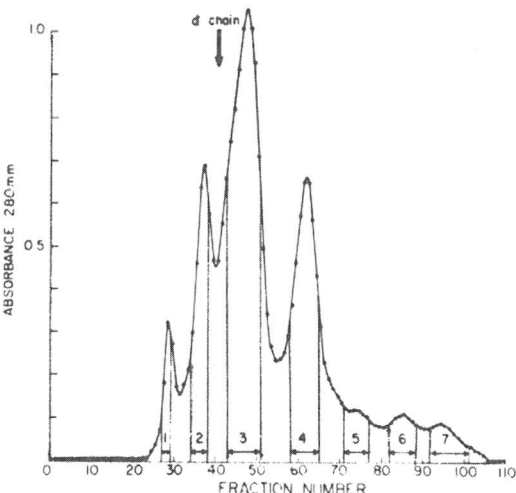

Figure 4. Gel filtration of totally S-sulfonated fraction 1
of CNBr-cleaved S-IgA (Fig. 2). The arrow indicates the
elution position of S-sulfonated α chain without CNBr
treatment.

Small amounts of two peptides which were detected in
fractions 5 and 6, were derived from the α chain, as
determined by comparison with the elution profiles of CNBr
cleaved, totally S-sulfonated α and L chains. Results of
this study indicated that SC and J chain were not mutually
connected by disulfide bonds. It is intriguing to consider
that material containing J chain was released from both IgA
proteins by CNBr without the cleavage of disulfide bonds.

Since it was reasonable to suspect that fragments of α
chain might be linked to J chain, detailed analyses were
performed on myeloma IgA to avoid any possible ambiguity
that might arise from using heterogenous S-IgA. J chain-
containing fraction II from Sephadex G-200 filtration of
CNBr-cleaved myeloma IgA was pooled from several consecutive
runs and a small amount of contaminating peptides was removed
by DEAE-ion-exchange chromatography. Subsequent gel filtration through Sephadex G-75 and G-25 in 5M guanidine·HCl
(Fig. 5 - fraction Al) and disc electrophoreses in SDS and
at pH 9.4, demonstrated the homogeneity of the material
present in the fraction Al. Peptide maps of J chain and Al

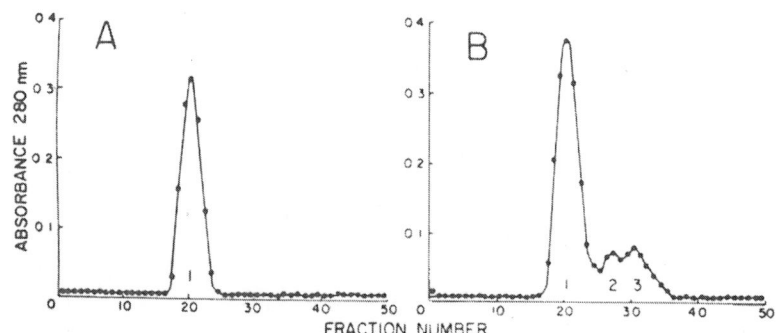

Figure 5. Gel-filtration through Sephadex G-25 (column
1.6 x 3 cm) in 5M guanidine·HCl of purified (see text) J
chain-containing fraction obtained from myeloma IgA by
CNBr treatment before (A) and after reduction and alkylation
(B).

were almost identical. The molecular weights of 17,000±100
for Al as compared to 15,600±200 for isolated J chain, were
determined by sedimentation equilibrium in 5M guanidine·HCl.
When the results of amino acid and carbohydrate analyses
(Table 1) were related to the molecular weights of Al and
J chain, a slight increase in the number of aspartic acid,
threonine, glycine and alanine residues were noted in Al.

Table 1. Amino acid and carbohydrate analyses of J chain and Fractions A1, B1-B3, CNBr fractions of J and α Chains. Expressed in Residues/Mole

	J Chain	A1	B1	B2	J CNBr fr.2	B3	α CNBr fr.2
Cys	6.1	7.7	5.3	1.0	1.0	0.7	0.8
Asp	20.8	23.7	18.3	3.1	3.0	1.1	1.0
Thr	11.7	13.6	9.9	2.8	2.8	1.1	1.0
Ser	8.9	9.5	7.1				
Glu	14.8	18.1	13.8	1.8	1.1	1.2	1.2
Pro	7.7	8.3	5.7	2.6	3.0		
Gly	2.4	3.8	2.2	0.7	0.1	1.3	1.2
Ala	5.9	7.0	4.5	3.1	3.0	0.8	1.2
Val	9.1	9.7	7.3	1.2	1.1	1.1	1.1
Met	0.8						
Hsr		1.2	1.1				
ILe	5.8	5.9	4.5				
Leu	7.6	8.4	6.7	1.4	1.5		
Tyr	5.2	4.7	4.1	0.9	1.4	0.7	0.5
Phe	1.1	1.1	1.1				
Lys	5.0	5.6	5.0				
His	1.1	1.3	1.2				
Arg	9.2	10.1	8.0				
number of amino ac.	124	140	106	18-19	18	8	8
Fuc	1	1	1				
Man	2	2-3	2				
Gal	1	1	1				
GlcNH$_2$	3	2-3	2				
S.A.	1	N.D.	N.D.				
Mol. wt.	15,000	17,000	13,400	2,000	1,900	860	860

The higher molecular weight and the differences in amino acid composition in fraction A1 suggested possible association with other peptides. This was confirmed by gel filtration of totally reduced and alkylated material in A1 on Sephadex G-25 (Fig. 5-B). To determine the origin of peptides in fractions obtained from this filtration, totally reduced and alkylated J and α chains were cleaved with CNBr and the resulting products were separated on an identical column of Sephadex G-25. These and previous fractions (Fig. 5B) were compared according to their amino acid and carbohydrate compositions, electrophoretic mobility, and peptide maps. The first and largest fraction (B1) had a molecular weight of 13,400; its peptide maps and the amino acid and carbohydrate compositions were similar to those of J chain (Table 1). When recalculated in respect to molecular weight, one homoserine residue was found in this fraction. Fraction B1 obviously represented a large N-terminal segment because peptides B2 and B3, which were further purified by rechromatography on a larger Sephadex G-25 column (1.6 x 60 cm), were devoid of homoserine. A peptide from fraction B2 and a peptide released from J chain by CNBr treatment were identical in the following respects: electrophoretic mobility, elution position on Sephadex G-25, and amino acid composition. The peptide in fraction B3 was found among products from CNBr cleavage of α chain. To isolate this peptide, α chain was totally reduced and alkylated, treated with CNBr, and then subjected to repeated gel filtration on Sephadex G-25. The elution position on Sephadex G-25, electrophoretic mobility, and amino acid compositions were alike in both peptides. Equimolar quantities (with the exception of tyrosine) of 8 amino acids were obtained (Table 1), and these proved identical in composition to those from the C-terminal octapeptide of α chain, previously analyzed and sequenced by Prahl et al. (16) and Chuang et al. (22).

DISCUSSION

Our results suggest that J chain is linked by disulfide bonds to the penultimate cysteine residue of the C-terminal octapeptide of α chain. Based on the amino acid analysis and molecular weight of fragment A1, which was released by CNBr treatment of IgA, most probably only two octapeptides would be associated with J chain. The C-terminal portion of J chain (composed of approximately 18 amino acids) was released as a result of cleavage of disulfide bonds. This indicated that the single cysteine residue present was involved in the intra-J chain disulfide bond rather than in the inter-chain linkage of J- to α chain. As described, a fragment with similar properties was released from S-IgA by CNBr cleavage and had no SC attached. This suggests that SC is not linked to polymeric IgA through J chain but is linked directly to the α chain(s). It is reasonable to speculate that during the process of polymer assembly, in which J chain seems to be instrumental (23), a disulfide-bond-exchange-reaction occurs, which results in the attachment of J chain to the penultimate cysteine. As a consequence, free -SH groups might be formed on α chain that

would subsequently react with -SH group(s) of SC.   Grey
et al. (24) reported that this penultimate cysteine residue
forms a labile intra-heavy chain disulfide bond with
cysteine in a large CNBr fragment in both monomeric and
polymeric immunoglobulins.   If this is true, by breaking
this disulfide bond as a consequence of J chain attachment
to the C-terminal portion, a cysteine residue on a large
CNBr fragment of α chain would be available for SC binding.
This hypothesis seems consistent with our results, wherein
SC released by CNBr cleavage was connected to a large
CNBr fragment rather than being associated with other
C-terminal octapeptides that were possibly available.

The C-terminal octapeptide of the α chain is a part of
19 amino acid residues that extend beyond the carboxy-
terminal ends of γ and ε chains (22,25); μ chain is
identical in this respect to α chain (Fig. 6) and both

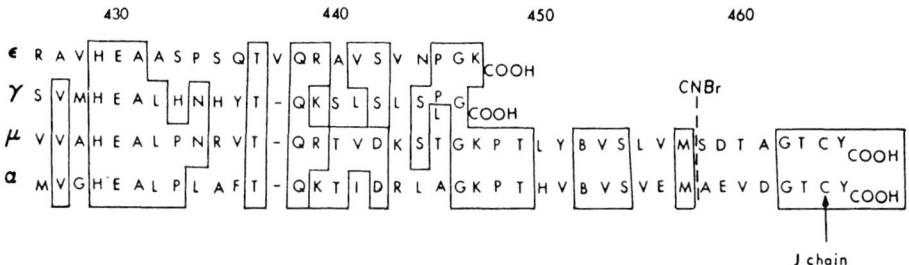

Figure 6.   Comparison of sequences of amino acids in
C-terminal segments of ε, γ, μ, and α chains.

chains show a high degree of sequence homology (22). A
fragment released by CNBr cleavage of IgM contained J chain
and exhibited properties similar to those of polymeric IgA;
it is tempting to suggest that the extension of α and μ
chains of polymeric immunoglobulins is the necessary
prerequisite for polymer formation. Because all polymer
forms of immunoglobulins contained only a single J chain,
this polypeptide, rather than binding all heavy chains,
might merely initiate the polymerization by the mechanism
suggested above or by still another means.

CONCLUSIONS

1) The presence of SC may enhance the stability of S-IgA,
against dissociation implemented by reduction of disulfide
bonds.

2) SC and J chain are not connected by disulfide bonds, although J chain might mediate SC attachment.

3) J chain is linked to the penultimate cysteine residue of the C-terminal octapeptide of α and probably μ chains.

Acknowledgement: This investigation was supported by US PHS research grants AI-10854, AI-10664, and DE-02670.

REFERENCES

1. Halpern, M.S. and Koshland, M.E., Nature 228: 1276, 1970.
2. Mestecky, J., Zikan, J. and Butler, W.T., Science 171: 1163, 1971.
3. Mach, J.-P., Nature 228: 1278, 1970.
4. Radl, J., Klein, F., Vanden Berg P., de Bruyn, A.M. and Hijmans, W., Immunology 20: 843, 1971.
5. Brandtzaeg, P., Nature New Biol. 243: 142, 1973.
6. Radl, J., Schuit, H.R.E., Mestecky, J. and Hijmans, W. this symposium, 1973.
7. Lawton, A.R., III, in The Secretory Immunologic System (Edited by Dayton, D.H., Jr, Small, P.A., Jr, Chanock, R.M., Kaufman, H.E. and Tomasi, T.B., Jr.) p. 55, U.S. Dept. of Health, Education and Welfare, PHS-NIH, Washington, D.C., 1971.
8. Mestecky, J., Kulhavy, R. and Kraus, F.W., Fedn Proc. 30, Abstr. No. 1527, 1971.
9. Meinke, G.C. and Spiegelberg, H.L., Fedn Proc. 30, Abstr. No. 1526, 1971.
10. Knight, K.L., Lichter, E.A. and Hanly, W.C., Biochemistry 12: 3197, 1973.
11. Kobayashi, K., Immunochemistry 8: 785, 1971.
12. van Munster, P.J.J., Stoelinga, G.B.A., Clamp, J.R., Th Gerding, J.J., Reijnen, J.C.M. and Voss, M., Immunology 23:249, 1972.
13. Lamm, M.E. and Greenberg, J., Biochemistry 11: 2744, 1972.
14. Mestecky, J., Hammack, W.J., Schrohenloher, R.E. and Bennett, J.C., Prot. Biol. Fluids 20: 279, 1973.
15. Wilde, C.E., III and Koshland, M.E., Biochemistry 12: 3218, 1973.
16. Prahl, J.W., Abel, C.A. and Grey, H.M., Biochemistry 10: 1808, 1971.
17. Mestecky, J., Kulhavy, R. and Kraus, F.W., J. Immunol. 108: 738, 1972.

18. Tomana, M., Niedermeier, W., Mestecky, J. and Hammack,
     W.J., Immunochemistry 9:933, 1972.
19. Reisfeld, R.A. and Small, P.A., Jr., Science 152:1253,
     1966.
20. Schrohenloher, R.E., Mestecky, J. and Stanton, T.H.,
     Biochim. Biophys. Acta 295:576, 1973.
21. Tomana, M., Mestecky, J. and Niedermeier, W., J.
     Immunol. 108:1631, 1972.
22. Chuang, C.-Y., Capra, D.J. and Kehoe, J.M., Nature
     244:158, 1973.
23. Parkhouse, R.M.E. and Della Corte, E., this symposium,
     1973.
24. Grey, H.M., Abel, C.A. and Zimmerman, B., Ann. N.Y.
     Acad. Sci., 190:37, 1971.
25. Bennich, H., Milstein, C. and Secher, D.S., FEBS
     Letters 33:49, 1973.

MODULATION OF THE ASSEMBLY OF IMMUNOGLOBULIN SUBUNITS BY J CHAIN

Thomas B. Tomasi, Jr. and S. Hauptman

Department of Immunology, Mayo Medical School
Mayo Foundation
Rochester, Minnesota 55901

INTRODUCTION

Because J chain is present in polymeric and not monomeric immunoglobulin molecules and since it is released from
polymers when they are reduced to subunits, it has been suggested that J chain plays an important role in the assembly
of both IgA and IgM polymers. J chain has been reported (1)
to have a high half cystine content (10-12 per mole), and
there are, therefore, sufficient cysteine residues to undergo
disulfide bond formation with each of the subunits in a
pentameric immunoglobulin molecule. Consistent with this
thesis are quantitative estimates of the amount of J chain
in IgM and IgA suggesting that there is one J chain per mole
of polymer regardless of the polymeric size.

This paper presents evidence suggesting that J chain
may not be directly involved in all of the intersubunit disulfide linkages. The data are consistent with the hypothesis that J chain links 2 monomeric subunits in both the
IgM or IgA systems and that the remaining subunits then become directly disulfide bonded to one another through linkages which do not involve J chain.

MATERIALS AND METHODS

Four human IgM proteins were isolated from the serum of
patients with Waldenström's macroglobulinemia by euglobulin
precipitation (3-5 times) followed by chromatography on

111

Biogel P200 in .14M sodium chloride. Eight IgA myeloma proteins were isolated by precipitation with 18% and then 16%
sodium sulfate (W/V) followed by chromatography on Biogel
P200. In some cases starch-block electrophoresis or affinity
chromatography using an anti-$\alpha_2$macroglobulin immunoabsorbent
column was performed to remove $\alpha_2$macroglobulin. The IgM and
IgA proteins were judged to be homogeneous by immunoelectrophoresis and Ouchterlony gel diffusion employing several
anti-whole human sera.

Reduction was carried out according to Morris and Inman
(2) at a protein concentration of 5-8 mg/ml using mercaptoethylamine (MEA) in concentrations ranging from .01 to .03M
for one hour at 37°C followed by alkylation with .013 to
.036M iodoacetamide for 15 min. at 4°C. In some experiments,
reduction was also performed with .01M DTT for two hours at
37°C and alkylation with .025M iodoacetamide.

Polyacrylamide gel electrophoresis was performed in 5%
gels according to the method described by Ornstein and Davis
(3,4). The samples were applied in 8M urea, but the gel
buffer did not contain urea. The gels were stained with
Coomassie blue in 12% TCA and scanned in a recording densitometer (Clifford Instruments). Polyacrylamide gel diffusion
was carried out by placing the unstained gels in 2% agar and
the antisera in lateral troughs.

Analytical ultracentrifugation was performed in a Spinco
Model E ultracentrifuge at 52,000 rpm at 20°C using schlieren
optics. $s^{\circ}_{20,w}$ were calculated by correcting sedimentation
coefficients to water at 20°C and extrapolating to zero concentrations. Molecular weights were determined by the high
speed sedimentation equilibrium method described by Yphantis
(5) using the photoelectric scanner. Two species plots of
the equilibrium data were carried out according to Roark and
Yphantis (6) as previously described in this laboratory (7).
A partial specific volume ($\bar{v}$) of .717 was assumed for IgM
in accordance with previously reported values (8).

An antiserum to J chain was produced in a rabbit by
immunization with J chain bands cut from unstained, polyacrylamide gels containing a reduced alkylated IgA myeloma.
The antiserum was absorbed with reduced and alkylated Fab
fragments obtained by peptic digestion of the same myeloma
protein. This antiserum reacted in gel diffusion with reduced alkylated IgM and IgA but not with the unreduced

proteins. In polyacrylamide gel diffusion a reaction was
seen only in the area of the J chain bands, following electrophoresis of either reduced (.01M DTT) IgM or IgA.

RESULTS

Although there were some variations between proteins,
it was found that when IgM was reduced with .02M MEA about
40% of protein was reduced to IgM subunits (IgMs), as determined by measuring the areas under the respective 7S and 19S
peaks on analytical ultracentrifugation. Sephadex G200
chromatography of the .02M MEA reduced and alkylated IgM
protein was performed on a column which was previously
marked with proteins of known size, including 19S IgM, 7S
IgG, and 2S L chain monomers. Pool I (void volume fractions)
consisted of the "19S", Pool II of the "7S", and Pool III
of the "2S" (L-J) region of the column. Pool I was found
to have an $s^o_{20,w}$ of 18S compared to 18.5S for the unreduced
IgM. The molecular weight of the IgM in Pool I was one
million. It was at first assumed that the 19S peak seen on
ultracentrifugation of Pool I represented residual IgM which
was unsplit by the reducing conditions employed. However,
when Pool I was centrifuged in 4M guanidine or 1M propionic
acid, dissociation to smaller subunits occurred. Similarly,
on electrophoresis in 5% gels, Pool I penetrated the gel bed
whereas the native unreduced IgM did not penetrate the gel
significantly. These data suggested that the 19S IgM remaining after MEA treatment consisted of noncovalently
bonded subunits. The various sedimentation coefficients and
molecular weights measured are shown in Table I. The boundary
of Pool I in 4M guanidine split into two peaks late in centrifugation, and it is important to note that the sedimentation coefficients of both components (2.7S and 2.1S) are
close to that of the 7S marker (2.3S) and considerably lower
than that of the native unreduced IgM (6.9S). Thus far all
attempts at separating the two components present in Pool I
have been unsuccessful.

Polyacrylamide gel diffusion performed on Pool I revealed that the L-H disulfides had not been split by the
.02M MEA as previously reported by Morris and Inman (2).
Moreover, complete reduction with .01M DTT revealed that J
chain was present in Pool I, and densitometer tracings
showed the same percentage of J chain in Pool I as in the
native 19S IgM. Reduction of Pool II with DTT did not show
J chain, whereas Pool III demonstrated typical J chain bands

Table I. Sedimentation coefficients and molecular weights of
IgM and 2-mercaptoethylamine reduction products.

Protein	Solvent	Sedimentation Coefficient*	Molecular Weight
Native IgM	.1M Guanidine	18.5S	950,000
Native IgM	4M Guanidine	6.9S	-
Pool I**	.1M NaCl	18.0S	1,000,000
Pool I	4M Guanidine	2.7S,2.1S	181,000-90,000
Pool II**	.1M NaCl	7.4S	164,000
Pool II	4M Guanidine	2.8S	-
IgG	4M Guanidine	2.3S	-

*Sedimentation coefficients in .1M NaCl were extrapolated to
 infinite dilution from plots of s vs. c. Sedimentation coefficients in 4M guanidine were not corrected but were all
 measured at the same protein concentration (6 mgm/ml).
**Pools represent Sephadex G-200 fractions of MEA reduced
 IgM as described in the text.

after reduction. That Pool III contained J chain was confirmed by polyacrylamide gel diffusion using an anti-J chain
antiserum.

    IgA polymers larger than 10S were isolated from the as-
cending limb of the void volume peak after chromatography of
a myeloma IgA containing large amounts of higher polymers on
Sepharose 4B. As shown in Fig. 1, reduction with .02M MEA
resulted in the disappearance of polymers higher than 10S
and the appearance of 10S and 7S bands. The position of the
gel bands corresponding to 10S and 7S IgA proteins were
marked by electrophoresis of ultracentrifugally homogeneous
preparations of 10S and 7S IgA. We have repeatedly observed
that the higher polymers of IgA are sensitive to .01-.03M
MEA, whereas the 10S dimer is resistant to this treatment.
When the higher polymers were reduced with MEA and separated
into the 10S and 7S species by Sephadex G-200 chromatography,
it was found that J chain was present in the 10S but not in
the 7S subunit.

    J chain was isolated from serum IgA and IgM by water
precipitation as previously described (7). Two species plots
of the equilibrium data obtained on these preparations showed
two populations of molecules, one with a molecular weight of
about 15,000, the other of approximately one-half this value.

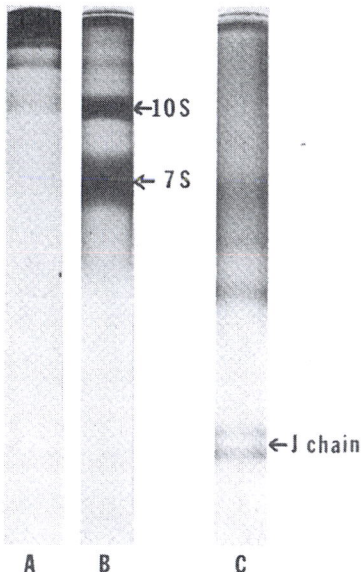

Fig. 1.   Polyacrylamide gel electrophoresis of higher poly-
          mers of IgA: Unreduced (Gel A), reduced with .02M
          MEA (Gel B), and reduced with .01M DTT (Gel C).

During the course of these experiments, it was observed
that after reduction of the isolated IgA proteins with .02M
MEA, two additional fast migrating bands were present.
Using specific antisera in polyacrylamide gel diffusion it
was found that the two bands represented albumin and α1 anti-
trypsin (α1AT) (see Fig. 2).   Both the α1AT and albumin were
covalently bonded to the IgA since they were not released by
electrophoresis in 10M urea.   The albumin and α1AT bands
seen on gel electrophoresis following MEA reduction diminished markedly and in some cases disappeared following .01M
DTT reduction.   Employing purified preparations of human albumin it was shown that reduction with .01M DTT resulted in
considerable aggregation, and most of the polymers of albumin produced, migrated near the top of the gel but one band
was present in the "J chain region" as shown in Fig. 3.
Gel diffusion of an IgA protein reduced with .01M DTT also
demonstrates that antigenic determinants of both α1AT and
albumin are located within, or close to, the "J chain region."
When an IgA protein containing α1AT and albumin was reduced
with .01M DTT and chromatographed on Sephadex G100 in 1M
acetic acid or in 4M guanidine, the albumin and α1AT were
both found in the H-chain peak as shown in Fig. 2.

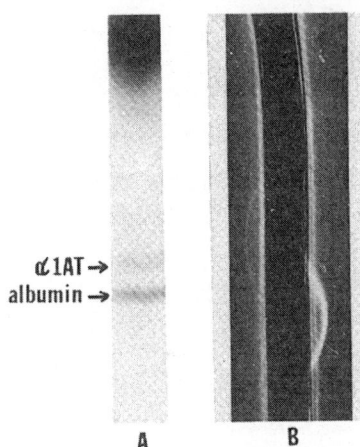

Fig. 2.   (A) Polyacrylamide gel of H-chain peak obtained by
          chromatography of reduced and alkylated IgA on
          Sephadex G100 in 4M guanidine   (B) Polyacrylamide
          gel diffusion developed with anti-α1AT (on the
          left) and anti-albumin (on the right).

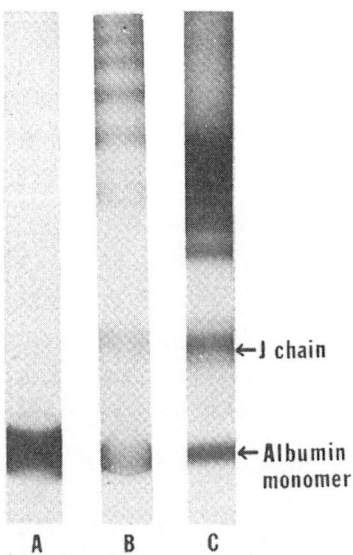

Fig. 3.   Polyacrylamide gel electrophoresis of monomer
          albumin (gel A), monomer albumin reduced with .02M
          DTT (gel B) and an IgA myeloma reduced with .02M
          DTT (gel C).

After finding αlAT and albumin bound to all 8 isolated
IgA proteins we subsequently studied the whole sera from 49
patients having monoclonal IgA proteins by immunoelectrophoresis, employing antisera to albumin and αlAT. Positive
binding was characterized by a double precipitin arc with
bound αlAT or albumin being present in the cathodal portion
of the arc and unbound or free αlAT or albumin in their usual
anodal positions. Fig. 4 shows a typical double arc seen
with an IgA myeloma sera which bound αlAT. Using this technique, 73% of the IgA myeloma sera showed binding with αlAT
whereas 65% showed complex formation with albumin. Most of
the sera demonstrated binding with both albumin and αlAT.
When antisera containing antibodies to both αlAT and albumin
were employed, complete crossing of the arcs occurred suggesting that these proteins were complexed to different IgA
molecules.

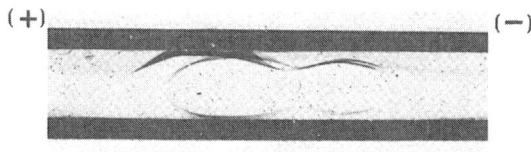

Fig. 4.   Immunoelectrophoresis of an IgA myeloma serum
          (center well) developed with an antiserum having
          antibodies to both αlAT and albumin (top trough)
          and an antiserum which is specific for αlAT (lower
          trough).

DISCUSSION

The data demonstrated that a noncovalently bonded pentamer of IgM can be produced by light reduction with MEA and
that the pentamer contained J chains in the same proportion
as the native IgM molecule. IgA polymers (higher than 10S)
reduced with MEA under the same conditions dissociated to
a 10S dimer containing J chain and a 7S monomer lacking J
chain. These results suggest the following interpretations:
J chain interacts with the 7S monomer or more likely links
two such units together as a relatively stable dimer as
shown for IgA. Complexing J chain so alters the conformation
of the subunits that they are then able to interact with
other subunits not containing J chain through noncovalent
forces. These forces are responsible for bringing the
subunits into close enough apposition to allow the remaining

Consistent with this thesis is the observation that J chain
isolated from either IgA, or IgM has a molecular weight of
about 15,000. The nature of the smaller species present in
these preparations,which were detected only after two-spe-
cies analysis, is presently under study (see also Ref. 7).
Wilde and Koshland (9) have also reported that human J chain
has a molecular weight of approximately 15,000. As pointed
out by these workers, using this molecular weight rather than
the previously obtained values of 25-30,000 suggests that J
chain has 7 to 8 half cystines rather than 10-12. Thus,
the number of cysteines is not sufficient to allow a single
bond to be formed with each heavy chain in the pentameric
immunoglobulins.

   If the above speculation is correct it should be possible, following MEA reduction of IgM, to isolate a dimer consisting of two IgM proteins containing covalently bonded J
chain. Thus far we have been unsuccessful in our attempts to
definitely isolate an IgM dimer. Also, in the IgA system,
one would expect, according to this theory, to be able to
identify a noncovalently bonded polymer analogous to that
found with IgM. Gel electrophoresis experiments after reduction with varying concentrations of MEA have thus far failed
to produce a noncovalently bonded polymer, but further work
is required with the use of ultracentrifugation. It may be
that the secondary forces between the IgA subunits are relatively weak and that electrophoresis in a sieving gel results
in dissociation.

   The significance of the binding of α1AT to IgA is presently unknown. It may have little or no biological significance and simply may be another example of the propensity of
IgA proteins to complex with other molecules. However, it is
possible that the observed association between IgA and α1AT
has an important biological implication. For example, α1AT
may protect IgA against proteolysis. Alternatively, IgA
could determine the transport of α1AT into secretions. We
have recently found that human colostrum and gastrointestinal
fluids contain relatively large amounts of α1AT compared with
other serum proteins of similar size. This suggests the
possibility of selective transport. On immunoelectrophoresis,
however, the α1AT in these secretions is in the unbound
(anodal) form. When an isolated IgA monoclonal protein containing bound α1AT is incubated with either colostrum or
intestinal fluids, the α1AT is removed from the IgA and now
migrates anodally. Whether this process is enzymatic,

reductive, or by some other unknown process, is presently
under investigation. However, since removal of α1AT from
IgA occurs within 15 minutes and at 4°C, proteolytic cleavage seems unlikely.

Regardless of the importance of the binding of α1AT to
IgA the observed binding phenomenon does have some practical
significance. We do not at present, for a variety of reasons, believe that J chain and α1AT or albumin are identical.
The chemistry of these molecules is quite distinct as are
their synthesis and distribution. In the IgM system we have
found that only one of ten monoclonal IgM proteins contains
α1AT while all had typical J chain bands. Finally, we have
found that after removal of albumin and α1AT from IgA by MEA
reduction and chromatography on Sephadex G200, that the dimer
of IgA contains typical J chain bands (two in number). However, despite the above, the fact remains that after reduction with DTT, α1AT and albumin determinants are found in
the J chain region. It is possible, therefore, that one or
both of these proteins may be responsible for some of the
multiple bands typically seen in the J chain area. We believe that J chain typically has two bands. When three or
four bands are present, as is sometimes observed, these
additional bands may represent α1AT, albumin, or both.

Another problem results in the "contamination" with
α1AT and albumin during structural studies on IgA proteins.
For example, if J chain is isolated by preparative polyacrylamide electrophoresis, albumin and α1AT may contaminate
these preparations. On the other hand, when IgA is separated
into L and H chains by classical methods, these proteins contaminate the H chain peak. Although accurate quantitation
of the amount of α1AT and albumin has not been undertaken
with a large number of IgA proteins, with certain IgA preparations sufficient amounts of these proteins are present
to be chemically significant in structural studies.

REFERENCES

1. Morrison, S.L. and Koshland, M.E., Proc. Natl. Acad.
    Sci. 69:124, 1972.
2. Morris, J.E. and Inman, F.P., Biochemistry 7:2851, 1968.
3. Ornstein, L., Ann. N.Y. Acad. Sci. 121:321, 1964.
4. Davis, B.J., Ann. N.Y. Acad. Sci. 121:404, 1964.
5. Yphantis, D.A., Biochemistry 3:297, 1964.
6. Roark, D.E. and Yphantis, D.A., Ann. N.Y. Acad. Sci. 164:
    66, 1969.

7.   Kang, Y.S., Calvanico, N.J. and Tomasi, T.B., Jr., J. Immunol. In press.

8.   Chen, J.P., Reichlin, M. and Tomasi, T.B., Jr., Biochemistry $\underline{8}$:2246, 1969.

9.   Wilde, C.E. and Koshland, M.E., Biochemistry $\underline{12}$:3218, 1973.

DISCUSSION

Dr. Franklin (Initial Discussant) - I would like to take a few minutes to tell you of some of the studies that have been done by Dr. Mendez in our laboratory which confirm and extend those of Dr. Mestecky. Figure 1 shows the separation on Sephadex G-200 in 1M HAc, 5M guanidine of a cyanogen bromide digest of a polymeric IgA λ myeloma protein. The separation is similar to the one Dr. Mestecky just showed you. Utilizing both acrylamide gel electrophoresis as shown in the insert and Dr. Mestecky's antiserum to J chain,

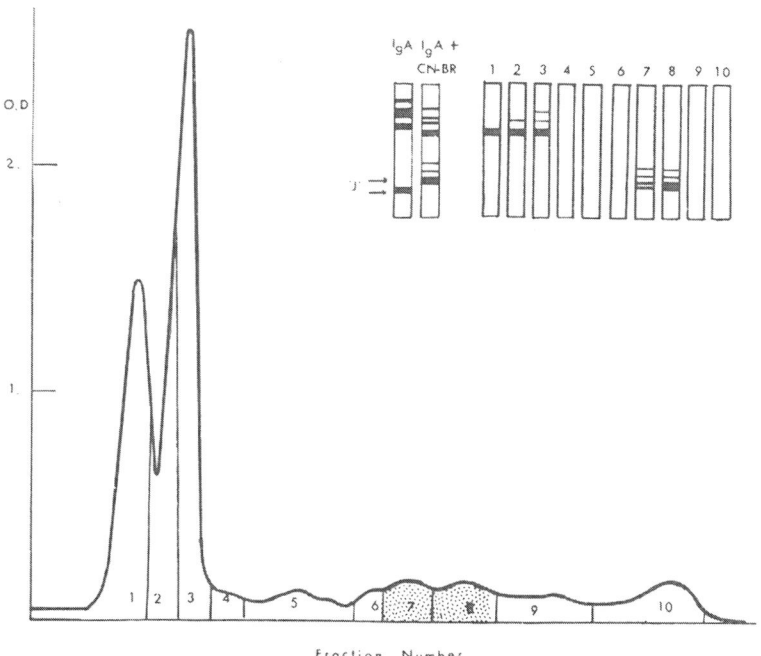

Figure 1. Fractionation of the CNBr digest of a human myeloma protein Prot (IgA$_1$, λ) on a Sephadex G-200 column in 1M acetic acid 5M guanidine. Three hundred mg of protein were dissolved in 5 ml of 1M acetic acid 5M guanidine and applied to a (130 x 3 cm) column. Four ml aliquots were collected. The diagrams of polyacrylamide disc gels in urea (top) identified the J chain in pools 7 and 8.

we were able to localize the cyanogen bromide fragment that
contained the J chain to fractions 7 and 8 of the elution
pattern.   In order to characterize the α chain peptide that
is bound to the J chain and also the peptide in the J chain
which binds to the α chain, we took advantage of the diagonal electrophoresis technique since it permits identification of both partners of a disulfide bridge.   Figure 2 shows
the results.   For those of you who are not acquainted with
this technique, I would like to briefly describe it.   As a
first step, the protein or the peptide is digested with pepsin and trypsin and subjected to high voltage electrophoresis

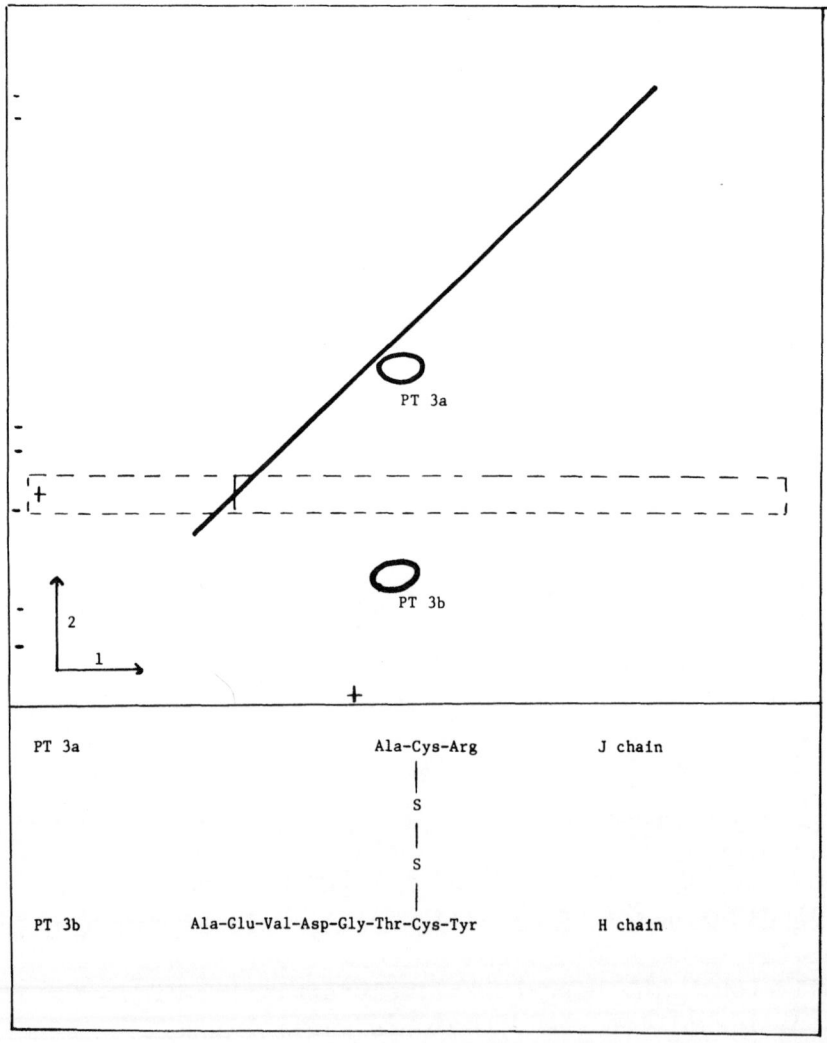

Figure 2.   Diagram of diagonal map electrophoresis at pH 3.5
of a peptic-tryptic digest of the CNBr fractions containing
the J chain.

in the horizontal direction. Under these conditions, the
disulfide linked peptides will remain together in the same
region of the strip. You then take this strip and oxidize
it to break the disulfide bridges. This introduces an additional negative charge into those peptides that were disulfide bridged. Then you take this strip, sew it onto a larger paper, and subject it to a second electrophoretic separation in a direction perpendicular to the original. As you
would expect, all the peptides that have not been altered
by oxidation retain the same relative mobility and migrate
along a straight line. The only peptides that deviate from
the straight line are those that have acquired an additional
negative charge, namely those containing cysteic acid residues that were induced after oxidation. When we subjected
the J chain containing peak to this kind of procedure, about
four or five peptides moved off the diagonal. Two peptides
were present in high yield. One of these, peptide 3TB, is
the same one that Dr. Mestecky showed you, namely the carboxy
terminal octapeptide of the α chain with the sequence Ala-
Glu-Val-Asp-Gly-Thr-Cys-Tyr. The peptide lying in the same
region of the diagonal, PT3a, and therefore presumably bound
to it is a peptide with alanine NH_2 terminal and a composition Ala, Cys, Arg. Since it is a tryptic peptide its sequence must be Ala, Cys, Arg. We have previously isolated
this peptide in low yield from the J chain of IgA (1) and
consequently this must be the peptide from the J chain that
is bound to the carboxy-terminal peptide of the α chain.
While we have not isolated all the peptides from the map,
the only α chain peptide that we have been able to find so
far is the carboxy terminal one. If this is the sole disulfide bridge that can be identified, then the J chain would
have to be bound to only a single α chain in each polymer.
However, the possibility that Ala, Cys, Arg could occur more
than once in the J chain, or that additional bridges could
exist can not be excluded at this time and is currently under
study. For this reason, it appears a bit premature to propose a definitive model for the polymers of IgA and IgM.

REFERENCES

1. Mendez, E., Frangione, B. and Franklin, E. C., Structure
    of Immunoglobulin A. Amino acid sequence of cysteine-
    containing peptides for the J chain. Biochemistry 6:
    1119-1123, 1973.

GENERAL DISCUSSION

Dr. Inman - I would like to address this to Dr. Tomasi. We found that the IgM partially dissociated with MEA gave rise to IgM$_S$ subunits with some covalently attached J chain. Similar results were found when sodium sulfite was used to cleave disulfide bonds but the point to be made is that the ultracentrifuge patterns of the residual IgM$_S$ did not indicate the presence of IgM$_S$ dimers. We have found, however, what might be IgM$_S$ polymers of less than pentameric size in IgM$_S$ synthesizing cells which would be in keeping with what you suggested. The question I would like to ask you is this -- if J attachment to one IgM$_S$ subunit intracellularly results in inducing polymerization, then I think that one would end up on the last IgM$_S$ of the pentamer with a free sulfhydryl residue. If that is the case then how would you propose that the last link between the IgM$_S$ of the last part of the pentamer and the J chain is made?

Dr. Tomasi - I'm not quite sure, Dr. Inman, that I understand your question. I am proposing that the J chain links two subunits together as a dimer.

Dr. Inman - What I was thinking was that when the J chain was put on, the two subunits didn't attach simultaneously, but one went on and this induced polymerization of the rest and finally the fifth one was added. That would also result in a J chain between two IgM$_S$ residues.

Dr. Tomasi - I'm proposing that it is the initial formation of the dimer by the J chain which induces a conformational change and then allows the other subunits to approach and to bond first noncovalently and subsequently disulfide bonds would be formed in the circular pattern which I illustrated. This may or may not be catalyzed by an interchange enzyme.

Dr. Parkhouse - I would like to make three remarks which are pertinent to Dr. Tomasi's presentation. The first is that we have experiments which lead us to the same conclusion that

he drew in relation to the initial formation of a dimer and
our experiments are quite simply as follows: Following
partial reduction of mouse IgM, if you run it on a sucrose
gradient you get a reasonably large 19S peak. If you now put
that 19S peak on an SDS gel you find that it is composed of
a heterogenous collection of subunits, some monomer, a
little HL protomer and some dimer. As you proceed to increase the reducing conditions, when you lose the dimer
form, you also lose the formation of the 19S peak. Thus the
covalently linked 7S subunit shows no tendency to associate
to a high molecular weight form unless dimeric IgM is present
and this is very much in keeping with what Dr. Tomasi has
told us. The second point is that he will be pleased to
know that trimer IgA does in fact have a circular array of
subunits. The third point is that mouse IgM also contains
covalently attached albumin.

Dr. Heremans - It seems to me that a little confusion is
creeping into this discussion. We have been hearing a
discussion whether one or two alpha chains are linked to
the J chain, but may I draw your attention to the fact that
there are four alpha chains to account for in the IgA dimer?
So, would please Dr. Mestecky, Dr. Franklin and Dr. Tomasi
or anybody else who has data on it care to specify whether
they think that the J chain is linked to one, two, three or
four alpha chains?

Dr. Mestecky - I think it is attached to two alpha chains.
Our evidence is that the molecular weight of the J chain in
our set-up anyway, is 15,600 and after cyanogen bromide
cleavage,J chain plus fragments of alpha chain is 17,000
so that there would be room for two fragments of alpha chain
only, not more.

Dr. Heremans - I was making the point that there ought to
be in a complete enzymatic digest as many different "mixed"
peptides and by a mixed peptide I understand a stretch of
J chain disulfide-linked to a stretch of alpha chain as there
are covalent binding sites between one J chain and the four
possible candidates for binding in an IgA dimer. So,
provided that the amino acid sequence of the J chain is not
repetitive, each of these mixed peptides should be different
and therefore they ought to be separable. So my question
is, how many different mixed peptides have you got?

Dr. Bennett - Well, perhaps those other spots on Dr. Franklin's map would add something to it.

Dr. Franklin - I don't think so. We've analyzed partially some of the other spots and they all seem to come from the J chain and not the alpha chain. I think the question is not whether J chain is linked to one, two or four, but rather if, every heavy chain is linked to a J chain or not. I think the number of cysteines in the J chain alone tells you that in IgM this is not possible so it really doesn't matter too much whether it is one, two, three or four.

I wonder, Dr. Mestecky, if your evidence indicates that there is a single J chain per dimer of IgA that you studied.

Dr. Mestecky - In this protein, yes.

Dr. Tomasi - The model I am proposing is quite similar to the model that you proposed and that is, J chain linked to two alpha chains and two disulfides are free for binding of other molecules. I am proposing that that's supposedly the same sites that the J chain is bound to, on the opposite side, if you will, as shown.

Dr. Koshland - I really should give my talk now because I could give you some of the answers to your questions but I don't want to give the talk twice. I would like, therefore, to ask Dr. Brandtzaeg a quick question. Did he try blocking the secretory component binding with the anti-J?

Dr. Brandtzaeg - You ask if we tried to block the SC-combination with an anti-J. No, we did not. We confirmed that our J-chain preparation reacted with anti-J, which was a gift from Dr. Mestecky; but we don't have enough anti-serum to do the blocking experiments.

Dr. Radl - I have a question for Dr. Brandtzaeg. We have been lucky to be able to investigate a unique material. It was milk from a mother with a selective IgA and IgG deficiency. This milk contained only IgM in rather high concentrations, in the 19S form only. Part of it was combined with the secretory component but the SC was completely released at acid pH. My question is: in the 19S IgM preparations of Dr. Brandtzaeg, what percentage of these molecules can combine with the secretory component and whether this secretory component is covalently bound to IgM.

Dr. Brandtzaeg - We have isolated secretory IgM from parotid secretions and also from normal colostrum. We have found that between 60 and 70% of the IgM in these secretions contain secretory component; but this is after isolation. Before isolation it is completely saturated with secretory component since we can add radioactive SC to the whole secretion and get no combination with 19S IgM. So apparently the association between SC and IgM is much more loose than between SC and IgA; probably because, as I pointed out in my talk, disulfide exchange giving stabilization by covalent bonds takes place much more readily in the IgA-SC complexes than in the IgM-SC complexes. So, I think that you have much fewer disulfide bonds involved in the stabilization of secretory IgM than in secretory IgA.

Dr. Radl - Was there any covalent binding or not?

Dr. Brandtzaeg - You can enhance slightly the reactivity of the I determinant also in secretory IgM by reducing the molecule, so I think there is a slight structural stabilization by covalent bonds in that molecule, too; but it cannot be compared to what you have in secretory IgA. Moreover, all SC cannot be released from IgM-SC complexes by acid urea.

Dr. Heremans - I have one remark to what Dr. Tomasi said. Dr. Kunkel who is sitting next to me just reminded me of something. These complexes between α1 anti-trypsin and IgA that you have been mentioning, I have also found and described them, I think 13 or 14 years ago. That is buried in the deeper geological layers of immunologic literature. At the same time I also found complexes between IgA and haptoglobin and transferrin. I was wondering why you hadn't observed these in your studies. All these things became dissociated when I reduced my preparations.

Dr. Tomasi - I am aware of the case you described with the binding of what you called at that time α1 glycoprotein. It was not known to be α1 anti-trypsin at this time. I am not aware that you followed upon this with a large series of studies and this was a single case to my knowledge. We did not find any evidence for the binding of other proteins (other than α1 anti-trypsin and albumin) in this panel of about 50 sera. Incidentally, this binding can be picked up very easily in the whole sera simply by noting the double gull arc. 75% of our sera has this with α1 anti-trypsin.

MECHANISM OF IMMUNOGLOBULIN POLYMER ASSEMBLY[*]

Marian E. Koshland and Charles E. Wilde III

Department of Bacteriology and Immunology

University of California, Berkeley

INTRODUCTION

Recent studies on polymeric immunoglobulins have demonstrated the presence of a small polypeptide chain, the J chain, in addition to the heavy and light chains that comprise the monomer units (1,2). The presence of J chain in covalent disulfide linkage within these polymers and its absence from all forms of monomeric immunoglobulins strongly suggests that J plays a fundamental role in establishing and maintaining the polymeric state. In order to understand this role, several questions must be answered. First, what is the stoichiometry of J chain in the various polymeric forms? Second, is J chain linked to every heavy chain in the polymer, or merely to one or two? Third, is J an obligatory requirement for correct polymer formation, or can normal covalent polymers be assembled in the absence of J chain? When this information has been obtained, a mechanism for the assembly of immunoglobulin polymers can be developed.

MOLECULAR WEIGHT OF J CHAIN

The determination of J chain stoichiometry required an accurate value for the molecular weight of J. Initial studies using SDS-polyacrylamide gels and gel filtration showed that J had the same mobility as light chains (1,2). On this basis, J was assumed to have a comparable molecular weight. However, once J was isolated in sufficient amounts

129

to permit centrifuge studies of molecular weight, the value
of 25,000 was thrown in doubt. For example, O'Daly and
Cebra (3) found a molecular weight of 15,000 for rabbit J
by equilibrium centrifugation, and subsequently, Schrohenloher et al.(4), using a guanidine solution, and our laboratory (5), using non-dissociating buffers, obtained similar values for human J chain. The discrepancy between the
values of 25,000 and 15,000 could not be attributed to
charge effects nor to carbohydrate content. An explanation
was provided by velocity sedimentation analysis (5). The
data obtained for J chain are compared in Table 1 with the
values for three other proteins (6) with molecular weights
in the range of 13,000-25,000. The $s_{20,w}$ and $D_{20,w}$ of J

Table 1   The Unusual Physical Properties of J Chain

protein	mol. wt.	$s_{20,w}$	$D_{20,w}$	axial ratio
J chain	15,000	1.28	6.96	17.9
Ribonuclease	13,700	1.64	11.9	2.1
Lysozyme	14,100	1.87	10.4	4.3
Chymotrypsinogen	23,200	2.54	9.5	3.0

chain were found to be much lower than those of ribonucle-
ase, lysozyme and chymotrypsinogen, and the derived axial
ratio was much higher, indicating that J is a very elongated molecule. This expanded conformation accounted for
the anomalous molecular weight of 25,000, since other elongated proteins have been shown to migrate at slower than
expected rates during gel filtration and electrophoresis (7).

STOICHIOMETRY OF J CHAIN

The determination of the correct molecular weight of J
chain allowed its composition to be expressed in residues
per mole. Using this information, two quantitative methods
were developed for determining the stoichiometry of J chain.

The first method (8) utilized the large differences between J and light chains in the contents of seven amino acids.
To prepare a fraction containing light and J chains, IgA
polymers were reduced, alkylated with ^{3}H-iodoacetic acid and
chromatographed on Sephadex G-200 equilibrated with sodium
decyl sulfate as a denaturing agent. This procedure was

shown to give a quantitative separation of the light-J mixture from heavy chain. The control of pure light chains was prepared from the IgG of the polymer donor by the same method. The J content of the polymer was then determined by comparing the amino acid composition of the light-J fraction with that of the pure light chain fraction. For each of the seven critical residues, the factor was calculated by which the light chain content was diluted by J to give the observed content in the light-J mixture. The average of these factors and the known number of light chains per polymer allowed the determination of the number of J chains per polymer.

This method was applied to colostral IgA which had been separated into a dimer and a tetramer-enriched fraction by successive sucrose density gradient centrifugations. From the amino acid analyses, the J content of the dimer was calculated to be 1.02 ± 0.06 moles of J per mole of dimer (Table 2).

Table 2   Stoichiometry of J Chain in Dimer IgA

Amino acid	Light[a]	J chain[a]	J-L mixture[a]	Moles of J/dimer
arg	6.2	14.5	7.3	0.97
asp	15.5	33.7	17.8	0.97
ser	27.3	11.5	25.2	0.94
gly	15.5	3.2	13.5	1.21
ileu	5.4	13.3	6.3	0.85
phe	7.1	2.0	6.3	1.24
CMCys	5.0	12.0	5.9	0.98
			Mean	1.02 ± 0.06

[a]Residues/23,000 g. After 20 hours of hydrolysis.

The J content obtained for the tetramer-enriched preparation was 1.32 ± 0.2, but when a correction was applied for residual dimer contamination, this value dropped to 1.01 moles of J per mole of tetramer. Thus only one J chain was found per SIgA polymer independent of the size of the polymer. This finding explains earlier observations (3) of less than one mole of J per mole of unfractionated colostral IgA, since the latter has been shown by centrifuge studies to be a mixture of two polymeric forms, dimer and tetramer (8).

As the ratio of J to light chain decreases with higher polymerization, the amino acid dilution method becomes less accurate, and thus the determination of the IgA tetramer

stoichiometry was judged to be at the limit of confidence
of the method. To determine the stoichiometry of J chain
in IgM, therefore, an alternate method (9) was developed
which utilized the radiolabelling of thiol groups. A Waldenströms IgM was completely reduced in 10 M urea to its
component chains and alkylated with ^{3}H-iodoacetic acid. Samples of the mixture were electrophoresed on alkaline urea
polyacrylamide gels. The gels were sliced and the radioactivity determined by scintillation counting. As the electrophoretic pattern in Figure 1 shows, the alkylated chains
differed sufficiently in net charge to permit a clean separation and a determination of the total tritium counts in each
chain. Yields were calculated from the ^{3}H-carboxymethylcys-
teine contents and the known numbers of half-cystines in each
chain; values of 14, 5, and 6 were used for μ, light and J
chains respectively. Typical results are shown in Table 3,
where 0.94 moles of J were recovered for every 10 moles of μ
or light chains. The average yield from nine experiments was
0.96 ± 0.03 moles of J per pentamer.

Table 3   Stoichiometry of J Chain in Pentamer IgM

chain	total ^{3}H cpm	Total μmoles (x 10^{-3})		Chains/pentamer
		^{3}H-CMCys	Chain	
μ	13,074	17.23	1.23	10
L	4,651	6.13	1.23	10
J	524	0.690	0.115	0.94

NATURE OF POLYMER LINKAGE

Since J chain contains 6 half-cystine residues, the
finding of one J per polymer limits the number of possible
J-heavy chain intersubunit bonds to six, and the number per
monomer to one in the larger polymers such as IgM. If J chain
serves as a bracelet (5) to link each monomer unit, then one
J-μ bond would be broken for every monomer released upon reductive cleavage. If, on the other hand, the J chain serves as a
clasp (5) between two monomers, the number of J-μ bonds broken
would not correspond to the number of monomers released. To
distinguish these possibilities, a method (9) of stepwise
reduction and differential radioalkylation was developed
which permitted the cleavage of J chain disulfides

to be correlated with the extent of depolymerization. The
method consisted of two steps: I. limited reduction with
dithioerythritol (DTE) and alkylation with ^{14}C-iodoacetic
acid, followed by II. complete reduction and alkylation with
[3]H-iodoacetic acid. The amounts of reduction products formed
in step I were assayed by velocity sedimentation analysis.
The chains formed in step II were separated by alkaline
urea polyacrylamide gel electrophoresis and their radioactivity was determined. The total ^{3}H and ^{14}C label provided a measure of chain yield and the ^{14}C label per chain
provided a measure of the half-cystines alkylated after
the limited reduction step. An example of the gel electrophoretic patterns is given in Fig. 1.

When these methods were applied to a human monoclonal
IgM, the results shown in Fig. 2 were obtained. The data
cannot be explained by a bracelet model of J linkage to

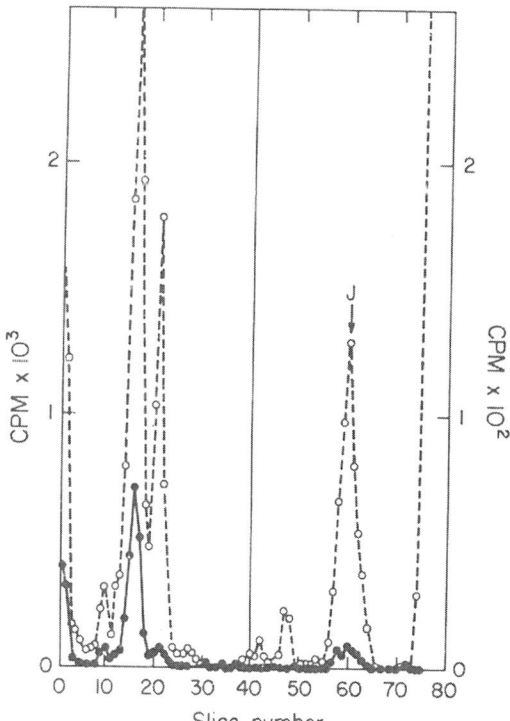

Fig. 1. Electrophoresis of completely reduced and alkylated
IgM on urea 4.2% polyacrylamide gels, pH 9. ●—● = [14]C cpm
from cysteines alkylated in limited reduction step. O– –O =
[3]H cpm from cysteines alkylated in complete reduction step.

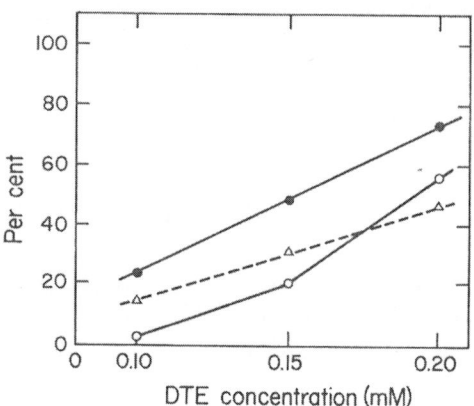

Fig. 2.   Correlation of disulfide cleavage with depolymerization.   Δ--Δ = % monomer yield.   O—O = % of J chain and
●—● = % of μ chains containing 1 ^{14}C-CMCys per chain.

monomers. After reduction with 0.1 mM DTE, 39.2% of the
pentamer was cleaved, 14.3% to monomer. This cleavage was
accompanied by the incorporation of one carboxymethylcysteine
(CMCys) into 27.7% of the μ chains, but into only 3.6% of the
J chains. Similarly, after reduction with 0.15 mM DTE, the
number of J half-cystines labelled was much less than the
ratio of one per monomer required by the bracelet model. At
0.2 mM DTE, the rapid increase in the ^{14}C-CMCys of J was
shown to reflect the release of J chain and the consequent
reduction of intra-J bonds.

To pinpoint the location of J in the pentamer, the dimers formed after limited reduction with 0.1 mM DTE were
isolated by elution from SDS-polyacrylamide gels and examined
by the differential labelling method (Fig. 3). Analyses of
the μ chain showed that 43% contained one ^{14}C-CMCys, in good
agreement with the theoretical value for the dimer of 50%.
Analyses of the J chain showed that it was present in 63%
of the dimers and contained no detectable amounts of [14]C
label. The most plausible explanation of these data is a
clasp model of linkage in which J is disulfide bonded to
adjacent monomers and the remaining J half-cystines form
intrachain bonds.

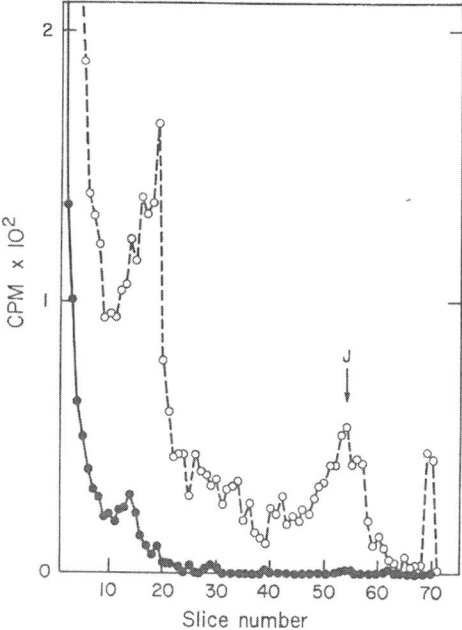

Fig. 3. Electrophoresis of completely reduced and alkylated
IgM dimer on urea 5% polyacrylamide gel, pH 9. See legend
under Fig. 1 for explanation of symbols.

REASSEMBLY OF IgM

Evidence for the requirement for J chain during polymerization was obtained from reassembly studies conducted on
a human Waldenströms IgM. The IgM pentamer was dissociated
into its monomer subunits and J chain by reduction in 20 mM
mercaptoethylamine. Under the conditions used all the intersubunit disulfide bonds were reduced, and in addition, an average of 0.35 intrasubunit μ-μ bonds per monomer. However,
the monomers remained intact by the criteria of gel filtration in 1 M acetic acid. The dissociation of J was complete
within the limits of detection. No J chain was observed when
the monomers were completely reduced and alkylated and examined for J by either electrophoretic or immunological methods.

The mixture of reduced monomers and J chain was allowed
to reoxidize by extended dialysis against buffers containing
progressively lower mercaptoethylamine concentrations. The
controls consisted of reduced monomers that had been freed of
J chain by gel filtration through Sephadex G-200 equilibrated

with 20 mM mercaptoethylamine. The reoxidized proteins were
then examined in the Spinco Model E ultracentrifuge for the
presence of polymeric material. Maximal reassembly was achieved using high protein concentrations, 15–20 mg/ml, and
0.1 M sodium acetate buffer, pH 5.5. In the mixture of monomer and J chain reoxidized under these conditions, approximately 40% of the material cosedimented with native 19s IgM;
in the monomer control, approximately the same amount of
polymer was formed, but it was heterodisperse, sedimenting
both ahead of and behind the IgM control.

To characterize the structures of these reformed polymers,
they were separated from the residual monomer by gel filtration and examined in the ultracentrifuge in the presence of
6 M guanidine-HCl. The polymers formed in the presence of J
chain again cosedimented with native IgM, indicating that they
were covalently linked. In contrast, the polymers obtained in
the absence of J were converted to material that cosedimented
with IgM_s, and were therefore non-covalent aggregates.

The J content of the reassembled polymers was analyzed
by alkaline urea polyacrylamide gel electrophoresis (Fig. 4)
both before and after complete reduction and alkylation.

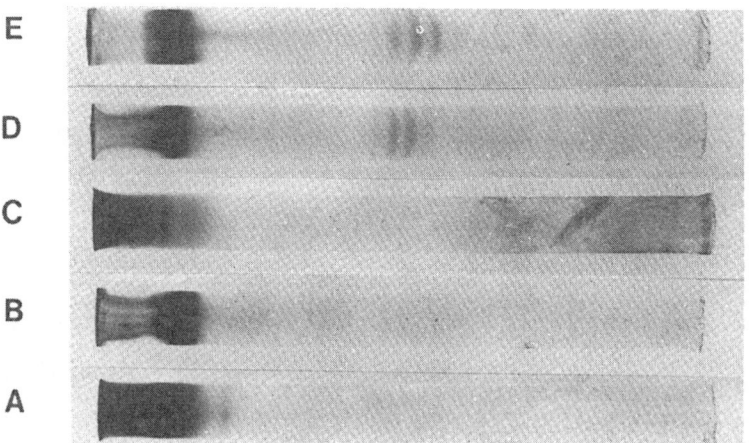

Fig. 4. Electrophoresis of reassembled polymers on urea 4%
polyacrylamide gels, pH 9. A and B = reoxidized IgM_s. C
and D = reoxidized IgM_s + J chain. E = IgM control. A, C
unreduced; B, D, E completely reduced and alkylated.

No J chain bands were observed in the unreduced polymers
(Fig. A and C). The characteristic J bands appeared only
following complete reduction and alkylation of the polymers
reassembled in the presence of J chain (Fig. 4). Furthermore, the amount of J chain released from these polymers
appeared nearly equivalent to that released from native IgM
(Fig. 4E). These results indicate that J chain is indeed
required for IgM polymer formation, and that it is covalently
incorporated into the reassembled polymers.

MODEL FOR POLYMER ASSEMBLY

The studies reported here provide strong evidence for a
clasp model of J linkage. Moreover, the finding that some
of the μ-μ intersubunit bonds are more susceptible to reduction than the μ-J bonds indicates that the J clasp provides
the nucleus for polymerization rather than the closure of
the polymer. On this basis a series of sequential disulfide
exchanges can be postulated to explain the assembly process.
The first intermediate would be formed by an exchange between
a J chain thiol and a monomer heavy-heavy bond, yielding a
J-heavy disulfide and a free-SH in the opposing heavy chain.
According to the available evidence, the potential intersubunit half-cystines are either reversibly blocked (10) or
are linked in an intrasubunit heavy-heavy bond (11). In
rapid succession, a similar reaction would occur between a
second J thiol and another monomer subunit to produce a
J-linked dimer. The heavy chain thiols generated could then
either be oxidized to form dimers or induce additional exchanges with other monomers to form larger polymers. The two
initial thiols on J chain may reflect its native intracellular
state or the first step in the disulfide exchange catalyzed
by an external oxidation-reduction system.

Since any disulfide-sulfhydryl interchange is an equilibrium reaction, an efficient yield of product depends on push-
ing the reaction to completion. Two such means are available,
an excess of monomer reactant and a rapid removal of polymer
product. The studies on cells synthesizing polymers suggest
that both means are operating. The intracellular immunoglobulin consists of a large monomer pool and little or no polymers of any size, while the extracellular immunoglobulin is
predominatly in the form of correctly completed polymers
(10,12). In contrast, no significant amounts of free J chain
have been detected within cells, indicating that the supply
of J is the rate-determining step in polymer assembly.

Any model for assembly must take into account the differences in the size of secreted polymers. Although it is possible that the relative concentrations of monomer and J chain affect the degree of polymerization, their relative pool sizes make this explanation unlikely. It is much more likely that several other interrelating factors are involved. For example, in IgM, steric constraints upon the intersubunit disulfide bridges may prevent closure of any non-pentameric form. In IgA, these constraints may not be so stringent so that the varying degree of polymerization mainly reflects the relative rates of assembly and secretion.

*Supported by USPHS Grant AI-07079-07

REFERENCES

1. Halpern, M.S. and Koshland, M.E., Nature 228:1276, 1970.
2. Mestecky, J., Zikan, J. and Butler, W.T., Science 171: 1163, 1971.
3. O'Daly, J.A. and Cebra, J.J., Biochemistry 10:3842, 1971.
4. Schrohenloher, R.E., Mestecky, J. and Stanton, T.H., Biochim. Biophys. Acta 295:576, 1973.
5. Wilde, C.E. and Koshland, M.E., Biochemistry 12:3218, 1973.
6. Tanford, C., Physical Chemistry of Macromolecules, Wiley, New York, N.Y., 1967.
7. Andrews, P., Meth. Biochem. Anal. 18:1, 1970.
8. Halpern, M.S. and Koshland, M.E., J. Immunol. in press.
9. Chapuis, R.M. and Koshland, M.E., Proc. Natl. Acad. Sci., in press.
10. Askonas, B.A. and Parkhouse, R.M.E., Biochem J. 123:629, 1971.
11. Feinstein, A., Munn, E.A. and Richardson, N.E., Ann. N.Y. Acad. Sci. 190:104, 1971.
12. Halpern, M.S. and Coffman, R.L., J. Immunol. 109:674, 1972.

ASSEMBLY AND SECRETION OF IMMUNOGLOBULIN A

R.M.E. Parkhouse and E. Della Corte

National Institute for Medical Research
London, England

INTRODUCTION

Immunoglobulins, like other secreted glycoproteins, are synthesised on membrane-bound polyribosomes, released into the cysternae of the endoplasmic reticulum and pass to the outside via the Golgi apparatus. During passage through the cell there is a stepwise addition of carbohydrate at different subcellular sites, and a general rule is that mannose and hexosamine are added early, whereas fucose and galactose are added late (1,2).

A unique feature of IgA among immunoglobulins is its molecular weight heterogeneity (3-9). The degree of polymerisation is characteristic and stable for a given myeloma protein (4,9) raising the question of what controls this variable degree of polymerisation. It is particularly interesting that myeloma cells which secrete polymeric IgA certainly contain all the biochemical machinery for polymerisation and yet still secrete a proportion of monomer form.

The molecular heterogeneity of secreted IgA contrasts with the uniform pentameric product formed by IgM-secreting cells, in spite of the fact that polymerisation in both cases occurs from monomeric (H_2L_2) subunits just before, or at the time of secretion (10-15). At this time, J chain (16,17) is incorporated into IgM (18) and polymeric, but not monomeric, IgA (18,19).

139

In order to explain control of polymerisation we have investigated the role played by carbohydrate addition, J chain and an enzyme catalysing disulphide interchange (20).

MATERIALS AND METHODS

Mouse Plasma Cell Tumours secreting IgA (MOPC 315 and 5647) and IgM (MOPC 104E and TEPC 183) were obtained from Dr. M. Potter and maintained by subcutaneous transfer.

MOPC 315 Myeloma Protein was purified from serum (21) without reduction, and the purified protein consisted predominantly of monomer and dimer molecules.

J chain was isolated from MOPC 315 protein by reduction followed by preparative acrylamide gel electrophoresis (22). The protein sample was not alkylated following reduction.

Myeloma Cell Suspensions were labelled in vitro with radioactive leucine, mannose, galactose or fucose as previously described (23,24). Radioactive intracellular and secreted myeloma proteins were determined by precipitation with rabbit anti-(MOPC 315) myeloma protein and added homologous carrier protein (10). To determine molecular sizes, such antibody-antigen precipitates were analysed by electrophoresis in sodium dodecyl sulphate - polyacrylamide gels (SDS gels, 11). The presence or absence of J chain in radioactive secreted and intracellular myeloma protein was determined by electrophoresis of reduced and alkylated specific antibody-antigen precipitates in alkaline urea gels (AU gels, 18). Radioactive intracellular monomer IgA and radioactive secreted monomer and dimer IgA were prepared from the labelled cell suspensions by sucrose density gradient centrifugation (25). No carrier protein was added to the isolated radioactive IgA samples, so that the purified material is always high specific activity immunoglobulin.

Reduction and Reconstitution Experiments. J chain (0.2-0.8 mg/ml), was reduced at room temp for 60 min with 10mM DTT and then added to a solution of radioactive immunoglobulin for a further hour. During reduction of the immunoglobulin, J chain was present at 80μg/ml and DTT was 1-5mM. As controls, J chain was either omitted or replaced by other proteins. Part of the reduction mixture was alkylated with iodoacetamide in order to assess the extent of reduction of radioactive immunoglobulin; the remainder

was separated from the reducing agent by filtration through
Sephadex G-25 and then incubated at 37° for 30 min with or
without the disulphide exchanging enzyme (2.5mg/ml). All
samples were analysed on SDS gels. The enzyme was purified
from beef liver and given to us by Dr. R.B. Freedman (Biol.
Lab., Univ. Kent, Canterbury, England).

RESULTS AND DISUCSSION

Secretion and Addition of Carbohydrate

The incorporation of leucine into intracellular and
secreted MOPC 315 myeloma protein follows the now well
established kinetics for immunoglobulin synthesis and
secretion, there being an immediate incorporation into intracellular immunoglobulin and a lag period of about 30 min
prior to the appearance of secreted protein. The average
time taken for synthesis and secretion of the myeloma protein
was found to be approximately 2 hr. In similar incorporation
experiments with radioactive mannose, galactose and fucose
(24), analysis of intracellular and secreted molecular forms
of IgA, together with kinetic data, support the contention
that there is a stepwise addition of carbohydrate residues
to immunoglobulin during the process of secretion. In
common with other mouse myeloma proteins, mannose is added
early in biosynthesis whereas fucose is added late, about
the time of secretion. Analysis of galactose incorporation
into MOPC 315 myeloma proteins shows that a substantial
proportion of galactose must be added early, although some
may be incorporated later. This is not the case in previously studied immunoglobulins, the galactose being added late
in biosynthesis, and may simply reflect structural features
of the MOPC 315 myeloma carbohydrate i.e., the location of
certain galactose residues close to the core of the carbohydrate prosthetic groups. Alternatively, the sites of the
carbohydrate addition may vary among the different myeloma
tumours.

Following labelling of MOPC 315 cells with radioactive
leucine for 4 hr the major secreted products of the cell are
monomer and dimer, whereas the intracellular IgA is largely
monomer (24). This observation demonstrates that polymerisation of the monomer occurs just before, or at the time,
the molecule is secreted. During the period studied, 0.5-4
hour, there was no change in the monomer: dimer ratio of the
secreted 3H-leucine - labelled myeloma protein. Thus there

is no progressive polymerisation or degradation in the
culture fluid, and the rates of secretion of monomer and
dimer are identical.

Since polymerisation of intracellular 7S subunits and
addition of fucose occur simultaneously, close to the time
of secretion, perhaps these two processes are correlated.
We therefore considered the possibility that secreted
monomers and polymers were different with the respect to
carbohydrate, there being, for example, more (or less) fucose
in the monomer than the dimer. That this is not the case
was shown by the incorporation of radioactive mannose,
galactose, fucose and leucine into secreted monomer and dimer
IgA (Table 1). It is clear that the radioactivity ratios
of monomer to dimer were identical irrespective of the
isotopic precursor used to label the immunoglobulin. We can
conclude that there are no obvious compositional differences
in carbohydrate between IgA monomers and dimers secreted by
a myeloma cell suspension, and would therefore argue that
control of IgA polymerisation does not reflect regulation
at the level of carbohydrate addition. A definite role for
the carbohydrate remains controversial. If it is required
to label the protein for secretion, then it is surprising
that there are examples of secreted proteins which do not
contain carbohydrate (26). Perhaps the addition of fucose
controls the release of immunoglobulin from cells to the
exterior milieu, but as yet there is no evidence for this.

Requirement for J chain and a Disulphide -
Exchanging Enzyme for polymerisation

Prior to the discovery of J chain we had been able to
polymerise IgM from intracellular 7S monomers (IgMs) as well
as from subunits of secreted 19S IgM obtained by reduction
(27,28). Isolated radioactive intracellular IgMs showed
no tendency to polymerise unless first treated with a

Radioactive precursor	Leu	Mann	Gal	Fuc
Monomer: dimer ratio	0.61	0.63	0.60	0.63

Table 1. Incorporation of leucine, mannose, galactose and
fucose into secreted monomer and dimer forms of MOPC 315.
Secreted immunoglobulins were precipitated with anti-(MOPC
315, myeloma protein), electrophoresed in SDS gels and the
ratio of monomer to dimer was obtained by integrating the
areas under the peaks of $\alpha 2$ and $\alpha 4$.

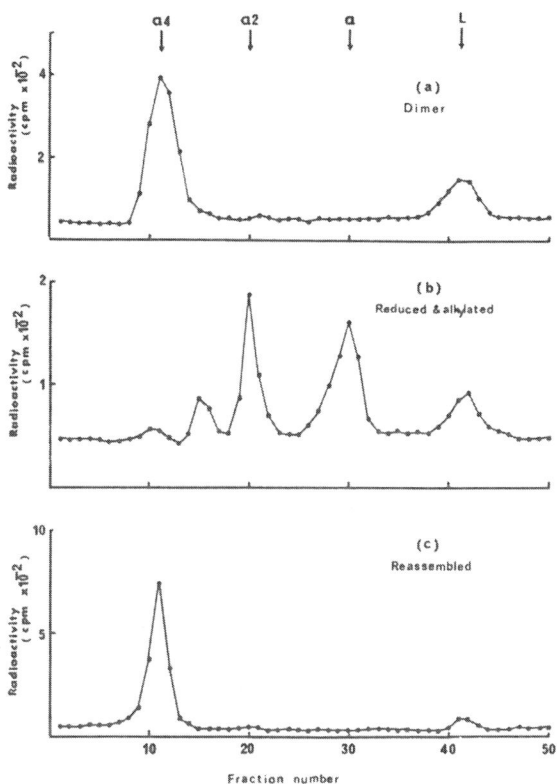

Fig. 1. Polymerisation of reduced, secreted dimer IgA
(MOPC 315). The isolated radioactive dimer (a) was reduced
with 5mM DTT in the presence of J chain. A portion was
alkylated (b), whilst the remainder was filtered through
Sephadex G-25 and incubated with the disulfide exchanging
enzyme (c). Analysis by SDS gels.

reducing agent, suggesting that the cysteine residues
responsible for inter-subunit linkage were blocked within
the cell. Under optimal conditions removal of the reducing
agent caused 70% of the subunits to be assembled into 19S
(pentameric) IgM. The polymerisation only occurred in the
presence of reduced carrier IgM isolated from serum.
Similarly reassembly of reduced 19S IgM occurred at high,
but not low, protein concentrations. In identical
experiments with IgA, we never observed polymerisation of
subunits obtained by reduction of polymer molecules (29).
Using the same methodology we now show that IgA subunits
can be polymerised providing J chain and a disulfide
exchanging enzyme are supplied.

Purified secreted radioactive dimer IgA from MOPC 315

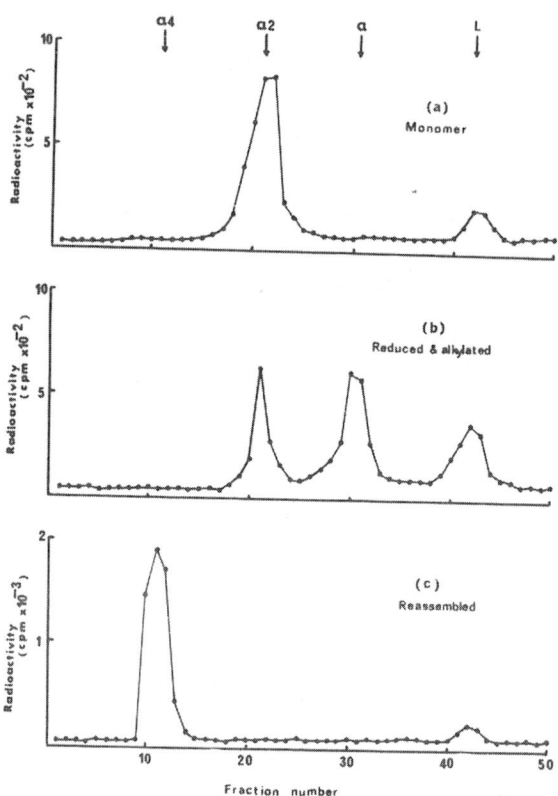

Fig. 2. Polymerisation of intracellular monomer IgA (MOPC 315). The isolated protein (a) was reduced and then alkylated (b) or polymerised (c) as indicated in the legend to Fig. 1 Analysis by SDS gels.

(Fig. 1a) was depolymerised by reduction (Fig. 1b). In the absence of any carrier protein, removal of the reducing agent by passage through Sephadex G-25 did not result in any reassembly, even when the sample was incubated with the disulphide exchanging enzyme. If isolated J chain was present in the reduction mixture, then polymerisation to the dimer form was total (Fig. 1c), but only occurred when the Sephadex G-25 eluate was incubated with the enzyme. Thus polymerisation only occurred when J chain and the enzyme were provided. For simplicity in presentation, the negative controls are omitted from the figures.

Similarly, secreted radioactive monomer IgA or radioactive intracellular monomer IgA (Fig. 2) yielded entirely dimer IgA after reduction (Fig. 2b), passage over Sephadex G-25 and enzyme treatment (Fig. 2c). Again both J chain

and the enzyme were necessary for polymerisation of the
reduction mixtures. The data obtained with the secreted
monomer are not shown.

A remarkable specificity in polymerisation was demonstrated. Not only did reduced albumin or IgG fail to induce
or interfere with polymerisation of IgA, but reduced IgG
could not be polymerised when J chain and the enzymes were
supplied. The specificity of polymerisation was further
emphasised by an experiment in which 14C-leucine-labelled
secreted IgM (MOPC 104E) and 3H-leucine-labelled secreted IgA
(MOPC 315) were mixed, reduced and reassembled without the
formation of hybrid molecules (25).

Although we have demonstrated that polymerisation occurs
in the presence of added J chains, it is critical to demonstrate that, J chain is incorporated into the reassembled
polymer molecule. In order to establish this point we have
taken advantage of the fact that subunits of IgM can be
polymerised at high concentrations of carrier IgM in the
reduced mixture (27,28). For IgM the endogenous J chain is
sufficient for reassembly.

Radioactive IgM was mixed with carrier IgM at 2 mg/ml
and reduced with 5mM DTT. A portion was alkylated, whilst
the remainder was reassembled into IgM by filtration through
Sephadex G-25 and incubation with the disulphide exchanging
enzyme. The reduce-alkylated and reassembled samples were
electrophoresed in AU gels in order to determine the amounts
of free J chain.

Furthermore, to check for selective loss of J chain, the
reassembled IgM was reduced again with 5mM DTT and the released J chain was measured on an AU gel. It is evident
that reduction releases comparable amounts of radioactive
J chain from IgM before (0.62% total radioactivity Fig. 3a)
or after (0.66% total radioactivity Fig. 3b) reassembly. In
the reassembled 19S IgM (Fig. 3c), J chain could not be
detected and must therefore have been entirely incorporated
into the polymer molecules. The chain is not therefore
simply a catalyst for polymerisation and appears to be an
essential structural requirement for polymeric immunoglobulins.

It is interesting that intracellular and secreted
monomer subunits of IgA can be completely polymerised.

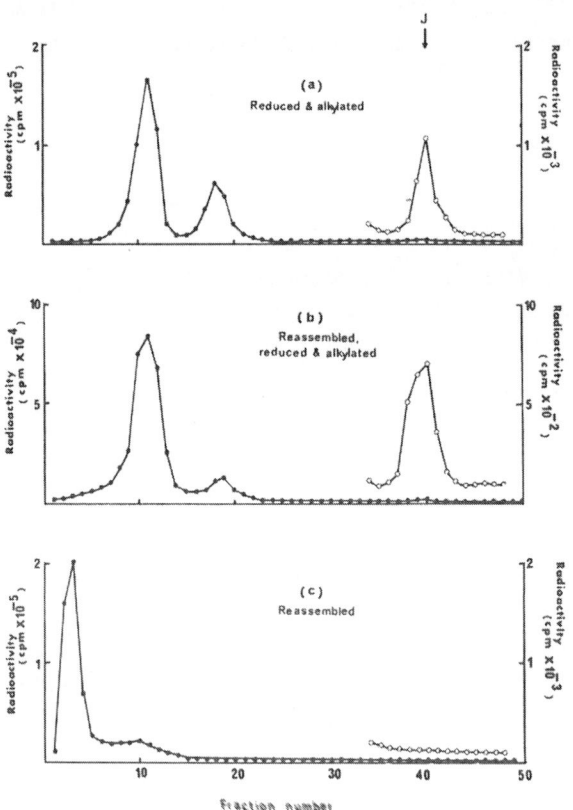

Fig. 3.   Incorporation of J chain into reassembled IgM (MOPC 104E).   The sample was reduced (a) and then polymerised (c) as indicated in the legend to Fig. 1, except that carrier IgM replaced J chain in the reduction mixture.   A sample of the reassembled material was again reduced and alkylated (b) Analysis by AU gels.

Apart from indicating a manadatory role for J chain in assembly, these findings question a role for carbohydrate in polymerisation and demonstrate unequivocally that secreted IgA monomers are certainly capable of further assembly.   The similarity in carbohydrate composition between secreted IgA monomers and dimers has already prompted the suggestion that carbohydrate does not control polymerisation.   Perhaps the strongest argument against carbohydrate addition as a controlling factor is the observation that intracellular monomers could be completely polymerised to dimers.   In similar experiments with IgM-producing mouse myeloma cells we also observed complete conversion of intracellular 7S subunits of IgM to the 19S form (25), and yet the intracellular monomer molecules of both IgA and IgM are deficient in fucose and galactose (13,23,24).

Control of Polymerisation by J chain

Since the IgA producing cell contains the biochemical machinery for polymerisation and since secreted (or intra-cellular) IgA monomer can be polymerised in vitro, we thought the amount of intracellular J chain might be a critical factor. Thus myeloma cell lines secreting IgA (5647 and MOPC 315) and IgM (TEPC 183) were incubated with radioactive leucine for varying periods of time, and secreted radioactive immunoglobulins were precipitated with specific antisera for gel analysis.

The radioactive secreted products were as follows: TEPC 183 secreted 19S IgM (90%), 7S IgM (2%) and free light chains (8%); MOPC 315 secreted monomer (32.3%), dimer (51.3%) and trimer (16,4%) IgA; 5647 secreted monomer (15%), dimer (34.3%) and trimer (50.7%) IgA. In both IgA producing cell lines the relative concentrations of secreted molecular forms remained constant over the period 1-4 hr.

Determination of J chain revealed a striking difference between cells secreting IgM and IgA (Fig. 4). Secreted radioactive IgM contained a constant fraction of radio-activity in J chain at all times. With secreted IgA, on the other hand, the proportion of radioactivity in J chain, was relatively high in immunoglobulin collected after short periods of culture, but decreased as the time of incubation was prolonged. Similar results were obtained when "pulse-chase" type experiments were done (29). For IgM-secreting cells, therefore, there is a balanced synthesis of 7S sub-units and J chains. In cells secreting IgA. however, the results demonstrate that the pool of intracellular J chain is less than the intracellular pool of 7S IgA.

The balanced synthesis of immunoglobulin subunits in IgM-secreting cells thus determines the fact that the major secreted molecule is the pentamer. As previously suggested (18), the occurence of 7S IgM in sera from a variety of pathological conditions may simply reflect a deficiency in J chain synthesis. The absence of polymeric forms of IgM other than the pentamer must indicate that this is the most thermodynamically stable assembly form.

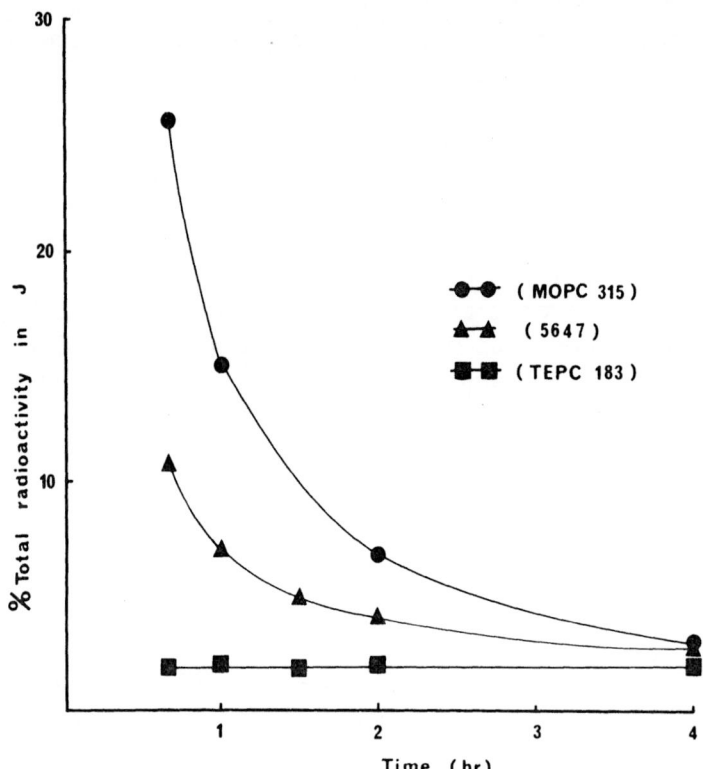

Fig. 4.   Radioactivity in J chain as per cent total secreted radioactive Ig. To determine the fraction of radioactivity in J chain, secreted IgA was precipitated with antibody, reduced and alkylated and analysed by AU gels.

In IgA secreting cells the size of the intracellular J chain pool is limiting and is less than the requirement for complete polymerisation. The major factor which determines whether an intracellular monomer molecule is secreted as such or is polymerised with the addition of J chain is therefore the amount of intracellular J chain. When this is limiting, monomer will be secreted.

Acknowledgements: We would like to thank Iain Hunter for valuable and expert assistance, and the Biochemical Journal for permission to publish the figures.

REFERENCES

1.   Bevan, M.J., Parkhouse, R.M.E., Williamson, A.R. and Askonas, B.A., Progr. Biophys. Molec. Biol. 25:131, 1972.
2.   Hughes, R.C., Progr. Biophys. Molec. Biol. 26:189, 1973.
3.   Vaerman, J.P., Fudenberg, H.H., Vaerman, C. and Mandy, W.J., Immunochemistry, 2:263, 1965.

4. Fahey, J.L., J. Clin. Invest., 42:111, 1963.
5. Levin, W.C., Ritzmann, S.E., Seeuwen, J.P. and Nanninga, L., Clin. Chim. Acta., 10:12, 1964.
6. Fahey, J.L., J. Exp. Med., 114:399, 1961.
7. Cummings, N.A. and Franklin, E.C., J. Lab. Clin. Med., 65:8, 1965.
8. Vaerman, J.P., Johnson, L.B., Mandy, W.J. and Fudenberg, H.H., J. Lab. Clin. Med., 65:18, 1965.
9. Abel, C.A. and Grey, H.M., Biochemistry, 7:2682, 1968.
10. Parkhouse, R.M.E. and Askonas, B.A., Biochem. J., 115: 163, 1969.
11. Parkhouse, R.M.E., Biochem. J., 123:635, 1971.
12. Parkhouse, R.M.E., Febs. Lett., 16:71, 1971.
13. Parkhouse, R.M.E., Transplant Rev., 14:131, 1973.
14. Bevan, M.J., Europ. J. Immunol., 1:133, 1971.
15. Bargellesi, A., Periman, P., and Scharff, M.D., J. Immunol., 108:126, 1972.
16. Halpern, M.S. and Koshland, M.E., Nature, 288:1276, 1970.
17. Mestecky, J., Zikan, J. and Butler, W.T., Science, 171: 1163, 1971.
18. Parkhouse, R.M.E., Nature New. Biol. 236:9, 1972.
19. Halpern, M.S. and Coffman, R.J., J. Immunol. 109:674, 1972.
20. Fuchs, S., DeLorenzo, F. and Anfinsen, C.B., J. Biol. Chem., 242:398, 1967.
21. Goetzl, E.J. and Metzger, H., Biochemistry, 9:1267, 1970.
22. Parkhouse, R.M.E., Manuscript in preparation, 1973.
23. Parkhouse, R.M.E. and Melchers, F., Biochem. J., 125: 235, 1971.
24. Della Corte, E. and Parkhouse, R.M.E., Biochem. J., In the press, 1973a.
25. Della Corte, E. and Parkhouse, R.M.E., Biochem. J., In the press, 1973b.
26. Winterburn, P.J. and Phelps, C.F., Nature 236:147, 1972.
27. Parkhouse, R.M.E., Askonas, B.A. and Dourmashkin, R.R., Immunology, 18:575, 1970.
28. Askonas, B.A. and Parkhouse, R.M.E., Biochem. J., 123: 629, 1971.
29. Parkhouse, R.M.E., Virella, G. and Dourmashkin, R.R., Clin. Exp. Immunol. 8:581, 1971.

SPECIAL CHARACTERISTICS OF THE IgA2 SUBCLASS

L.M. Jerry* and H.G. Kunkel**

Department of Experimental Medicine,
McGill University, Montreal, Canada* and
Rockefeller University, New York, N.Y., 10021**

Although in man IgA is a relatively minor fraction of
circulating serum immunoglobulins, lately it has been the
object of a burgeoning research effort. Mainly this is due
to the realization that IgA is the principal immunoglobulin
in external secretions, where it is the prime mediator of
local humoral immunity on mucous membrane surfaces. In
addition, the genetics of human IgA has been advanced by the
discovery of genetic markers on the IgA2 subclass. The Am_2
marker is linked to and behaves like the Gm markers of IgG
which have been so thoroughly studied. The other marker
involves the presence or absence of the light-to-heavy
interchain disulfide bridges in IgA2 proteins. The absence
of these bridges in one of the genetic variants is
associated with unusual structural properties.

PROPERTIES OF THE IgA SUBCLASSES

In 1966 human IgA was divided on the basis of marked
antigenic differences into two subclasses called IgA1 and
IgA2 [1,2,3]. Some antisera made in rabbits, goats and
monkeys against human IgA myeloma proteins recognized
certain of them as antigenically deficient to others.
Because the antigenic differences between the two IgA subclasses seemed to be greater than those which distinguish
the IgG subclasses, it was surprising that early attempts to
produce an antiserum directed specifically against the minor
IgA subclass failed [1]. Later, an antiserum made in a

cynomologus monkey against the IgA2 myeloma protein Her
showed specificity for the IgA2 subclass, and permitted its
quantitation in serum and secretions (6). This antigenic
distinction resides on the Fc region of the heavy chains (1).
In man, then, the heavy chain constant regions of IgA are
controlled by at least two cistrons (1,4). The distribution
of kappa and lambda light chain types does not differ in the
two subclasses (4). The IgA2 subclass constitutes some 7 -
14% of normal serum IgA (5), and has been called the He,
minor or deficient subclass. The IgA1 subclass has been
called the Le or major subclass. In the sera of 24 young
male adults IgA1 had a mean concentration of 1.81 mg/ml and
IgA2, of 0.22 mg/ml (5). IgA2 myeloma proteins tend to occur
at higher average concentrations in pathological sera (4).
In external secretions the IgA2 subclass was found in higher
relative concentrations compared to serum (6).

The IgA subclasses differ in structural properties.
Because of different sialic acid content, IgA2 myeloma
proteins often show a faster electrophoretic mobility
towards the anode at pH 8.6, although occasional IgA1
proteins are equally fast (1,4). The total carbohydrate
content of IgA averages 7 to 8%, and most of it is attached
to the Fc portion of the heavy chains. While the amount is
independent of the heavy chain subclass and light chain type,
it differs in composition between the two IgA subclasses (7).
Both subclasses contain all the sugars found in most immunoglobulins (galactose, mannose, fucose and sialic acid), but
differ in amino sugar content. IgA1 has one galactosamine
and two glucosamine-containing peptides (8). The galactosamine peptide is attached to the hinge region (8,9). IgA2,
in contrast, has two glucosamine peptides, neither of which
lies in the hinge region. As a group IgA paraproteins are
sensitive to proteolytic hydrolysis, but IgA2 paraproteins
are three to four times more susceptible to pepsin hydrolysis
than IgA1 proteins (10). While the C-terminal octapeptide
sequences are identical (11) the IgA subclasses show
differences in the primary structure of the hinge regions
(12). The hinge regions of two human IgA1 myeloma proteins
showed identical amino acid sequences, and consisted of a 30
residue fragment containing 3 cysteines, 12 prolines and
carbohydrate containing galactosamine. The hinge region of
IgA2 showed marked homology, being identical in the first
eight and the last five residues, and containing 3 cysteines,
8 prolines but no carbohydrate. The hinge of IgA1, however,
was unique in that the carbohydrate was associated with a

stretch of 15 residues consisting of two identical stretches
of seven or eight amino acids, suggesting a gene duplication.
IgA2 by contrast had a gap of 12-13 residues in exactly the
area which shows the duplication in IgA1. The heterogeneity
in interchain disulfide bridging has also allowed the IgA
subclasses to be identified by chemical typing using high
voltage electrophoresis of peptic-tryptic digests of the
partially reduced proteins (13).

   IgA subclasses also differ in their metabolism (5).
In 14 turnover studies the average biologic half-life for
radioiodinated IgA1 myeloma proteins was 5.9 days and only
4.5 days for IgA2. The fractional catabolic rates were 24%
of the intravascular pool per day for IgA1 and 34% for IgA2.
About 55% of the total body pools of both subclasses was
intravascular. IgA1 had a synthetic rate of 24 mg/kg per
day and IgA2 of 21.3 mg/kg per day. Thus the low serum
concentration of IgA2 results mainly from its low synthetic
rate, but its higher fractional catabolic rate is a
contributing factor.

   The IgA subclasses are further distinguished by the
presence of the Am_2 (+) or $A_2m(1)$ genetic marker on the Fc
region of IgA2 heavy chains (14,15). The genetic locus
which codes for IgA2 heavy chain constant regions in both
serum and secretions occurs in two allelic forms. Am_2 (+)
heavy chains carry the marker and Am_2 (-) chains do not. No
such markers have been described as yet on IgA1. Like the
Gm markers, the Am_2 genetic marker differs greatly in
incidence in different population groups (14). Caucasians
carry predominantly the Am_2 (+) marker, while the Negroid
and to a lesser extent the Mongoloid races tend to be Am_2 (-).
The Am_2 marker follows Mendelian inheritance through families
(14,15), and is closely linked to the Gm system of IgG (14).
A similar close linkage between markers of the IgG_2 (Ig-1
cistron) and the IgA (Ig-2 cistron) genetic loci occurs in
mice (17). Recently a second genetic marker $A_2m(2)$ has
been located on the constant region of the Fd fragment of
IgA2 heavy chains (16). Mating of a homozygous $A_2m(1)$
individual with a homozygous $A_2m(2)$ individual gave rise to
only heterozygous offspring, indicating that $A_2m(1)$ and
$A_2m(2)$ are alternative alleles. The antisera used for Am_2
genetic typing come from isoimmunized individuals who have
selective IgA deficiency (14,15). These iso-antibodies may
show specificity for the IgA class, for its two subclasses
or for the Am_2 genetic marker (18), and have been

implicated as a major cause of anaphylactoid transfusion
reactions (19-21). The isoantibodies are frequently non-pre-
cipitating and require hemagglutination techniques for their
detection (14,15). The addition of 3% polyethylene glycol
to precipitate soluble antigen-antibody complexes (22,23)
allows the conversion of this isoantibody system to a precipitating one which can be handled more simply in gel
diffusion in Ouchterlony plates (24). Isoantibodies directed
against class and subclass antigens (which cause the fatal
anaphylaxis)are easily recognized, and sometimes the iso-
antibodies with Am_2 specificity (which cause urticarial
reactions) can be detected as well. Thus a simple and
clinically applicable screening method to detect isoantibodies in IgA deficient individuals may become possible.

The striking difference between the IgA subclasses is
the phenomenon of dissociability which characterizes IgA2
proteins. In the presence of denaturants such as acid, urea,
guanidine or detergent, IgA2 myeloma proteins dissociate
spontaneously into disulfide-linked heavy (H_2) and light (L_2)
chain dimer subunits without requiring prior reduction (6).
This phenomenon implies that the disulfide bridges joining
the light to the heavy chains are absent in IgA2 proteins.
Not all IgA2 paraproteins, however, are dissociable (25,26).
Only those belonging to the genetic type Am_2(+) do so.
IgA2 paraproteins of the Am_2(-) type have heavy and light
chains which are linked by disulfide bonds just as in IgA1
and all other human immunoglobulins. The presence or absence
of the light-to-heavy (L-H) interchain bridge in human IgA2
is an expression of a particular allotype. The peptides
containing the L-H disulfide bridges in human IgA genetic
variants have been isolated by cystine diagonal mapping (27).
Sequences at the heavy chain end of the L-H bridge of IgA1
and Am_2(-), IgA2 proteins are homologous, indicating an
identical location of the L-H bridges in molecules of the
two subclasses. There is also a difference in the degree of
noncovalent interaction between the subclasses (40). IgA1
proteins which have H-L disulfide bridges have weaker non-
covalent interactions, while the IgA2 proteins which lack
the H-L disulfide bonds have stronger interchain noncovalent
binding. Similar dissociable immunoglobulins have been
described in lower vertebrates. IgA paraproteins produced
by plasmacytomas induced in BALB/c mice lack light-to-heavy
interchain disulfide bridges and are potentially dissociable
(28). Recently, Warner et al (29) have shown that 3 out of
3 NZB-derived IgA paraproteins possessed L-H disulfide

bridges, as did 5 out of 10 (BALB/c x NZB)F₁ hybrid-derived proteins. The existance of L-H disulfide bridges in the hybrid-derived proteins completely correlated with the presence of Ig-2^e (NZB type) IgA allotype antigens. Thus in mice, as in man, the differences in L-H covalent bonding in IgA molecules are allotype associated. Ovine colostral IgA has been found also to be dissociable, and for this reason it has been designated IgA2 by analogy with man (30). More recently Vaerman (31) has found dissociable colostral IgA in dogs, horses, pigs and man, indicating that dissociable IgA molecules may be more widespread among vertebrates than previously thought. Finally, the IgM-like 6.6S antibody obtained from the sea lamprey, Petromyzon marinus, in response to immunization with bacteriophage f2, lacks all interchain disulfide bridges. Under denaturing conditions it dissociates spontaneously into free heavy and light chains (32). Because of these observations in several species such dissociable molecules might represent primitive immunoglobulins in the evolutionary sense (6).

PROPERTIES OF GENETIC VARIANTS OF HUMAN IgA2

Not only does dissociability indicate that the L-H interchain disulfide bridges are absent in the Am₂(+) IgA2 molecule, but it also implies that the light chains are present within the molecule as a disulfide-bonded dimer. Dissociability is unaffected by the presence of an alkylating agent, indicating that an artifact of disulfide interchange is not involved. That this arrangement of light chains may also be applicable to IgG is suggested by experiments of Grey (33). When partially reduced and alkylated human gamma chains were recombined with reduced but not alkylated light chains, the reconstituted reoxidized IgG protein possessed 65% of its light chains in the form of L-L disulfide-linked dimers. This suggests that the C-termini of light chains in IgG are positioned sterically in the molecule such that they are capable of forming an L-L disulfide bond under these unusual experimental conditions.

Although one might expect this difference in disulfide bridging in these IgA2 genetic variants to produce some structural distinctions between them, no differences in their overall conformation have been detected (26). They are identical in size and shape as judged by their sedimentation properties. Despite the fact that papain

digestion produces an Fc fragment from dissociable IgA
paraproteins derived from BALB/c mice (34), the use of
several enzymes under various conditions of digestion have
failed to produce an Fc fragment or to distinguish the
genetic variants in any way. Rabbit antisera to F(ab')$_2$
fragments have not detected the differences in H–L bridging.
Nor do the sensitive techniques of optical rotatory dis-
persion and circular dichroism detect the alteration in
disulfide bonding.

Dissociable Am$_2$(+) IgA2 molecules, however, do show
unique features in recombination experiments and in their
response to mild reduction (26,35).   In the case
of IgG, disulfide-linked covalent light chain dimers
do not recombine with dimer heavy chains (26,35,36).
However, the dissociation of Am$_2$(+) IgA2 myeloma proteins
is reversible in that the Am$_2$(+) variant can be reassembled
from covalent heavy and light chain dimers (26,37). IgA1,
IgG and Am$_2$(-) IgA2 proteins in which the L-H interchain
disulfide bridges are intact can not be recombined in this
fashion. Since preparations of Am$_2$(+) covalent heavy chain
dimers recombine well with a mixture of kappa and lambda
covalent light chain dimers from pooled human IgG, the heavy
chains are implicated as the site of the structural
peculiarity which allows this variant to reversibly dissociate.
The Am$_2$(+) variant also shows a unique response to mild reduction (26,37). 0.02M cysteine will selectively cleave the
disulfide bridge which links the light chain dimer within
the molecule, so that after denaturation the light chains
are released predominantly as monomer. The inter-heavy-
chain disulfide bridges, however, remain intact. As in the
case of IgM (38), this procedure also converts polymers of
IgA into 7S subunits through cleavage of the intersubunit
disulfide bridges (26,37).

STABILIZATION OF DISSOCIABLE IgA2 BY SECRETORY COMPONENT

In human colostrum IgA is the predominant immunoglobulin,
and the IgA2 subclass is relatively enriched compared to
serum (6). Yet when secretory IgA (SIgA) was isolated from
human colostra containing significant amounts of Am$_2$(+)
IgA2 by antigenic analysis, it did not dissociate after the
fashion of its serum counterpart to the degree expected
(26,39). This anomaly may be explainable by the observation
that in vitro both bovine and human secretory components

will bind to and stabilize potentially dissociable $Am_2(+)$ IgA2 myeloma proteins, so that they will no longer dissociate into subunits in the presence of denaturants (26,39). Human secretory component stabilizes more efficiently than does the bovine protein; however, in both instances an excess of secretory component is required.

Enough data are available to allow formulation of a hypothesis as to the mechanism of the stabilization reaction. Both bovine and human secretory components will stabilize $Am_2(+)$ IgA2 polymers, but only human secretory component will stabilize the monomer (24). This interaction with the monomer is unique to the $Am_2(+)$ variant and likely depends on its unusual disulfide bridging. Binding to $Am_2(-)$ IgA2 or IgA1 monomers does not occur. At least in this instance J chain need not be present for secretory component binding, since none of the monomer IgA genetic variants contain J chain (24). Secretory component reacts with the whole myeloma protein and not with just subunits thereof. In the reaction with IgA2 monomer, species with one and with two moles of IgA2 monomer per mole of secretory component are formed (39). The site of the reaction appears to involve the heavy chains close to the region of the L-L dimer within the molecule (26). Secretory component reacts with the heavy and not the light chains, and it will stabilize the $F(ab')_2$ fragment of a pepsin digested $Am_2(+)$ molecule, which retains its interchain disulfide bridges intact (26). Stabilization takes place through covalent disulfide bonding since it can be blocked with iodoacetic acid (39) and by prior complete reduction and alkylation of the secretory component. Since secretory component fails to interact with the light chain dimer in vitro, stabilization is visualized most easily by postulating that secretory component, through an interaction with the $C\alpha1$ domains, may induce the formation of L-H interchain disulfide bridges in the IgA2 molecule. These bridges might or might not be homologous with those normally found in the $Am_2(-)$ variant.

While the lack of L-H bridges in $Am_2(+)$ IgA proteins could be due to a deletion of the requisite heavy chain cysteines, the mechanism proposed for stabilization by secretory component implies that these cysteines are present but unreactive. Preliminary evidence to support this contention is available. When monomer $Am_2(+)$ IgA2 is dissociated into subunits by gel filtration in acid, the

heavy chain dimers spontaneously aggregate on the column
(26). This aggregation can be prevented by the addition of
iodoacetamide to the buffer, suggesting the presence of
buried cysteine(s) which become reactive after denaturation
and dissociation of subunits. In Am_2 (+) IgA2 myeloma
proteins L-H interchain disulfide bridges can be induced to
form under certain conditions (39). After partial
reduction of these proteins, and also following their
reconstitution and reoxidation from reduced heavy and light
chains, a band with the mobility of an L-H species appears
in SDS acrylamide gel electrophoretograms. The band
disappears after further reduction and alkylation. When
secretory component is removed from human SIgA by reduction
followed by gel filtration in neutral buffers, the
resulting IgA portion of the molecule still shows little
dissociation despite the presence of large amounts of Am_2 (+)
IgA2 detected antigenically. Finally, cystine diagonal maps
of peptic-tryptic digests of Am_2 (+) IgA2 myeloma proteins
after interaction with secretory component, show the
appearance of peptides similar in position to those known
to be derived from the L-H bridge in the IgA variants
possessing it (24). Proof of the ability of secretory
component to induce L-H bridge formation in Am_2 (+) IgA2
proteins, however, must await identification of the peptides
on the diagonal maps by composition and sequence.

It has been suggested that secretory component may
function to stabilize the IgA2 dimer against reductive and
proteolytic attack in the hostile environments of external
secretions (41). The stabilization of potentially
dissociable IgA2 proteins by secretory component lend
further support to this view, and might confer a selective
advantage on the molecule, thus explaining the enrichment
of the IgA2 subclass in secretions compared to serum.

ACKNOWLEDGEMENTS

The authors wish to thank Ms. L.S. Adams and Mr. C.W.
Sylvester for expert technical assistance, and the La Leche
League International for supplying human colostrum.

REFERENCES

1. Kunkel,H.G. and Prendergast,R.A., Proc.Soc.Exptl.Biol.
    Med., 122:910,1966.
2. Vaerman,J.-P. and Heremans,J.F., Science 153:647,1966.
3. Feinstein,D. and Franklin,E.C., Nature 212:1496,1966.
4. Vaerman,J.-P., Heremans,J.F. and Laurell,C.-B.,
    Immunology 14:425,1968.
5. Morell,A., Skvaril,F., Noseda,G. and Barandun,S., Clin.
    Exptl.Immunol., 13:521,1973.
6. Grey,H.M., Abel,C.A., Yount,W.J., and Kunkel,H.G.,
    J.Exptl.Med., 128:1223,1968.
7. Grey,H.M., Adv.Immunol. 10:51,1969.
8. Abel,C.A. and Grey,H.M., Fed.Proc., 28:495,1969.
9. Ko,A., Clamp,J.R., Dawson,G. and Cebra,J., Biochem.J.,
    105:35p,1967.
10. Shuster,J., Immunochemistry 8:405, 1971.
11. Prahl,J.W., Abel,C.A. and Grey,H.M., Biochemistry 10:
    1808, 1971.
12. Frangione,B. and Wolfenstein-Todel,C., Proc.Nat.Acad.
    Sci.USA 69:3673,1972.
13. Frangione,B. and Franklin,E.C., FEBS Letters 20:321,
    1972.
14. Kunkel,H.G., Smith,W.K., Joslin,F.G., Natvig,J.J. and
    Litwin,S.D., Nature 223:1247,1969.
15. Vyas,G.N. and Fudenberg,H.H., Proc.Nat.Acad.Sci., 64:
    1211,1969.
16. Wang,A.C., van Loghem,E. and Shuster,J., Fed.Proc., 32:
    1003 Abs,Part 1,1973.
17. Herzenberg,L.A., Cold Spring Harbor Symp.Quant.Biol.
    29:455,1964.
18. Kunkel, H.G., Jerry, L.M. and Smith, W.K., Immunopathology
    6:151, 1971.
19. Vyas, G.N., Holmdahl, L., Perkins, H.A. and Fudenberg,
    H.H., Blood 34:573, 1969.
20. Vyas,G.N. and Fudenberg,H.H., New Eng.J.Med. 280:1073,
    1969.
21. Schmidt,A.P., Taswell,H.F. and Gleich,G.J., New Eng.J.
    Med. 280:188,1969.
22. Harrington,J.C., Fenton,II,J.W. and Pert,J.H.,
    Immunochemistry, 8:413, 1971.
23. Eby,W.C., Kim,B.S., Dray,S., Young-Cooper,G.O. and
    Mage,R.G., Immunochemistry, 10:417, 1973.
24. Jerry,L.M., Unpublished data.
25. Jerry,L.M., Kunkel,H.G., and Grey,H.M., Proc.Nat.Acad.
    Sci.USA 65:557,1970.

26. Jerry,L.M., Doctoral thesis, The Rockefeller University, New York, 1971.
27. Mihaesco,E., Seligmann,M. and Frangione,B., Nature New Biol. 232:220,1971.
28. Abel,C.A. and Grey,H.M., Biochemistry 7:2682, 1968.
29. Warner,N.L. and Marchalonis,J.J., J.Immunol. 109:657, 1972.
30. Heimer,R., Jones,D.W. and Maurer,P.H., Biochemistry 8:3937, 1969.
31. Vaerman,J.-P., Doctoral thesis, Catholic University of Louvain, Louvain, 1970.
32. Marchalonis,J.J. and Edelman,G.M., J.Exptl.Med., 127: 891,1968.
33. Grey,H.M., J.Immunol. 102:848,1969.
34. Askonas,B.A. and Fahey,J.L., J.Exptl.Med., 115:641, 1962.
35. Gally,J.A. and Edelman,G.M., J.Exptl.Med. 119:817,1964.
36. Stevenson,G.T. and Dorrington,K.J., Biochem.J., 118: 703,1970.
37. Jerry,L.M., and Kunkel,H.G., J.Immunol. 109:982,1972.
38. Miller,F. and Metzger,H., J.Biol.Chem., 240:4740,1965.
39. Jerry,L.M., Kunkel,H.G. and Adams,L., J.Immunol., 109: 275,1972.
40. Tomasi,T.B. and Grey,H.M., Progr.Allergy 16:81,1972.
41. Tomasi,T.B. and Bienenstock,J., Adv.Immunol., 9:1,1968.

GENETICS AND EVOLUTION OF HUMAN IMMUNOGLOBULIN A

An-Chuan Wang and H. Hugh Fudenberg

University of California School of Medicine

San Francisco, California   94143

INTRODUCTION

In contrast to all other immunoglobulin classes which occur predominantly in serum, IgA occurs as the most preponderant class in exocrine secretions(1). This makes the evolutionary study of IgA of particular interest since IgA may encounter some pressure from natural selection not encountered by other immunoglobulins.

Two antigenically distinguishable subclasses of human IgA currently designated as IgA1 and IgA2 have been described (2-5). The existence of these subclasses was confirmed by chemical typing methods (6,7). By means of starch gel electrophoresis in the presence of 8M urea, Grey et al. (8) demonstrated that the inter-heavy-light chain disulphide bond characteristic of all immunoglobulins including the IgA1 subclass is absent in the IgA2 subclass. Subsequently, Jerry et al. (9) showed that not all IgA2 proteins lack this disulphide bond; it appears to be unique to only one of the genetic variants of the IgA2 proteins. Thus far, no genetic marker has been discovered for the IgA1 subclass. The first genetic marker on IgA2 subclass was described independently by Vyas and Fudenberg (10) who termed it Am(1) and by Kunkel and his colleagues (11) who designated it Am(2). Subsequently, it was shown that Am(1) and Am(2) are related to an identical antigenic determinant (12). The second genetic marker on IgA2 proteins was described by van Loghem, Wang and Shuster (13). Since these allotypic markers are associated with α2 chains, the terminology $A_2m(1)$ and $A_2m(2)$ is used for them herein.

MATERIALS AND METHODS

Sera were collected from several patients with IgA multiple myeloma, random samples from Caucasians, Negroes, Orientals, Melanesians, New Guinea Papuans, Eskimos, American Indians and Australian aborigines and the following primates: chimpanzee, gorilla, orangutan, gibbon, anubis baboon, gelada baboon, rhesus monkey, bonnet monkey, pig-tailed monkey, stump-tailed monkey, Macaca cynomologus , Cercopithecus aethiops, Cercocebus fulginosus, Erythrocebus pates, Callicebus, Cebus capucinus, Saimiri sciurea, Aotes trivirgatus, Logothris, Saguinus oegitus, Lemur fulvus, Nycticebus concang and Galago senegalenesis braccatus. The $A_2m(1)$ and $A_2m(2)$ allotypes were detected by a hemagglutination inhibition procedure modified from the method of Gold and Fudenberg (14). Fresh human type 0, Rh positive red blood cells were coated with purified IgA molecules. IgA proteins in approximately 0.5 to 2 mg per ml were mixed with an equal volume of a solution of 0.05% $CrCl_3$ in 0.9% NaCl. An equal volume of washed and packed red cells were added immediately. The mixture was left at room temperature for 4 minutes then washed three times with 20 to 40-fold volumes of saline. These coated cells were then mixed together with monospecific antisera directed toward $A_2m(1)$ or $A_2m(2)$ determinants and sera to be tested at various dilutions on a microtiter V-plate. After 30 minutes, the plate was centrifuged at 3,000 RPM and scored for agglutination or inhibition.

IgA myeloma proteins were isolated from sera by precipitation with 18% sodium sulfate, ion-exchange chromatography with DEAE cellulose (DE-52, Whatman), and gel filtration with Sephadex G-200 (15). Purified IgA proteins were examined for their electrophoretic behavior on starch gel in the presence of 8M urea by the method of Grey et al. (8).

RESULTS AND DISCUSSION

Typing for A_2M markers was done on sera of many primates including four species of apes (Hominoidea), ten species of Old World monkeys (Cercopithecoidea), six species of New World monkeys (Ceboidea) and three species of Prosimians. Neither the $A_2m(1)$ nor the $A_2m(2)$ allotypic marker is present in any of these species. This result indicates that $A_2m(1)$ and

$A_2m(2)$ genetic markers appeared very late, apparently after man and ape diverged in evolution.

Population studies were carried out on random serum samples from many ethnic groups. Results are shown on Table 1. Gene frequencies were calculated assuming the $A_2m(1)$ and $A_2m(2)$ are alternatives in a bi-allelic system (13). The gene frequency of the $A_2m(2)$ allele is highest among the African population decreases in the Asian population and is lowest in the European population. This result is in agreement with earlier work (13,16) and is compatible with the idea that $A_2m(2)$ was not present originally in Caucasians. Further, the $A_2m(2)$ allotype in Caucasians appears to be associated with either the Oriental Gm (a,z,b,s,t), $A_2m(2)$ or the Negro Gm (a,z,b), $A_2m(2)$ haplotype (16). Thus, the presence of $A_2m(2)$ in Caucasians appears to be due to admixture with Orientals and Negroes. This type of gene distribution furnishes further support for the concept that human species originated in Africa followed by migration to other portions of the world and suggest that $A_2m(2)$ was the original allele whereas $A_2m(1)$ was generated from $A_2m(2)$ by mutation (13). High frequencies of $A_2m(1)$ in other continents may have resulted from selective advantage. Europeans are almost homogeneous for $A_2m(1)$. This may have happened when this population passed through a bottle neck of numbers during one of the disastrous periods within the last 200,000 years (for example, the Würm Glacial) or if the $A_2m(1)$ allele (or a closely linked gene) had a higher fitness in the Eruopean environment.

Pedigree studies on informative families indicate that A_2m markers are linked to the Gm markers, confirming earlier work done by others (11, 13). This provides additional evidence for the concept that the gene coding for the C-region of $\alpha2$ chain and those for $\gamma1$, $\gamma2$ and $\gamma3$ chains are located on a single chromosome.

Chemical studies showed that both the reduced and alkylated heavy chain and the $F(ab')_2$ fragment prepared from an $A_2m(2)$ positive protein inhibited in the $A_2m(2)$ testing system but isolated light chains from the same protein did not. Therefore, the $A_2m(2)$ antigenic determinant (or determinants) is located on the C_H1 domain of the $\alpha2$ chain. Further, the inter-heavy-light chain disulphate bond which is present in $A_2m(2)$ protein but absent in $A_2m(1)$ proteins is not enough to account for all the differences between the $A_2m(1)$ and $A_2m(2)$ antigens, additional difference must exist.

Table 1. Gene frequencies of A_2m markers

Population	$A_2m(1)$	$A_2m(2)$
African-Negroes	0.23	0.77
Southern-Chinese	0.30	0.70
American-Negroes	0.36	0.64
Melanesians	0.54	0.46
Japanese	0.54	0.46
New Guinea Papuans	0.82	0.16
Eskimos	0.87	0.13
Australian aborigines	0.95	0.05
American-Indians	0.96	0.04
Caucasians	0.98	0.02

As mentioned earlier, the human $A_2m(1)$ proteins which lack an inter-heavy-light chain disulphide bond evolved very late, apparently after man and ape diverted. However, IgA molecules lacking this bond have been observed in mouse (17, 18), rabbit (19) and several other mammalian species (20). These observations raise the question whether the IgA molecules lacking the inter-heavy-light chain disulphide bond in different species are homologous to one another (21), and point out to the need for additional serological and biochemical studies on these proteins.

Acknowledgments: This work was supported in part by grants from the U.S.P.H.S. (AI-09813 and HL-05677), a grant from the National Science Foundation (GB-38153X) and a grant from the American Cancer Society (IM-16G). We thank Mrs. E Raines, Mrs. S. San Juan and Miss Wei-Lan Ma for their excellent technical assistance, and Dr. J. Shuster for supplying the anti-$A_2m(2)$ antiserum.

REFERENCES

1.   Tomasi, T.B.Jr. and Bienenstock, J., Adv. Immunol. 9: 1, 1969.
2.   Vaerman, J.P. and Heremans, J.F., Science 153:647, 1966.
3.   Kunkel, H.G. and Prendergast, R.A., Proc. Soc. Exp. Biol. Med. 122:910, 1966.
4.   Terry, W.D. and Robert, M., Science 153:1007, 1966.
5.   Feinstein, D. and Franklin, E.C., Nature 212:1496, 1966.

6. Zakin, M.M., Fine, J.M., Perrat-Laine, D., Boff, G.A. and Amouch, P., Rev. Europ. Etudes Clin. Biol. 16:1012, 1971.

7. Frangione, B. and Franklin, E.C., FEBS Letters 20:321, 1972.

8. Grey, H.M., Abel, C.A., Yount, W.J. and Kunkel, H.G., J. Exp. Med. 128:1223, 1968.

9. Jerry, L.M., Kunkel, H.G. and Grey, H., Proc. Natl. Acad. Sci. 65:557, 1970.

10. Vyas, G.N. and Fudenberg, H.H., Proc. Natl. Acad. Sci. 64:1211, 1969.

11. Kunkel, H.G., Smith, W.K., Joslin, F.G., Natvig, J.B. and Litwin, S.D., Nature 223:1247, 1969.

12. van Loghem, E. and de Lange, G., (in preparation).

13. van Loghem, E., Wang, A.C. and Shuster, J., Vox Sang. 24:481, 1973.

14. Gold, E.R. and Fudenberg, H.H., J. Immunol. 99:859, 1967.

15. Wang, A.C., Goodman, J.W. and Fudenberg, H.H., J. Immunol. 103:1149, 1969.

16. Schanfield, M.S. and Fudenberg, H.H., in a symposium on Social study of human biosocial interrelations in population adaptation. (in press).

17. Abel, C.A. and Grey, H.M., Biochemistry 7:2682, 1968.

18. Seki, T., Appella, E. and Itano, H.A., Proc. Natl. Acad. Sci. 61:1071, 1968.

19. Cebra, J.J. and Small, P.A., Biochemistry 6:503, 1967.

20. Vaerman, J.P., Studies on IgA immunoglobulins in man and animals, Thesis, Sintal-Louvain Pub., 1970.

21. Wang, A.C. and Fudenberg, H.H., J. Immunogenetics, (in press).

PHYSICAL-CHEMICAL CHARACTERISTICS OF J CHAINS OBTAINED FROM IgM

F. P. Inman

University of Georgia, Department of Microbiology

Athens, Georgia 30602

Although the subject of these meetings centers around the biology and chemistry of IgA, I would like to summarize some research done with J chains prepared from human Waldenström's IgM. J chains obtained from IgM molecules are, by most criteria, essentially identical to those originating from IgA. In this work IgM was treated with 0.25M Na_2SO_3 (1) and the J chains were isolated from acrylamide gels after electrophoresis (2).

The molecular weight of the protein was determined by electrophoresis on 4% polyacrylamide gels equilibrated with 1% sodium dodecylsulfate (3). The apparent molecular weight of the single band of protein was 27,000 (Table 1). To ascertain that this was a minimum molecular weight, J chains also were suspended in 5M guanidine-HCl, pH 6.1, for 21 days before electrophoresis. This time two sets of triplet bands were noted, and the three bands in each set migrated close together. The proteins in the set comprising most of the J chain material had molecular weights of 15,400, 14,900 and 14,300 (Table 1). The other set had bands of molecular weight 28,600, 26,200 and 24,000. These data indicated the J chain existed as a dimer in 1% sodium dodecylsulfate solution. The dimer was largely dissociated to the monomeric form after prolonged exposure to 5M guanidine-HCl solution.

Table 1.   Molecular weight of J chains from IgM

Method	Molecular weight
A. Polyacrylamide-gel electrophoresis	
1. 1% Sodium dodecylsulfate[1]	27,000
2. 5M Guanidine-HCl[2]:	
Triplet set one	14,300;
	14,900;
	15,400
Triplet set two	24,000;
	26,200;
	28,600
B. Sedimentation equilibrium	
1. Saline-borate[3]	29,600
2. 5M Guanidine-HCl[4]:	
Mean avg. min. mol. wt.	15,200
Mean avg. wt. avg. mol. wt.	17,400

[1] J chain was suspended in 1% sodium dodecylsulfate.

[2] J chain was exposed to 5M guanidine-HCl, pH 6.1 for 21 days before electrophoresis. It was dialyzed overnight in 1% sodium dodecylsulfate-sodium phosphate solution (6) for electrophoresis.

[3] J chain was suspended in 0.16M NaCl-0.001M sodium borate, pH 8.

[4] J chain was suspended in 5M guanidine-HCl for 14-28 days before molecular weight determination.

The molecular weight was determined also by the sedimentation equilibrium method (3). For J chain in saline-borate solution the average weight average molecular weight was approximately 29,600 (Table 1). Some aggregation was detected. In addition, J chain protein was suspended for 14 days or longer in 5M guanidine-HCl solution. The mean average minimum molecular weight was about 15,200 and the mean of the lowest values of the average weight average molecular weights was approximately 17,400. These data are consistent with those obtained by electrophoresis in indicating that the J chain existed in a dimeric form in nondissociating solutions. After extensive dialysis in guanidine-HCl solution, however, most of the protein dissociated to the monomeric form. The molecular weight of the monomer was about 15,000 while that of the dimer was about 30,000.

The sedimentation constant ($S^0_{20,W}$) of the protein in nondissociating solution was found to be 2.49S (Ricardo, M. J. and Inman, F. P., unpublished data). Based on the molecular weight determinations this constant must be that of the dimer form of this J chain. In contrast, a sedimentation coefficient of J_α chains at low concentration recently was reported to be 1.28s (4). The molecular weight of that protein was approximately 15,000 in nondissociating solution. Therefore, the latter sedimentation coefficient must be that of the monomer form.

An attempt was made to determine the shape of the J_μ chain. Its molecular radius appeared to be about 22.5 x 10^{-8} cm (Ricardo, M. J. and Inman, F. P., unpublished data), but because of difficulties encounted with the technique this figure probably is subject to revision. None the less, one calculated a frictional ratio of 1.65, and disregarding the effect of hydration, this is equivalent to an axial ratio of approximately 13 for a prolate elipsoid or 17 for an oblate elipsoid (5). Therefore, it was concluded that J_μ chain in the dimer form is more linear than globular in shape. This conclusion is not inconsistent with that of Wilde and Koshland (4) who concluded that the J_α chain, apparently in monomer form, is an elongated molecule.

Acknowledgment: Supported by a grant (GB-8449 A-1) from the National Science Foundation.

REFERENCES

1. Edelman, G. M. and Marchalonis, J. J., in Williams, C. A. and Chase, M. W. (eds.), Methods Immunol. Immunochem., Academic Press, New York 1:405, 1967.

2. Ricardo, M. J. and Inman, F. P., Biochem. J. 131: 677, 1973.
3. Ricardo, M. J., Brewer, J. M. and Inman, F. P., Biochem. J. (in press).
4. Wilde, C. E. and Koshland, M. E., Biochemistry 12: 3218, 1973.
5. Tanford, C., Physical Chemistry of Macromolecules, Wiley, New York, p. 326, 1961.
6. Weber, K. and Osborn, M., J. Biol. Chem. 244: 4406, 1969.

GENERAL DISCUSSION

<u>Dr. Grey</u> - A question for Dr. Parkhouse. Some of the data
that Dr. Jerry presented would suggest that the secretory
component might act in a manner similar to his reductase
enzyme that he uses to allow polymerization in conjunction
with J chain. I was just wondering whether he might conceivably have tried secretory component in place of the enzyme.

<u>Dr. Parkhouse</u> - The answer is no.

<u>Dr. Tomasi</u> - One comment regarding molecular weight of a
J chain. As I mentioned this morning, our data suggest that
the molecular weight of the monomer, by equilibrium ultracentrifugation, is about 15, to 16,000. The plots look like
a homogeneous molecule. However, if you do two species plots
which involves measurements of both weight average and number
average of molecular weight in the relations to the center
of rotation you find that there are two species: one of them
with a molecular weight of 7000, about half of the 15,000
figure. I don't know exactly the origin of these two species
but I'd be interested to know whether Drs. Inman or Koshland
or anyone else has done a similar analysis. The question I
have for Dr. Jerry is: I'm not quite clear, does he have
evidence that the LH bond induced by secretory component
occurs at the cysteine 131 or could that be another cysteine,
for example the possibility that one of the three inter-H
chain bonds are linked to the L chain. Could I get your
thinking on that point?

<u>Dr. Jerry</u> - The peptides in the map have the same position
as from LH bridge but they have to be sequenced and composition done in order to probe that; similar peptides from
different points could have similar positions on the map.
So we do not have evidence that particular cysteine is involved. But an LH bridge appears to be formed.

<u>Dr. Cebra</u> - My questions concern the initiation of polymer-
ization of subunits of polymeric immunoglobulin. I'd like
to ask Dr. Koshland whether she has been able to obtain
J chain and totally reoxidize it, so that it contains no free
SH groups. If so, does it form a ter-molecular complex with
IgM subunits - that is 2 IgM_s + 1 J-chain? I'd like to ask

Dr. Parkhouse if he's ever examined any variants of IgM or
IgA myelomas that have stopped producing heavy chains in an
effort to find out whether J-chains continue to be synthesized by such cell lines. If so, could these variant lines
be used as a source of 'native' J-chain to initiate the
repolymerization reaction with IgA or IgM subunits?

Dr. Koshland - No covalent or noncovalent complexes are
formed if both monomers and J are completely reoxidized
before they are recombined. However, if J is kept reduced
and recombined with oxidized monomers, polymers can be formed
in vitro. These results are in contrast with those of Dr.
Parkhouse, but the conditions of the experiments were
different. Instead of an excess of J, a large excess of
monomer was used, 20:1 on a molar basis. In other words only
enough J was present to polymerize one-fourth of the monomers
into pentamers. Under these conditions all the J was
covalently incorporated into polymer, since none could be
found without complete reduction and alkylation and the recovery was quantitative after such treatment. In the ultracentrifuge the reconstituted polymers appeared to be
primarily pentamers and tetramers with traces of dimers and
trimers. These experiments say that non-enzymatic polymerization can be achieved under certain in vitro conditions,
but the reaction may not necessarily represent the in vivo
process.

Dr. Parkhouse - We've not done exactly the experiment that
you asked, but we have looked at two aberrent IgA molecules.
It depends on what you call aberrent, but at any rate,we have
looked at 47A which secretes disulfide linked HL molecule and
MPCl which secretes only the monomeric species of IgA. Using
in vitro system I described, which requires addition of J chain
and the disulfide interchange enzyme, we looked to see if these
molecules could be polymerized, and the answer to the question
is no, they cannot. One interpretation of this, of course, is
that in these two molecules the peptide responsible for linking
to the J chain in ordinary polymerizible IgA is absent and we
are pursuing that.

Dr. Good - One can't sit here listening to this elegant
chemistry and not have some clinical or biological questions.
I wonder, if J chains have been looked for in relationship
to the phylogenetic development of the different species,
where one sees extraordinary variations of the polymerization
state of what we think is a molecule comparable to IgM. All

of these things must have an ontogenetic history. Do you
have any information on that score, and finally, what is the
consequence of the missing J chain as will turn up in human
diseases?

Dr. Mestecky - Dr. Vaerman will present evidence of the
existence of J chain in many different animal species. Dr.
Koshland found J chain in shark which is one of the lowest
animals that would contain polymeric immunoglobulins. We
examined birds and several other animals and they had J
chain, too. Clinically we have not seen any polymeric
immunoglobulin that would not have J chain.

Dr. Koshland - We have gone on with our studies of the shark
J and are isolating it from dogfish as well as the leopard
shark. When the shark J was tested in Ouchterlony analysis
with a rabbit antisera made to human J, a reaction of partial
identity was seen with the human J. Moreover, in a radio-
immune assay, the shark J inhibited the reaction between
human J and the rabbit anti-J antiserum. I thought that
this was a fabulous result until I went to talk to Dr. Allan
Wilson who is, of course, well known for his studies of
evolutionary development using immunological techniques. He
pointed out that we should be very careful about the interpretation of our shark data because we are looking at totally
reduced and alkylated J chains and with this kind of modified
denatured protein one can get all sorts of irrelevant cross
reactions. We are in the process, therefore, of repeating
the experiments using human and shark J which has been
isolated by reduction and allowed to reoxidize. Incidentally,
the amino acid compositions of shark and human chains are
fairly similar, but not as similar as might be expected from
the extent of their cross reaction.

Dr. Bennett - Dr. Koshland, do you know of anyone who has
looked at J chain from the standpoint of ontogeny as Dr.
Good mentioned, such as in molecular disease?

Dr. Koshland - No, I don't as a matter of fact. Great
project.

Dr. Good - The J chains are very primitive and we are
going to hear more about that. But does one find anything
to explain the extrordinary heterogeneity of IgM? There are
some species that have uniformly a monomeric IgM, others
dimeric IgM, others tetrameric IgM, pentameric and hexameric

IgM. Do you find any characteristic that would account for this difference in polymerization?

Dr. Bennett - Apparently not on the basis of J chain. It is there if the immunoglobulin is polymerized.

Dr. Kunkel - We have made a few efforts at making antisera to J chain and one of the things that we ran into, that might possibly explain Dr. Koshland's results, was that we got very strong antibodies to the iodoacetamide treated J chain, which did not react with iodoacetic acid treated J chain or J chain reduced with sodium sulfite or other agents. We have been interested in this problem so I would think that there is a possibility that Dr. Koshland's cross reaction with shark may relate to your use of iodoacetamide for alkylation. I think there, too, you can get specificity for this alkylating group that you put on.

Dr. Koshland - We have tested the antisera made against totally reduced and alkylated human J with human J which had been isolated in the reduced form and then allowed to reoxidize. The Ouchterlony analyses showed a strong line of precipitation with only a slight spurring of the reduced and alkylated J over the reoxidized sample. Thus, it would appear that most of the antibodies were not directed against iodoacetic determinants. On this basis, I would guess that the cross-reaction between shark and human J chain is real, but I wouldn't swear to it.

SESSION C

STRUCTURE

CHAIRMAN: JIRI MESTECKY

ISOLATION, PROPERTIES, AND STRUCTURE OF HUMAN IgA MYELOMA GLOBULINS[1]

Frank W. Putnam, Teresa Low, Victor Liu, Hans Huser, E. Raff, F. C. Wong, and J. R. Clamp

Department of Zoology, Indiana University
Bloomington, Indiana 47401

INTRODUCTION

For the past few years our work has been based on the principle that the characteristic covalent structure of 99% of all human immunoglobulins could be established by determining the amino acid sequence of five kinds of polypeptide chains: κ and λ light chains, and γ, μ, and α heavy chains. We reported the first complete sequence of κ (1) and λ (2,3) light chains. Others sequenced the γ chain (4,5) and we recently reported the complete sequence of the μ chain (6). The α chain is the last of the big five, and many laboratories are now engaged in its study.

The present status of the sequence of human α chains is as follows: Through the work of Wolfenstein-Todel, Mendez, Frangione and collaborators (7-10), Abel and Grey (11), and Moore and Putnam (12) we now know the sequence around all or nearly all the half-cystine peptides involved in disulfide bridges in the IgA molecule. This is a great advance, for in μ and γ the disulfide bridge peptides were the most difficult area to sequence. The carboxyl-terminal 40 residues of the α1 chain have been reported by Chuang et al. (13) and the same area has been determined by us. These data account for some 150 residues or about a third of the α1 chain. Also, amino-terminal sequences of the first 30 or so

[1]Supported by NIH CA08497, the Damon Runyon Fund (DRG-1134), and the American Cancer Society (NP-10).

residues of the V region of a number of unblocked α chains
have been determined by the sequencer technique in a number
of laboratories (14,15), and the complete sequence of the V
region of two α chains is being reported by Capra and co-
workers at this Symposium (16).

What then is holding up the complete sequence determination of human α chains? The basic problem is the inability to obtain a series of reproducible fragments by
methods of enzymatic or chemical cleavage; this results from
three problems: 1) the susceptibility of IgA to extensive
degradation by proteolytic enzymes such as papain, trypsin,
or pepsin which produce well-defined Fab and Fc fragments of
IgG and IgM, 2) the low content of methionine of the C region of α chains with the result that CNBr cleavage produces
one very large central fragment and a few small fragments at
the amino- and carboxyl-terminal ends, and 3) the failure as
yet to obtain specific cleavage of the α chain by use of
other chemical methods. In order to explore these problems
further we have undertaken comparative study of a series of
IgA1 and IgA2 myeloma proteins.

MATERIALS AND METHODS

For comparative structural study seven myeloma globulins were purified and characterized, five of the IgA1 subclass and two of the IgA2 subclass. Six of these (all but
Ha) were purified by the method described below. Some
properties of two of these (Ha and Ln) have been reported
(17). Because most methods for purification of IgA have
been on a small scale or have involved multiple techniques,
a large-scale method of purification was devised. The IgA
in defibrinated plasma is precipitated by adjustment to 1.8
M ammonium sulfate at pH 7 in the cold. The precipitate is
dialyzed against 0.01 M tris-HCl buffer, pH 8.0. A solution
containing from 1.5 to 2.0 g of protein is chromatographed
on DEAE-Sephadex A-50 and eluted with a linear gradient at
pH 8.0 (0.01 M tris-HCl buffer to 0.01 M tris-HCl——0.3 M
NaCl). The protein elutes as two major peaks (peak 1 and
peak 2 in Fig. 1). Tests with monospecific antisera indicated the first peak contains IgA and gives a weak reaction
for IgG but is essentially free of IgM, albumin, and other
major serum proteins, whereas the second peak though rich
in IgA contains some α-2-macroglobulin and albumin. The
IgA in peak 1 is largely 7S monomer; it has a purity of

Table I. Properties of Human IgA Myeloma Proteins[#]

Protein	Type[+]	$s_{20}(S)$	SDS Gel[@]	Amino Sugar[#] GlcNAc	GalNAc
Ha	IgA1λ	7.0[*],10.1, 12.6,15.0	Not tested	+	+
Bur	IgA1λ	6.9[*],8.0, 9.7,16.2	−	114	39
Shor	IgA1λ	6.8[*],12.5	−	102	46
Gra	IgA1λ	7.0[*],8.5,11.0	−	152	100
Rut	IgA1κ	9.0[*],12.8	−	+	+
But	IgA2λ,Am$_2$(−)	6.7[*],12.6,17.2	−	331	0
Lan	IgA2κ,Am$_2$(+)	9.5[*],11.2 13.0,17.0	+	204	0

[+]Serological typing done by F. Joslin.   [*]Major component.
[#]Values in nmoles/mg determined by J. R. Clamp.
[@]Dissociation in SDS gel.

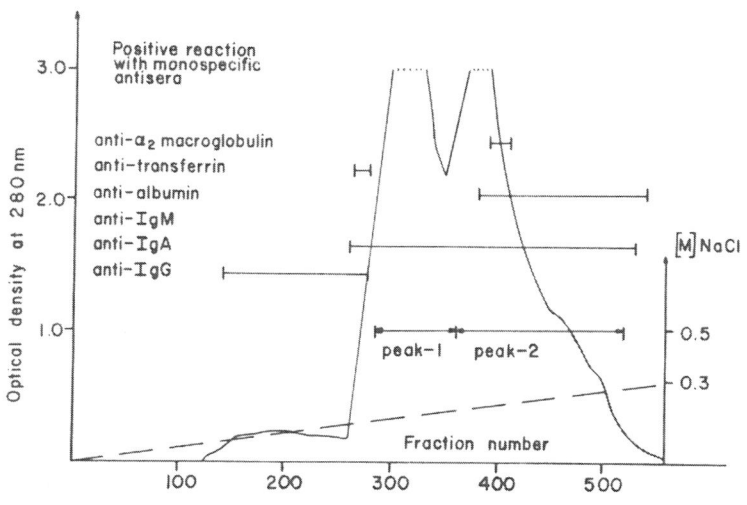

Figure 1. Purification of IgA on DEAE-Sephadex A-50.

about 98% and can be used for exploratory sequence study though further purification by gel filtration is desirable. The IgA in peak 2 consists mainly of polymers and has to be purified by gel filtration on Sephadex G-200 from which the protein elutes as two major peaks; the first largely contains polymers of IgA and the second mostly monomer. Although gel filtration separates most of the albumin, we were unable to remove all of the α-2-macroglobulin from the polymeric IgA fraction. Structural studies on IgA1 Bur were done on the monomeric form, which lacks J chain. The behavior of all six IgA proteins in the purification procedure is very similar and is apparently independent of their subclass. Table I summarizes the serological type and some of the physical and chemical properties of the seven IgA proteins.

RESULTS

Tryptic Peptide Maps and TNP Peptide Composition

For comparative structural study peptide maps were made of tryptic digests of the reduced-carboxymethylated α chains of two IgA1 proteins (Bur and Shor) and two IgA2 proteins (But and Ln). The maps were prepared by two-dimensional chromatography and electrophoresis at pH 3.7 (18) and were stained with ninhydrin and specific staining reagents or with trinitrobenzenesulfonic acid. The trinitrophenyl (TNP) peptides were eluted and their amino acid composition determined. Fig. 2 shows a map indicating by number the 35 peptides identified in the Bur α1 chain by this method. About half of these--the 17 dotted peptide spots--are common to more than two of the α chains. The two peptide spots shaded by diagonal lines are common to only two of the α chains, and the remainder appear to be unique for the Bur α1 chain. This identification is based on the position of the spot, its reactivity to specific staining reagents, and on the composition of the TNP peptides. The number of peptides identified on the map is close to the theoretical number of tryptic peptides for α1 and α2 chains (about 38 to 42 based on the arginine and lysine content) though it does not include the large glycopeptides that fail to separate at the baseline. Between any pair of α chains from 12 to 16 peptides were in common; about the same number were identifiable by composition with the tryptic peptides of the Ha α chain, which had been analyzed previously.

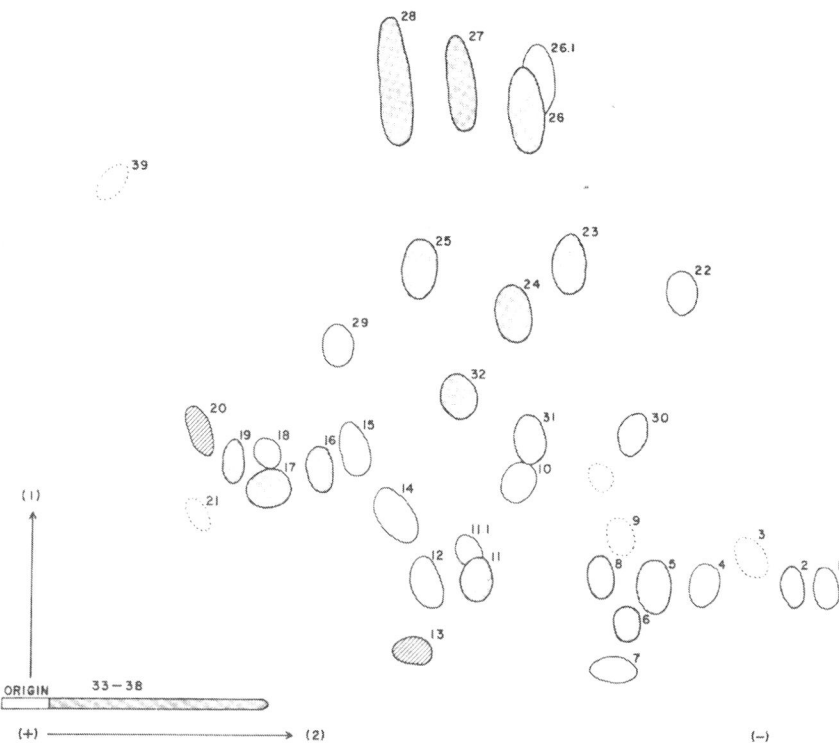

Figure 2. Tryptic peptide map of the Bur α1 chain. Shaded peptide spots are common to more than two α chains except for peptides 13 and 20 which were found in only two α chains.

Because about 10 V region peptides are expected for each heavy chain, neither the peptide maps nor the compositions of the TNP peptides enable a ready distinction between the α1 and α2 chains. At least 12 peptides appear to be common to the two subclasses. Only one peptide was detected in the pair of α2 chains that was absent in the pair of α1 chains and that one differed from an α1 peptide by a single residue. Thus, the α1 and α2 chain sequences must be identical over extensive portions of the C region. The puzzling thing is that only about half the peptides appear to be common even to two chains of the same subclass. Yet, one would expect about three-fourths of the peptides to be identical in a pair of α1 chains because the C region is thought to be about three times as long as the V region.

Disulfide Bridge Peptides

The total number of intra- and interchain bridges in
α1 and α2 heavy chains is still uncertain despite much study.
Assuming that the α1 heavy chain has about 450 amino acid
residues distributed nearly equally among four homology regions (one V_H and three C_H), the minimum number of half-cystines expected is about 14, namely, eight intrachain, one
heavy-light, perhaps two hinge region heavy-heavy bridges,
the C-terminal bridge, and at least one disulfide bridge to
the J (joining) chain and one to the secretory (S) piece.
Wolfenstein et al., (19) reported the sequence around 9
half-cystine residues in the α1 chain Pat. Moore and Putnam
(12) gave the sequence around 11 in the α1 chain of IgA1 Ha
for a minimum total of 13 different half-cystines in the α1
chain. Mendez et al. (9) have in press data about 19 different half-cystines in the α1 chain Oso, and since only one V_H
half-cystine is reported their total may be as high as 20.
This is an uncomfortably large number for a heavy chain with
an assumed molecular weight of about 54,000. The μ chain Ou,
which has a higher molecular weight and some 576 residues
distributed in 5 homology regions, has only 14 half-cystine
residues.

In our current studies of the disulfide bridges in the
α1 chain Bur, we have isolated and sequenced 10 tryptic peptides containing 15 half-cystine residues with a total of
almost 200 residues in sequence (Table II). In addition, we
have partially sequenced the C-terminal tryptic peptide which
is not listed in Table II. This total of 16 half-cystine
residues does not include the heavy-light interchain bridge
and two other half-cystine peptides reported by Mendez et al.
(9) but it does include both of the half-cystine residues in
the V_H bridge plus one half-cystine peptide presumably from
the C_H region of the α1 chain Bur that was not found by Mendez et al.(9). Many of the C region cystine peptides listed
for the α1 chain Bur in Table II have also been isolated by
us from other α1 or α2 chains. None of the tryptic peptides
in Table II is derived from light chains, nor do any appear
to be from J chain.

An exact ordering of the intrachain and interchain disulfide bridges is essential for further structural study of
α1 and α2 chains. The unusually high number of half-cystine
residues may arise from the presence of extra intrachain
bridges, additional interchain bridges, bridges to J chain

Table II

Disulfide Bridge Peptides of the C Region of α1 Chains

Protein	
Bur *+	Ser-Val-Thr-Cys-His-Val-Lys
Bur *+	Asx-Phe-Pro-Pro-Ser-Glx-Asx-Ala-Ser-Gly-Asx-Leu-Tyr-Thr-Thr-Ser-Ser-Gln-Leu-Thr-Leu
Bur	Pro-Ala-Thr-Glx-Cys-Leu-Ala-Gly-Lys
Bur *+	Leu-Ser-Leu-His-Arg-Pro-Ala-Leu-Glx-Asp-Leu-Leu-Leu-Gly-Ser-Glu-Ala-Asx-Leu-Thr-Cys (CHO)
Bur	Thr-Leu-Thr-Gly-Leu-Arg
Bur *+	Thr-Phe-Thr-Cys-Thr-Ala-Ala-Tyr-Pro-Glu-Ser-Lys
Bur *+	His-Tyr-Thr-Asx-Pro-Ser-Glx-Asx-Val-Thr-Val-Pro-Cys-Pro-Val-Pro-Ser-Thr-Pro-Pro-Thr (CHO)
Bur	Pro-Ser-Pro-Ser(Thr)Pro-Pro(Thr)Pro-Ser-Cys-Cys(His,Pro)Arg
Bur *+	Asp-Leu-Cys-Gly-Cys-Tyr-Ser-Val-Ser-Ser-Val-Leu-Pro-Gly(Cys)Ala-Glx-Pro(His,Asx)Lys
Bur *+	Lys-Gly-Asx-Thr-Phe-Ser-Cys-Met-Val-Gly-His-Glu-Ala-Leu-Pro-Leu-Ala-Phe(Thr,Glu)Lys
Bur	Ser-Glx-Cys(Ser,His)Val-Thr(Glx)Tyr-Gly-Ser-Thr-Val-Glx-Lys

Disulfide Bridge Peptides of the V Region of α1 Chains

Protein	
Bur	Leu-Ser-Cys-Thr-Ala-Ser-Ala-Phe-Asx-Leu-Ser-Asx-Tyr-Ala-Met(His,Trp)Val-Arg (CHO)
Bur	Thr-Glx-Asx-Thr-Ala-Val-Tyr-Tyr-Cys-Ala-Lys

*Also in Ha. +Also in Oso (Mendez)

or S piece, a fifth homology unit, or some combination of these factors.

Because of the frequency of hydrophobic, aromatic, and hydroxyamino acid residues on either side of the half-cystine, the sequence homology of heavy and light chains is greatest around the intrachain bridges. For example, the sequence Phe-Thr-Cys is present twice in the constant region of μ chains (C2μ and C3μ); in C3μ the sequence is Phe-Thr-Cys-Thr, the same as in one of the tryptic peptides of the α1 chain listed in Table II. Several other identical tetra-peptide sequences are found in the C-terminus of μ and α1 chains (see later), but so far none longer than this have been identified.

Tryptic and Chymotryptic Peptides

With more than 200 residues already sequenced in the tryptic peptides containing half-cystine, much of the most difficult work in sequencing the α chain has already been done. This has been facilitated by the use of radioactive labeling of the half-cystine residues during reduction-alkylation. In an attempt to isolate all of the tryptic peptides of the α1 chain we have fractionated a digest of the Bur α1 chain and purified the peptides by a combination of gel filtration, ion-exchange chromatography, and paper electrophoresis and chromatography. This work is still in progress. Chymotryptic peptides are being purified by similar procedures in order to secure overlaps of the tryptic peptides. To date, we have complete or partial sequence data on some 30 tryptic peptides including the disulfide bridge peptides and some chymotryptic peptides. These range in size from 2 to 38 residues and account for about 370 residues but many of the tryptic peptides still have to be overlapped. From this we are beginning to get a picture of the structure of the α1 chain on which we can base our future strategy.

The complete sequence determination of the α chain would be facilitated if large fragments suitable for automatic analysis with the sequenator could be obtained either by enzymatic cleavage of the whole IgA or by chemical cleavage of the α chain. However, all of the IgA proteins we have studied are degraded extensively by trypsin, papain, or pepsin under a variety of conditions. Thus, we have not yet obtained Fab and Fc fragments in good yield. Cleavage with CNBr yields several smaller N-terminal and C-terminal peptides

and one large central fragment. Three other chemical methods
of cleavage have been tried without much success as yet, i.e.,
cleavage at Asp-Pro with acid, cleavage at Asn-Gly with
hydroxylamine, and cleavage at tryptophan bonds.

Glycopeptides of IgA1

IgA immunoglobulins are unique among glycoproteins in
having two distinct types of linkage of carbohydrate to the
polypeptide chain, namely, an O-glycosidic linkage between
galactosamine and serine or possibly threonine (Type 1),
and an N-glycosidic linkage between glucosamine and asparagine (20). The latter is present both in a complex oligosaccharide (Type 2) and a simple oligosaccharide (Type 3).
In IgA1 proteins the galactosamine is attached to a serine
residue in the hinge region of the α1 chain. Because of the
repeating sequence of 7 to 8 residues in the hinge region,
the exact site of attachment is not established nor is it
sure whether the carbohydrate occurs once or twice in the
repeat area (7-10). The galactosamine-containing carbohydrate is characteristic of the IgA1 subclass and is absent
in IgA2. No exception to this rule has yet been found in our
work or by Dr. John Clamp (personal communication).

The number and distribution of oligosaccharide units in
human α chains is unknown but should differ for IgA1 and IgA2
and might vary within each subclass. In IgA1 Bur we have
evidence for 4 different glycopeptides (Table III) and there
may be a fifth elsewhere in the α1 chain. The Type 1 galactosamine oligosaccharide occurs in the hinge region. A Type
2 glucosamine oligosaccharide occurs in the leucine-rich
27-residue glycopeptide. We have evidence for a glucosamine
oligosaccharide in the COOH-terminus, and for another at
about position 28 in the V region.

Carbohydrate analysis of the glucosamine-containing
peptides we have isolated has not yet been completed by our
collaborator Dr. John R. Clamp, so we are unable to classify
them all as Type 2 or Type 3. The leucine-rich 27-residue
glycopeptide has a Type 2 core unit; it contains 4 residues
of glucosamine, 3 of mannose and 2 of galactose but lacks
fucose and sialic acid. Since the sialic acid in Type 2 carbohydrates is known to be in a terminal branched structure,
the absence of fucose suggests that this sugar is added
after the main branch structure of the oligosaccharide is
laid down.

Table III.   Glycopeptides of Human α1 Heavy Chains

Protein	Position	Region	Sequence	Amino Sugar
Bur Ha	Hinge	Cα	Pro-Ser-Thr-Pro-Pro-Thr-Pro (CHO over Pro[4])	GalNac
Bur Ha	27-residue peptide	Cα	Glu-Ala-Asn-Leu-Thr-Cys (CHO over Asn)	GluNac
Bur	C-terminus	Cα3	His-Val-Asn-Val-Ser-Val-Glu (CHO over Asn)	GluNac
Bur	N-terminus	V_H	Asn-Leu-Ser-Asx-Tyr (CHO over Asn)	GluNac

Although there are occasional reports of the presence of carbohydrate in the V region of human heavy chains, one oligosaccharide in IgA1 Bur is unique in being located so close to the amino terminus, i.e., at about position 28. This may not be so unusual as it seems; only half a dozen heavy chains have been sequenced by manual methods in this region, and in the automatic sequencing technique an asparagine residue bearing carbohydrate is likely to be missed. One would expect to find oligosaccharides attached at fixed points in the C region of all α chains wherever the obligatory sequence Asn-X-Ser/Thr occurs and also at similar sites whenever this sequence does occur in the V region of heavy chains (see Table III). The last glucosamine oligosaccharide in μ and α chains occurs at an homologous position (14 residues in from the C-terminus), but we have no evidence yet whether the other glucosamine oligosaccharides occur at homologous positions. Although the sites of attachment contain the obligatory structure, they are not identical in sequence.

Structural Homology of α, μ, γ, and ε Heavy Chains

Structural and evolutionary relationships among human heavy chains can be deduced now that the complete sequence is available for the γ1 (4,5) and μ (6) chains and partial sequence data for the ε (21) and α1 chains (9,12,13). Each has a characteristic sequence in the C region, but all human heavy chains share certain structural features such as the intrachain disulfide bridges and the pattern of repeating homology regions. The most unexpected finding from our sequence of the μ chain is that C regions of μ and γ1 chains have only 30-35% homology despite the great homology of the V_H regions of μ and γ1 chains of the same subgroup. The most characteristic aspect of the α1 chain structure is the hinge region consisting of a 38-residue tryptic peptide containing 14 pro-lines. No comparable sequence containing many prolines, a series of disulfide bridges, and carbohydrate is present in the μ chain. Yet, the COOH-terminal sequence of μ and α1 chains shows greater identity than any segment of equal length among the other heavy chains. We have independently determined the COOH-terminal sequence of the α1 chain for IgA1 Bur and have extended this further into the C region (Fig. 3). Our sequence for the penultimate CNBr fragment agrees with that of Chuang et al. (13). In the last 50 res-idues the μ and α1 chains have 55-60% identity including the C-terminal nonadecapeptide tail that is missing in the γ and ε chains. Although this is almost twice as great as the hom-ology between the other pairs of heavy chains (6,21), our preliminary data on the rest of the α chain do not support such a high degree of homology throughout the entire length of the C regions of the μ and α chains. Further study should give a clue to the mechanism of gene duplication or crossing over that led to the addition or deletion of homology re-gions resulting in heavy chains of different lengths.

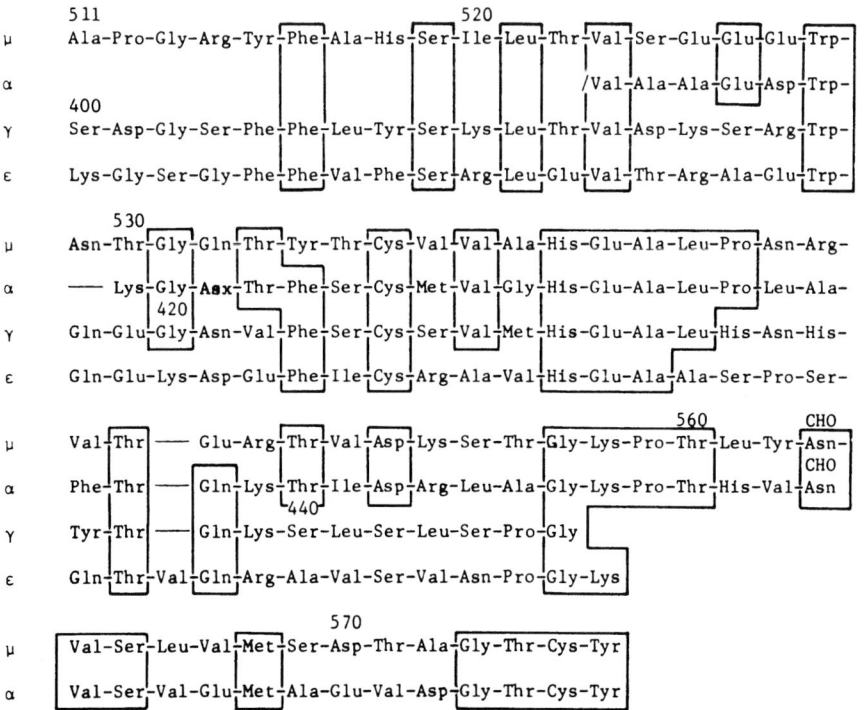

Figure 3. Homology of α, μ, γ, and ε chains.

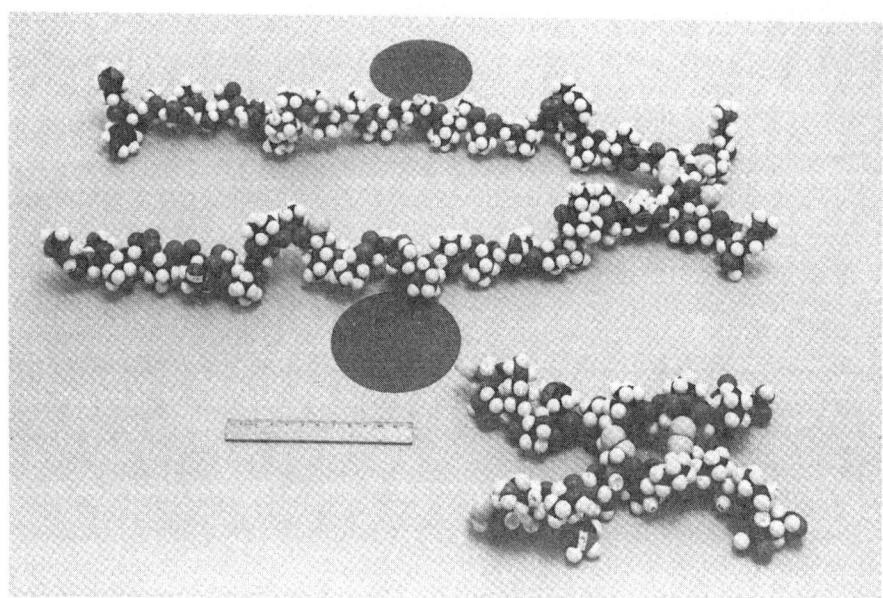

Figure 4. Molecular models of the dimeric form of the hinge
peptide of the human α1 heavy chain (upper model) and of the
hinge peptide of the human γ1 chain (lower model). Both
hinge peptides have three half-cystine residues and an abundance of prolines. The prolines impart a rigidity to the
backbone polypeptide chain by restricting its rotation. In
the α1 hinge peptide this results in a kinking of the chain.
In the γ1 hinge peptide the disulfide cross bridges produce
a rigid cyclic octapeptide with the sequence shown.

$$
\begin{array}{c}
\text{Cys - Pro - Pro - Cys} \\
| \qquad\qquad\qquad | \\
\text{Cys - Pro - Pro - Cys}
\end{array}
$$

This rigid point acts as a pivot for the flexible part of
the hinge region. Trypsin and papain cleave IgG in the
exposed region just before this pivot. The first half-
cystine in the α1 hinge region provides the disulfide bridge
to the light chain, and the other two are involved in heavy-
heavy interchain bridges. Only one of the half-cystines in
the α1 hinge has been shown to form an interchain bridge;
the other two appear to be involved in separate intrachain
bridges within the α1 chain. The black circles symbolize
the galactosamine oligosaccharide of the α1 chain, the exact
location of which is not known. The α2 hinge peptide lacks
this carbohydrate and has a deletion of about 13 residues and
also has a repeating proline sequence that causes a distor-
tion of the backbone.

REFERENCES

1. Putnam, F.W., Titani, K., and Whitley, E., Jr., Proc. Roy. Soc. (London) Ser. B (London), 166: 124, 1966.
2. Wikler, M., Titani, K., Shinoda, T., and Putnam, F.W., J. Biol. Chem., 242: 1668, 1967.
3. Putnam, F.W., Shinoda, T., Titani, K., and Wikler, M., Science 157: 1050, 1967.
4. Press, E.M., and Hogg, N.M., Biochem. J., 117: 641, 1970.
5. Edelman, G.M., Cunningham, B.A., Gall, W.E., Gottlieb, P.D., Rutishauser, U., and Waxdal, M.J., Proc. Nat. Acad. Sci. U.S., 64: 997, 1969.
6. Putnam, F.W., Florent, G., Paul, C., Shinoda, T., and Shimizu, A., Science in Press.
7. Wolfenstein-Todel, C., Prelli, F., Frangione, B., and Franklin, E.C., Biochemistry, in Press.
8. Wolfenstein-Todel, C., Frangione, B., and Franklin, E.C., Biochemistry, 11: 3971, 1972.
9. Mendez, E., Frangione, B., and Franklin, E.C., Biochemistry, in Press.
10. Frangione, B., and Wolfenstein-Todel, C., Biochemistry, in Press.
11. Abel, C.A., and Grey, H.M., Nature, 233: 29, 1971.
12. Moore, V., and Putnam, F.W., Biochemistry 12: 2361, 1973.
13. Chuang, C.-Y., Capra, J.D., and Kehoe, J.M., Nature 244: 158, 1973.
14. Köhler, H., Shimizu, A., Paul, C., Moore, V., and Putnam, F.W., Nature 227: 1318, 1970.
15. Wang, A.C., Pink, J.R.L., Fudenberg, H.H., and Ohms, J., Proc. Nat. Acad. Sci. U.S., 66:657. 1970.
16. Capra, J.D., Chuang, C.-Y., Kaplan, R., and Kehoe, M., This Symposium.
17. Bernier, G.M., Tominaga, K., Easley, C.W., and Putnam, F.W., Biochemistry 4: 2072, 1965.
18. Putnam, F.W., and Easley, C.W., J. Biol. Chem., 240: 1626, 1965.
19. Wolfenstein, C., Frangione, B., Mihaesco, E., and Franklin, E.C., Biochemistry 10: 4140, 1971.
20. Dawson, G., and Clamp, J.R., Biochem. J., 107: 341, 1968.
21. Bennich, H., Milstein, C., and Secher, D.S., FEBS Letters, in Press.

AMINO ACID SEQUENCE STUDIES OF HUMAN IgA MYELOMA PROTEINS

J. Donald Capra, Che-yen Chuang, Richard D.
Kaplan, J. Michael Kehoe
Department of Microbiology, Mt. Sinai School

of Medicine of the City University of New York
10 East 102nd Street, New York, New York 10029

The structure of the variable region of immunoglobulin
heavy chains has been a major interest of our laboratory
during the past four years. Recently, we have begun the
determination of the complete amino acid sequence of two IgA
myeloma proteins. Other sequence studies have permitted an
analysis of the distribution of heavy chain variable region
subgroups among the IgA immunoglobulins.

AMINO ACID SEQUENCE STUDIES ON IgA PROTEINS ZAP AND TUR

Most of the amino acid sequence studies have been performed on IgA1 myeloma proteins Zap (kappa type light chains)
and Tur (lambda type light chains), but some additional IgA1
proteins have been studied as well. The alpha chain of both
proteins contains three methionine residues in identical locations and thus each yields four cyanogen bromide (CNBr) fragments (H-1 through H-4). Both proteins contain a large V
region fragment comprising residues 1-85 (H-1) which is disulfide linked to residues 86 to 426 (H-2). H-3 and H-4 have
been completely sequenced in Zap (1) and H-3 and H-4 of protein Tur have been isolated and shown to have amino acid
compositions identical to the corresponding fragments from
protein Zap.

The majority of the sequence work reported here was performed on an updated Beckman automated sequencer. The details
of the procedures can be found in previous publications (1-4).
Generally, long sequencer runs from the N terminus of each

CNBr fragment were followed by tryptic and chymotryptic
digestion of the fragment. The resulting peptides were separated first on G-25 Sephadex in ammonium bicarbonate buffer,
and then on Dowex 50 x 4 using pyridine-formic acid buffer
systems. The composition of all peptides was determined, but
only those peptides which were not accounted for in the initial sequencer runs were subjected to further automated sequencing. Lysine peptides were treated with 4-sulfophenyl-
isothiocyanate prior to sequencing (5). Carboxypeptidase
digestion was used to establish the carboxyterminal residues.

The complete amino acid sequence of both Zap and Tur
H-1 fragments (residues 1-85) is shown in Figure 1. H-2 is
the largest CNBr fragment (residues 86-426). The amino acid
sequence of some of these peptides has been previously reported by others (6,7). Those portions of H-2 which have
been completed are shown in Figure 2. Figure 3 presents the
sequence of H-3 and H-4. [H-4 had been previously sequenced
by Prahl et al., (8)] Thus, a total of 214 of the 465
residues (nearly 50%) of the alpha chain have now been
assigned.

Figure 4 shows the V regions of both Zap and Tur and
compares their sequence with three other V_HIII myeloma proteins which have recently been sequenced in our laboratory.
Note that these two proteins differ by about as much as any

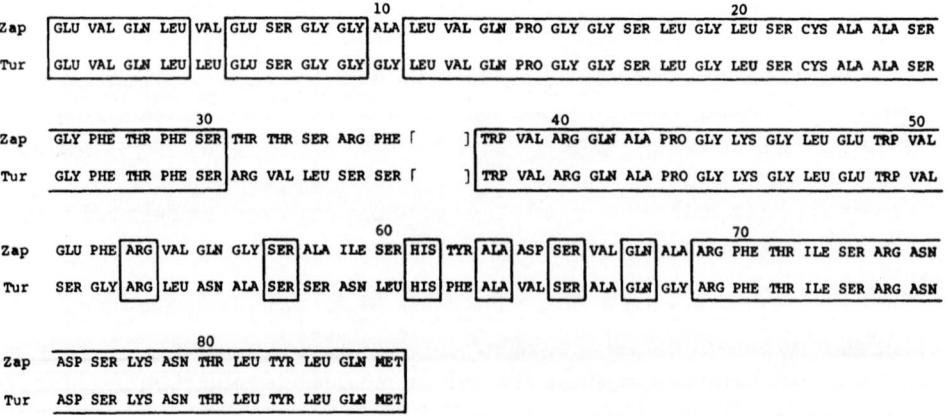

Figure 1: The amino acid sequence of Zap and Tur H-1.

```
TUR    LEU SER LEU GLN │ALA GLX ASX THR ALA│ LEU │TYR TYR CYS ALA ARG│ LEU SER VAL THR ALA VAL
ZAP    ASN THR GLY GLU │ALA GLX ASX THR ALA│ VAL │TYR TYR CYS ALA ARG│ THR ARG PRO GLY GLY TYR


TUR    ALA PHE │ASP VAL TRP GLY GLN GLY THR│ LYS │VAL SER│ SER ALA SER PRO THR SER LYS/VAL THR
ZAP    PHE SER │ASP VAL TRP GLY GLN GLY THR│ LEU │VAL SER│


TUR    VAL PRO CYS PRO VAL PRO SER THR PRO PRO THR PRO SER PRO SER THR PRO PRO THR PRO SER


TUR    PRO SER CYS CYS HIS PRO ARG/LEU SER LEU HIS ARG PRO ALA LEU GLN ASP LEU LEU LEU GLY


TUR    SER GLU ALA ASX LEU THR CYS THR LEU THR GLY LEU ARG/CYS MET
```

Figure 2: The partial amino acid sequence of H2, the largest CNBr fragment. Both Zap and Tur have been
completed to the V/C bridge, only protein Tur has
been sequenced beyond the bridge. The order of
the peptides is correct, but the number of residues between the / is presently unknown.

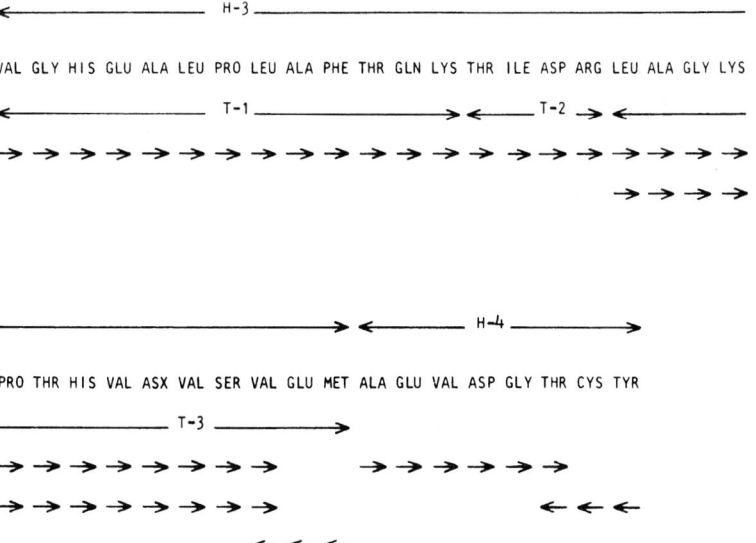

Figure 3: The amino acid sequence of H-3 and H-4.

```
                        10                              20
Tie  GLU VAL GLN LEU VAL GLU SER GLY GLY GLY LEU VAL GLN PRO GLY GLY SER LEU ARG LEU SER CYS ALA ALA SER

Was  _____ LEU _____

Jon  ASP_____ LYS _____

Zap  _____ ALA _____ GLY _____

Tur  _____ LEU _____


                        30                              40                              50
Tie  GLY PHE THR PHE SER THR SER ALA VAL TYR [      ] TRP VAL ARG GLN ALA PRO GLY LYS GLY LEU GLU TRP VAL

Was  _____ SER _____ ASP ___ MET ___ [      ] _____

Jon  _____ ALA TRP MET LYS [      ] _____

Zap  _____ THR SER ARG PHE [      ] _____

Tur  _____ ARG VAL LEU SER SER ⌐      ] _____


                        60                              70
Tie  GLY TRP ARG TYR GLU GLY SER SER LEU THR HIS TYR ALA VAL SER VAL GLN GLY ARG PHE THR ILE SER ARG ASN

Was  ALA ___ LYS ___ GLN GLU ALA ___ ASN SER ___ PHE ___ ASP THR ___ ASN _____

Jon  VAL _____ VAL ___ GLN VAL VAL GLU LYS ALA PHE ___ ASN _____ ASN _____

Zap  GLU PHE ___ VAL GLN _____ ALA ILE SER _____ ASP _____ ALA _____

Tur  SER GLY ____ LEU ASN ALA _____ ASN LEU ___ PHE _____ ALA _____


                        80                              90                              100
Tie  ASP SER LYS ASN THR LEU TYR LEU GLN MET LEU SER LEU GLU PRO GLX ASX THR ALA VAL TYR TYR CYS ALA ARG

Was  _____ ASN ARG _____ ALA _____

Jon  _____ ILE ___ VAL THR _____

Zap  _____ ASN THR GLY ___ ALA _____

Tur  _____ GLN ALA _____ LEU _____


                        110                             120
Tie  VAL THR PRO ALA ALA ALA SER LEU THR PHE SER ALA VAL TRP GLY GLN GLY THR LEU VAL THR

Was  PHE ARG GLN PRO PHE VAL GLN [      ] ___ PHE ASP ___ PHE _____

Jon  ___ VAL VAL SER THR ⌐      ⌐      ] SER MET ASP _____ PRO _____

Zap  THR ARG ___ GLY GLY TYR ⌐      ] _____ ASP _____ SER

Tur  LEU SER VAL THR ___ VAL ⌐      ] ALA PHE ASP _____ LYS ___ SER
```

Figure 4:   The complete V region sequence of five human
            myeloma proteins.

two other V_HIII proteins, and that the variable region
evidently ends at approximately the same point. Four regions
of the sequence show more variation than the rest of the V
region and have been termed hypervariable (9-12). Figure 5
presents these data in graphic form according to the method
of Wu and Kabat (13) including all the other human V region
data available to us. Again, four distinct regions of hyper-

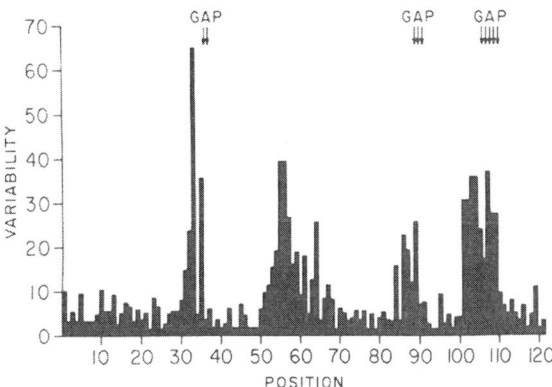

Figure 5:   Variability-factor values for all human V_H sequences determined by the method of Wu and Kabat (13).

variability are present. Such regions have been directly implicated in the antibody combining site (14-15).

Figure 6 compares the C terminal 40 residues of the alpha chain to other available C region sequences. The homology with the mu chain is especially striking, with 55% of the positions identical. Figure 7 presents an interpretation of the C region sequence comparison and suggests that the alpha chain is of recent evolutionary origin, and may have diverged from the mu chain about 200 million years ago, very early in mammalian evolution (16).

THE VARIABLE REGION SUBGROUP DISTRIBUTION AMONG HUMAN IgA
IMMUNOGLOBULINS

During the course of the above investigations we noted that several IgA myeloma proteins belonged to the V_HIII subgroup. Since it had been reported that this subgroup represented only about 20% of human immunoglobulin heavy chain variable regions (17), we solicited IgA myelomas from several colleagues and examined the distribution of the V_H subgroups among this group of proteins. Myelomas were unselected and essentially every protein sent was tested. In order to determine the V_H subgroup distribution in normal IgA, an anti-IgA immunoadsorbent column was prepared with CNBr activated sepharose (18). Separate experiments were performed using

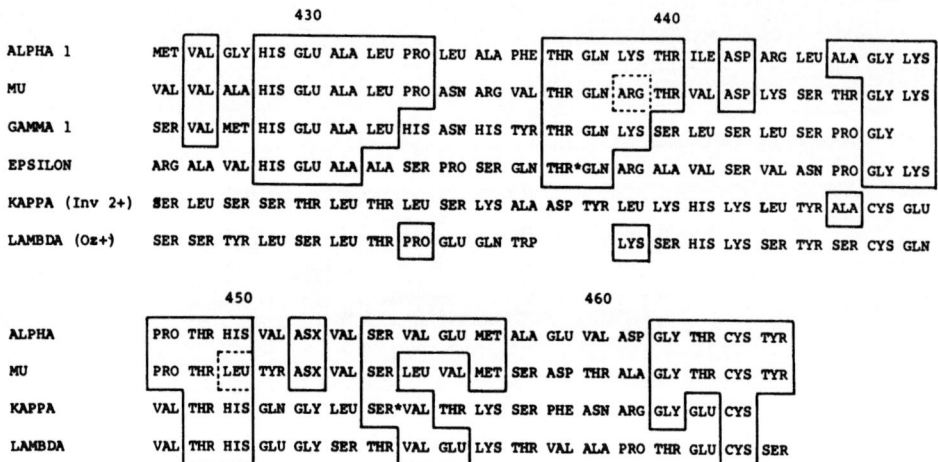

Figure 6:   A comparison of the C terminal 40 residues of
            the alpha chain to other available C region
            sequences.

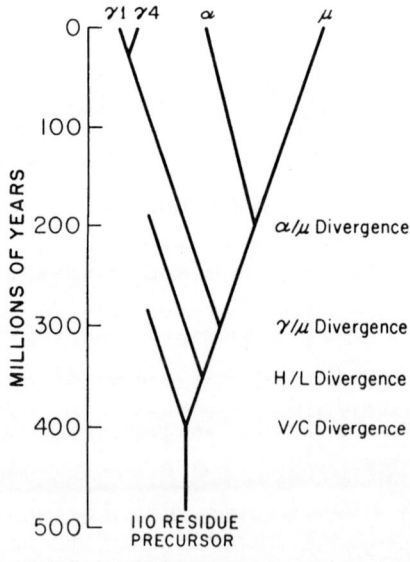

Figure 7:   Possible evolution of the alpha chain.

pooled human serum and a single human plasma. Results of
each were within experimental error. Quantitation of the
$V_H III$ subgroup was as previously described (17).

The results of a survey of 29 human IgA myeloma proteins
are presented in Table I which summarizes the myeloma data
and indicates our results on the distribution of the $V_H III$
subgroup in normal sera as well. The figures given for the
myelomas of the IgG or IgM class are clearly unreliable since
in the literature survey it was difficult to assess potential
biases in the protein selection criteria used by the various
authors. Our own limited experience would suggest that the
IgG and IgM classes both have less than 30% $V_H III$ with the
more correct figure probably being closer to 20%.

As illustrated in Table I, the presence of between 65
and 75% $V_H III$ subgroup in IgA contrasts distinctly with the
approximate value of 20% $V_H III$ seen in both IgG and IgM.

TABLE I

DISTRIBUTION OF THE $V_H III$ SUBGROUP AMONG
IMMUNOGLOBULIN CLASSES

	FROM MYELOMAS	FROM POOLED SERA
IgG	18% (5/28)*	20%
IgM	30% (8/26)*	ND
IgA	66% (19/29)	75%

*Literature plus our data

There are several possible explanations for the preponderance of $V_H III$ in IgA immunoglobulins, none of which seems
completely satisfactory to us at this point. One possibility
is that heavy chain subgroups are antigen dependent. Since
the bulk of IgA producing cells are gut-associated, it is
possible that the range of antigens present in the gut is
relatively restricted. The antigens might have a propensity
for selecting the $V_H III$ subgroup (as the best fit). Since
the $V_H III$ subgroup is already associated with IgA cells,
these antibodies would be IgA molecules with the $V_H III$ subgroup. There is in fact some data which suggest that this
might be the case. The mouse myelomas have been shown to be
predominantly $V_H III$ (19), and it is well known that most mouse
myelomas belong to the IgA class. In addition, all of the

specifically selected murine IgA myelomas with anti-
phosphoryl choline activity or anti-dextran activity are
V_HIII (20).

Another possibility to explain these data is that there
is genetic linkage between the V_HIII subgroup and the alpha
chain. If, in fact, the two gene hypothesis is correct, and
a translocation mechanism is operative, these data would suggest a degree of genetic linkage not previously expected.
Alternatively, if the two gene hypothesis is incorrect then
two possibilities must be considered: (1) There are multiple
copies of a single V-C gene (these data would then suggest
that there are more V_HIII-alpha genes than V_HI or V_HII-alpha
genes, or at least, that the V_HIII alpha genes are being utilized more extensively) or (2) There is only one V_HIII-alpha
gene and diversification occurs by somatic processes.

Finally, the predominance of the V_HIII subgroup could
be related to the cellular "switch" mechanism since IgA is
believed to be a product of a cell which has already pro-
gressed through the production of IgM and IgG. It is possible
that the presence of V_HIII favors the switch to IgA. The
presence of some human IgA molecules that do not contain the
V_HIII subgroup show, however, that the V_HIII subgroup is not
obligatory for the switch.

SUMMARY

Approximately 50% of the human alpha chain has now been
sequenced. Its variable region appears to be similar to
previously sequenced V regions from other immunoglobulin
classes. The V/C bridge is located at the same point as in
IgG and IgM molecules. The alpha chain constant region shows
striking similarities to the mu chain, and it is proposed
that IgA diverged from IgM only 200 million years ago. An
analysis of the distribution of $V_H$subgroups among IgA immunoglobulins indicates that, unlike the situation in the IgG and
IgM classes, the V_HIII subgroup predominates.

Acknowledgements: Aided by grants from the National Science
Foundation (GB 17046) and the U.S. Public Health Service
(AI 09810) and a Grant-in-Aid from the New York Heart
Association. J.D.C. is the recipient of National Institutes
of Health Career Development Award 6-K4-GM-35, C.C. was
supported by a fellowship from the American Bureau of Medical
Aid to China, R.D.K. was supported by a summer fellowship from

the New York Lung Association, and J.M.K. is an Established Investigator of the American Heart Association. Ms. Donna Atherton and Ms. Ellen Bogner provided expert technical assistance.

REFERENCES

1. Chuang, C., Capra, J.D. and Kehoe, J.M., Nature 244:158, 1973.
2. Capra, J.D. and Kunkel, H.G., Proc. Nat. Acad. Sci. 67: 87, 1970.
3. Capra, J.D., Nature New Biol. 230:61, 1971.
4. Capra, J.D., Kehoe, J.M., Kotelchuck, D., Walter, R. and Breslow, E., Proc. Nat. Acad. Sci. 69:431, 1972.
5. Inman, J.K., Hannon, J.E. and Appella, E., Biochem. Biophys. Res. Commun. 46:2075, 1972.
6. Frangione, B. and Wolfenstein-Todel, C., Proc. Nat. Acad. Sci. 69:3673, 1972.
7. Moore, V. and Putnam, F., Biochemistry 12:2361, 1973.
8. Prahl, J.W., Abel, C.A. and Grey, H.M., Biochemistry 10: 1808, 1971.
9. Milstein, C., Nature 216:330, 1967.
10. Kabat, E.A., Proc. Nat. Acad. Sci. 59:613, 1968.
11. Capra, J.D., Kehoe, J.M., Winchester, R.J. and Kunkel, H.G., Ann. N.Y. Acad. Sci. 190:371, 1971.
12. Kehoe, J.M. and Capra, J.D., Proc. Nat. Acad. Sci. 68: 2019, 1971.
13. Wu, T.T. and Kabat, E.A., J. Exp. Med. 132:211, 1970.
14. Kabat, E.A., Ann. N.Y. Acad. Sci. 169:43, 1970.
15. Ray, A. and Cebra, J.J., Biochemistry 11:3647, 1972.
16. McKenna, M.G., Ann. N.Y. Acad. Sci. 167:217, 1969.
17. Capra, J.D., Wasserman, R.W. and Kehoe, J.M., J. Exp. Med. 138:410, 1973.
18. Litman, G. and Good, R.A., Biochim. Biophys. Acta 264:89, 1972.
19. Hood, L., personal communication.
20. Potter, M., personal communication.

STRUCTURAL STUDIES ON A HUMAN IgA1 MYELOMA PROTEIN WITH A CARBOXY TERMINAL DELETION

Howard M. Grey, Jean-Pierre J. Despont,
Carlos A. Abel and Gerald M. Penn
From the Department of Medicine, National
Jewish Hospital and Research Center, Denver,
Colorado 80206, and the Children's Hospital,
Columbus, Ohio 43205.

INTRODUCTION

Low molecular weight variants of complete immuno-globulin molecules have frequently been described in multiple myeloma. The first such variant to be characterized was Bence-Jones protein, which has been shown to be free intact light chains. More recently, variants involving deletions of polypeptide chains have also been described. The deletions found, result in either a poly-peptide chain being secreted singly or in association with another polypeptide chain. Those deletions which involve significant portions of the Fd fragment of heavy chains have been defined as heavy chain disease proteins since the deletion results in the lack of any association with light chains (1, 2). These proteins appear to have normal Fc fragments and have been described for all the major immunoglobulin classes. Proteins with deletions in the Fc fragment have also been described in both man and mouse (3, 4). These proteins, because they possess intact Fd fragments, are found in association with light chains. In the mouse in situations when significant portions of the Fc fragment are deleted, these molecules may exist as L-H half molecules rather than a 4 polypeptide chain molecule due to the lack of significant interaction between the fore-shortened Fc fragments. Deletions involving small areas of the hinge region have also been described (5, 6).

In the present paper the structural abnormality associated with a human IgA myeloma protein is characterized
in relationship to this framework, and it will be shown that
this protein (Vo) had a deletion of more than 100 amino acid
residues involving the entire CH3 domain of the heavy
chains. Before presenting these data, however, it will be
necessary to consider some of our data on the cyanogen
bromide fragments and their alignments in normal-sized
α chains.

MATERIALS AND METHODS

IgA proteins were obtained from patients with multiple
myeloma and were isolated from their sera by starch block
electrophoresis and gel filtration. The polypeptide chains
from the isolated proteins were prepared by partial reduction and alkylation, followed by gel filtration in either 1 M
acetic acid or 6 M urea, 0.1 M formate buffer, pH 3.5.
F(ab')$_2$ fragments were prepared by pepsin digestion at
pH 4.1 for 16 hr at 37° C followed by gel filtration. The
molecular weights of heavy (H) and light (L) chains and Fd'
fragments were determined by polyacrylamide gel electrophoresis in the presence of sodium dodecyl sulfate (SDS).
Amino acid analysis was performed on an automatic amino
acid analyzer following hydrolysis with 5.7 N HCl for 24 hr
at 105° C. Hexosamines were measured using the short
column of the amino acid analyzer. Cyanogen bromide
(CNBr) cleavage of H chains was performed as previously
described (7), and separation by gel filtration was performed on Sephadex G-200 columns in 6 M urea formate, or
for the isolation of the smaller fragments on Sephadex G-50
in 0.05 M ammonia. Amino acid sequence analysis was
performed by utilization of carboxypeptidase A and B and
hydrazinolysis for C terminal analysis, and the Dansyl-
Edman method was used for N terminal sequence analysis.
Antigenic analysis on these proteins was performed utilizing
the immunodiffusion method with class and subclass specific antisera to IgA proteins which was raised in goats.
Hemagglutination inhibition assays were also performed

utilizing erythrocytes passively coated with suitable IgA myeloma proteins by the chromium chloride method. Isolation of 1/2 cystine containing peptides and quantitation of 1/2 cystine residues were performed utilizing ^{14}C iodo-acetamide for the alkylation procedure following either partial or complete reduction of disulfide bridges.

RESULTS

Cyanogen Bromide Fragments of Normal-sized α Chains

The α chains of six human IgA myeloma proteins (four IgA1 and two IgA2 proteins) were treated with CNBr, and after complete reduction and alkylation their fragments were isolated by gel filtration on Sephadex G-200 6 M urea formate, pH 3.5, or on Sephadex G-50 in .05 M ammonia. CNBr fragments were simultaneously analyzed by poly-acrylamide gel electrophoresis in the presence of SDS and by gel filtration to estimate the molecular weights. Three fragments were routinely observed, with 1-3 other frag-ments being observed in some proteins and not others. The three fragments routinely observed had molecular weights of 42,000 (F1), 4,000 (F2) and 1,000 daltons (F3). These fragments were observed in both IgA1 and IgA2 heavy chains. A fourth fragment with a molecular weight of 9,000 daltons (F4) was observed in some proteins, whereas in others this fragment was not observed, but two or three smaller fragments which were not isolated in pure form were observed instead. F1, the fragment having a molecular weight of 42,000, was studied in two α-2 chains for N terminal analysis. In protein Ke the N terminal residue was valine and in protein Ho the N-terminal sequence was Asn-Asn-Leu-X-Ala (kindly performed by Dr. J. W. Prahl). Carboxypeptidase A digestion of the F1 from both α-1 and α-2 chains released the same amino acid residues: (CAMcys, Phe, Ser) Hser. The kinetics of the amino acids released was such that it was not possible to make an unambiguous designation of amino acid sequence by this method. The C terminal tryptic peptides of F1 were isolated from the two α-2 chains, Ho and Ke. The amino acid composition of the C terminal peptides from both the F1 fragments of Ho and Ke were identical, being (Lys, Asp, Thy, Gly) (CAMcys, Phe, Ser) Hser. Digestion of this peptide with carboxypeptidase A resulted in similar data to that observed with the intact Fragment 1. These data suggest that the C terminal peptide of F1 is the same as peptide T7 TH3 sequenced by Moore and Putnam with the amino acid sequence of Phe-Ser-Cys-Met (8). These data indicate that Fragment 1, since it differs in its N terminal sequence between two proteins of the same subclass, begins in the variable region of the Fd fragment. The N terminal sequence of F1 from the α chain of protein Ho is most compatible with the sequence of the VH III protein sequenced by Hilchman and collaborators (protein Nie) (9), suggesting that the N terminal Asn residue of F1 occupies position 84 in the variable region. The α chains of protein Ho, from which these data were obtained, has an unblocked glutamic acid as N terminal residue and an N terminal sequence indicative of the VH III subgroup. Because protein Ho had an unblocked N terminal residue which was easily identifiable, further work on cyanogen bromide peptides was confined to this protein. In this particular protein the F4 fragment with a molecular weight of about 9,000 daltons was obtained. This fragment also had a glutamic N terminal and a homoserine C terminal residue. Since it was the only fragment obtained with this N terminal residue, it thereby could be assigned as the N terminal CNBr fragment of the heavy chain. Fragment (F2), which was isolated from this α-2 chain and several α-1 chains, contained 31 residues and an amino acid composition identical to a fragment isolated by Chuang et al. from several α-1 chains which appears to precede the C terminal octapeptide of the α chains (10). Finally, the F3 fragment is the C terminal octapeptide previously described by Prahl et al. (11). In summary, as shown in Figure 1, the alignment of the cyanogen bromide fragments from the N terminal to the C terminal end is F4, F1, F2, F3. In α-1 chains the F1 fragment contains the hinge region, and in all α-1 proteins studied galactosamine was found associated with this region, whereas α-2 proteins lacked this

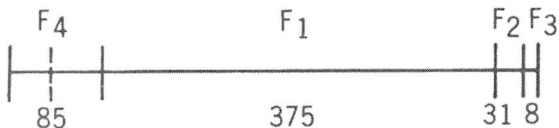

Figure 1. Alignment of cyanogen bromide peptides in human α chains.

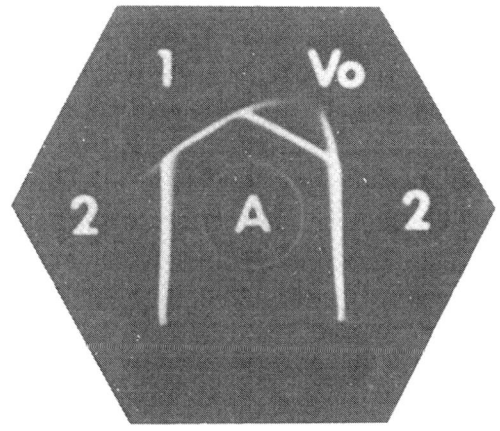

Figure 2. Agar gel diffusion of protein Vo (Vo), another IgA1 (1) and an IgA2 (2) myeloma protein against a sheep anti-human IgA1 antiserum (A).

glycopeptide. In all, twelve α - 2 proteins were studied in this regard, including a protein of the Am 2-allotype.

Structural Characterization of an IgA1 Myeloma Protein (Vo) with a Heavy Chain Deletion

The first indication that the IgA myeloma protein Vo had a deletion was obtained by immunodiffusion analysis of this protein compared with other IgA proteins. Figure 2

illustrates these results and shows the antigenic deficiency
of protein Vo compared to proteins of both IgA1 and IgA2
subclasses when reacted against a sheep anti-human IgA1
antiserum which was absorbed to render it class and Fc
fragment specific. It was not possible to subtype this
protein by immunodiffusion; however, using an absorbed
subclass specific antiserum in a hemagglutination inhibition
assay, it was possible to clearly type protein Vo as belonging to the IgA1 subclass. The L chains were of the λ type.
When this protein was subjected to gel filtration on G-200
Sephadex in phosphate buffered saline (PBS), the elution
profile showed that it had an elution volume slightly greater
than human IgG. This was the first indication that it had a
lower molecular weight than normal IgA since monomer
IgA is usually eluted slightly ahead of IgG. In keeping with
its being a monomer, when the completely reduced and
alkylated protein was electrophoresed on polyacrylamide
gel in SDS, no bands with the mobility of J chain were
observed. In order to further characterize the structural
abnormality in this protein, the molecular weights of both
H and L chains of protein Vo were compared with another
IgA1 myeloma protein, Pr. Molecular weights were determined by SDS acrylamide gel electrophoresis, and the
results are shown in Figure 3. While the L chains of both
proteins had the same mobilities, the H chains of protein
Vo had a significantly faster mobility than those of protein
Pr. The molecular weight of the H chain of Vo was calculated to be 42,000 compared with 58,000 for those of
protein Pr and other α chains. Similar molecular weight
determinations were performed on reduced and alkylated
$F(ab')_2$ fragments of proteins Vo and Pr. In Figure 4 the
mobility of L chains and Fd' fragments of these proteins
were compared and shown to be identical, the calculated
molecular weight of the Fd' being 27,000. These data
establish that structural deficiency in protein Vo is localized to the Fc fragment. The molecular weight data and
amino acid analysis of the H chains indicated that the α
chain of protein Vo had between 100 and 110 amino acid
residues less than normal-sized α chains. Quantitation
of stable and labile 1/2 cystine residues by the method of
[14]C iodoacetamide alkylation was performed. It was found

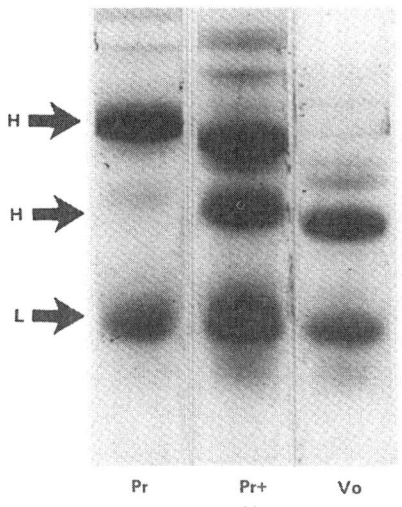

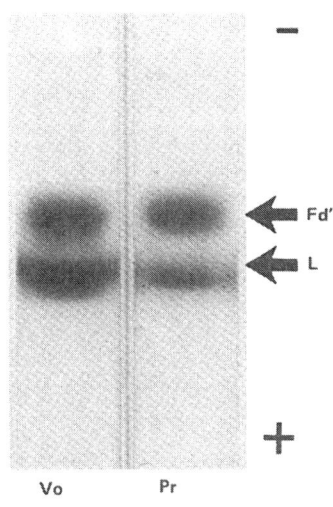

Figure 3. Polyacrylamide gel electrophoresis of completely reduced and alkylated protein Vo compared to another IgA1 protein, Pr. A mixture of both proteins is shown in the center.

Figure 4. Polyacrylamide gel electrophoresis of pepsin treated proteins Vo and Pr after complete reduction and alkylation.

that the α chain of protein Vo contained twelve 1/2 cystines instead of sixteen to seventeen present in normal α-1 chains. Of these twelve 1/2 cystines, six were labile and were alkylated following partial reduction. This compares with seven to eight labile 1/2 cystines normally found in α chains. This information indicated that there were three stable disulfide bridges present in protein Vo compared to the four usually found. By pepsin digestion and gel filtration using the method described by Steiner and Porter (9), it was possible to isolate the hinge peptide of protein Vo. Amino acid analysis of this peptide indicated that it was identical to hinge peptides characterized in other α-1 chains and that the interheavy hain disulfide bonds were intact.

As a next step in characterizing the o α chain, CNBr fragments were obtained in a manner similar to that

used for normal-sized α chains. Instead of obtaining
four or more fragments as has been described in the first
section in this paper, only two CNBr fragments were found:
a fragment with a molecular weight of 29,000 and a second
fragment with a molecular weight of 9,000. No fragments
comparable in size to the 31 residue fragment, F2, of
normal α chains or the C terminal octapeptide, F3, were
identified. Furthermore, digestion of protein Vo H chains
with either carboxypeptidase A or B yielded no amino acids.
The C terminal residue was subsequently identified by
hydrazinolysis as glycine. This is in contrast to the
results obtained with other α chains in which carboxypeptidase A readily releases tyrosine as a C terminal
residue and carboxymethyl cysteine as the penultimate
residue. Further analysis of the Fragments 1 and 2
obtained from protein Vo indicated that Fragment 1 had a
C terminal glycine residue, whereas Fragment 2 had a C
terminal homoserine. The N terminal of both the α chain
of protein Vo and of Fragment 2 were blocked. These data
then clearly indicate that the 9,000 dalton fragment
occupied the N terminal position in the H chain and extended
approximately 84 residues into the variable region and that
the large fragment, similar to the situation found in
normal α chains, extended approximately from position 85
in the variable region through most of the constant region,
but instead of consisting of 385 residues, it contained only
approximately 315 residues and occupied the C terminal end
of the α chain of protein Vo. Taken together then, these
data indicate that the α chain of protein Vo has an intact
Fd fragment as well as an intact hinge region and that it is
lacking 110 amino acid residues in the C terminal end of the
heavy chain which encompasses the last intrachain disulfide
bridge and includes most or all of the C terminal CH3
domain. Carbohydrate analysis indicated that there was one
glycopeptide missing in protein Vo which most likely comes
from this CH3 domain. Two other glycopeptides were
found in protein Vo, one was the galactosamine-containing
glycopeptide at the hinge region and the other a glucosamine-
containing peptide which, since it was not present in the Fd',
must be localized to the CH2 domain.

DISCUSSION

The finding of a myeloma protein of the IgA class with a deletion of the C terminal 100 amino acids of the heavy chain should afford a unique opportunity to study the possible structural and biologic importance of this portion of the heavy chain. The functions that we have been interested in studying in this regard are: the capacity of IgA to combine with J chains, its capacity to combine with secretory component, and its capacity to activate the alternate pathway of the complement system. Regarding the first two structural features associated with IgA, i. e., combination with J chain and secretory component, the data we have obtained thus far are negative, however, may be of interest to outline. The fact that the Vo protein is found solely as a monomer without any J chain in association with it is suggestive that the C terminal portion of the heavy chain may be involved in the polymerization process and the binding to J chain. This argument is strengthened by the experience that we and other investigators have had in the characterization of IgA myeloma proteins where it is extremely rare to find a protein that is entirely in monomer form. The finding of only monomer in the protein Vo therefore suggests that it is incapable of polymer formation due to the absence of some cirtical structure. We have attempted in vitro combination experiments with free secretory component and to date have been unsuccessful in this regard. However, since Vo is a monomer protein, and since it has been shown that monomer IgA proteins react very poorly with secretory component, until suitable means of aggregating protein Vo can be found, this experiment is not of any significance. Lastly, studies involving protein Vo with respect to its capacity to activate the alternate complement pathway have shown that protein Vo is as active as other IgA myeloma proteins and that most likely the portion of the IgA molecule necessary for complement activation is present in protein Vo and therefore is not a part of the CH3 domain. These last results were obtained in the laboratory of Dr. Hans Müller-Eberhard, and despite this fact, due to the difficulties with this system in general, these results would have to be judged as preliminary rather than definitive.

REFERENCES

1. Franklin, E. C., Frangione, B. and Cooper, S.:
    Ann. N.Y. Acad. Sci. 190:457, 1971.

2. Seligmann, M., Mihaesco, E. and Frangione, B.:
    Ann. N.Y. Acad. Sci. 190:487, 1971.

3. Seki, T., Appella, E. and Itano, H.A.: Proc. Natl.
    Acad. Sci. 61:1071, 1968.

4. DeCoteau, W. E., Calvanico, N.J. and Tomasi, T.B.:
    Clin. Immunol. Immunopathol. 1:190, 1973.

5. Fett, J.W., Deutsch, H.F. and Smithies, O.:
    Immunochemistry, 10:115, 1973.

6. Lopes, A.D. and Steiner, L.A.: Fed. Proc. 32:1003,
    1973.

7. Prahl, J.W., Abel, C.A. and Grey, H.M.:
    Biochemistry, 10:1808, 1971.

8. Moore, V. and Putnam, F.W.: Biochemistry, 12:
    2361, 1973.

9. Ponstigl, H., Schwarz, J., Reichel, W. and
    Hilschmann, W.: Z. Physiol. Chemie, 351:1591, 1970.

10. Chuang, C., Capra, J.D. and Kehoe, J.M.: Nature,
    244:158, 1973.

11. Steiner, L.A. and Porter, R.R.: Biochemistry, 12:
    3957, 1967.

THE HINGE PEPTIDE OF AN IgA2m(2) MYELOMA PROTEIN

Edith Mihaesco and R. Miglierina

Laboratory of Immunochemistry, Research
Institute on Blood Diseases, Hôpital
Saint-Louis, 75475 Paris Cedex 10, France

Human IgA proteins are divided into two antigenically
distinguishable subclasses known as IgA1 and IgA2 (1-3).   In
1969 Vyas and Fudenberg (4) and Kunkel et al. (5) described
independently a genetic marker associated with the minor
subclass IgA2.   This marker was called Am1 by the first
authors and Am2 by the latter.   Jerry et al. (6) reported in
1968 that two IgA2 myeloma proteins did not express this genetic marker and that these two proteins displayed the heavy-
light disulfide bridge which is lacking in the other IgA2
molecules [Am(2)+ in the Kunkel nomenclature].   Recently
Erna van Loghem et al. (7) described a new antigenic marker
antithetical to the first described marker and occuring in
these rare IgA2 proteins with the heavy-light bridge.   She
proposed to call this marker A2m(2) and the previous one
A2m(1).   We will adopt this nomenclature in our paper.   In
1971 we have described (8) an IgA2 myeloma protein (Rou.)
with κ light chains and heavy-light bridge which was typed
as negative for A2m(1) by Dr. Kunkel and which was more recently shown to be A2m(2)+ by Dr. Erna van Loghem.   We have
isolated the heavy-light bridge and showed that its sequence,
established by the dansyl-Edman procedure, was identical with
that of the heavy-light bridge of an IgA1 protein, indicating
an evolutionary relationship as was found in the different
subclasses of IgG.   In order to find out if the genetic variability described for the IgA2 is associated with differences
in the number or location of the interchain bridges, we have
studied the hinge peptide of the protein Rou.

MATERIALS AND METHODS

The myeloma polymeric protein Rou. was purified from the serum by zone electrophoresis in Pevikon at pH 8.6 followed by filtration through a 3.5 x 190 cm column of Sephadex G-200. The columns were eluted with 0.1 M Tris-HCl buffer pH 8, 1 M in NaCl and 1% in N-butanol. In order to avoid the α_2M-globulin contaminants the peak obtained in the Vo was again fractionated by Pevikon block electrophoresis. The isolated protein gave a single precipitin arc with a polyvalent antiserum in immunoelectrophoresis at 20 mg/ml.

Chemical Typing

Seven mg of protein Rou. were reduced (9) with DTT at a concentration of 5mM at room temperature and alkylated with ^{14}C iodoacetic acid 0.2 M, specific activity 0.7mCi/nmole. The labeled protein was digested with pepsin (Worthington,twice crystallized) at an enzyme to substrate ratio of 1/50 (w/w) in 5% formic acid for 15 hours at 37°C, followed by tryptic digestion with L-(1-tosyl-amido 2 phenyl) ethyl chloromethyl ketone trypsin (Worthington) in 0.2 M ammonium bicarbonate (pH 8.3) for 16 hours at 37°C, at an enzyme to substrate ratio of 1/50 (w/w). After digestion, the protein was run on paper high voltage electrophoresis at pH 3.5. The radioactive peptides were localized by autoradiography using Kodak Regulix X ray film HS2. An IgA1 and an IgA2, A2m(1)+ myeloma proteins were subjected to the same treatment and run on the same paper. The three proteins were of κ light chain type.

Enzyme Digestion, Partial Reduction and Alkylation

Protein Rou. (200 mg) was dissolved at a protein concentration of 20 mg/ml in 0.2 M ammonium bicarbonate pH 8.3 and digested with trypsin as previously described. The digest was freeze dried, dissolved in 5% formic acid and digested with pepsin. The soluble peptides were separated by chromatography on a column of Sephadex G-50 (2.5 x 190 cm) equilibrated with 1 M acetic acid at room temperature. Fractions of 4 ml were collected at a flow rate of 30 ml/hour. The eluates were monitored by absorbance of the fractions at 280 nm. When subtilisin-Carlsberg (Sigma) digestion was used, an enzyme-substrate ratio of 1/20 (w/w) was employed in 0.2 M ammonium bicarbonate pH 8.3 for 16 hours at 37°C. The different peaks obtained were then freeze-dried. The first

peak was further dissolved in 0.2 M Tris-HCl pH 8.6, reduced
with DTT and alkylated with ^{14}C iodoacetic acid as already
described.

Purification of Radioactive Peptides

The carboxymethyl cystein-containing peptides were purified on paper electrophoresis at pH 3.5 followed by electrophoresis at pH 6.5 and pH 2.1 (10). Mobilities at pH 6.5
were expressed as fractions of the distance between ε dinitro-
phenyl lysin and aspartic acid (11).

Amino Acid Analysis

Peptides were hydrolyzed at $110^{o}C$ for 20 hours with 6N
HCl containing 0.1% phenol and evacuated in sealed tubes.
Quantitative amino acid analyses were performed on a Jeol
model JLC 5AH automatic amino acid analyser. Values were
expressed relative to one of the residues taken as 1.0.
Amino sugars were quantitatively recognized in the short
column of the amino acid analyser.

N-terminal residues were identified with dansyl chloride
(12) and the derivatives were characterized as described by
Wood and Wang (13). Carboxyterminal residues were identified with carboxypeptidase ADFP Sigma and a mixture (1/1)
of carboxypeptidase A and carboxypeptidase B (Worthington).
The digestion was performed in 0.1 M ammonium bicarbonate
pH 8.3, for 30 min, 120 min and 24 hours at $37^{o}C$ at an
enzyme to substrate ratio of 1/20 (w/w). The digests were
freeze-dried and submitted to high voltage paper electrophoresis at pH 2.1.

RESULTS AND DISCUSSION

Figure 1 shows the high voltage electrophoretic pattern
of the radioactive bands containing the interchain S-S bonds
of the protein Rou. compared with those of the IgA1 and IgA2,
A2m(1)+ proteins. The only band common to all 3 proteins is
the carboxyl end of the κ light chain running with the glutamic acid. The band corresponding to the heavy-light cysteinyl peptide is present in the IgA1 and the IgA2m(2) proteins but is lacking in the IgA2m(1)+ variant. The heavy-
heavy cysteinyl peptides have the same mobilities in the
IgA1 and IgA2m(2) proteins, whereas the mobility of this peptide differs slightly in the A2m(1) type.

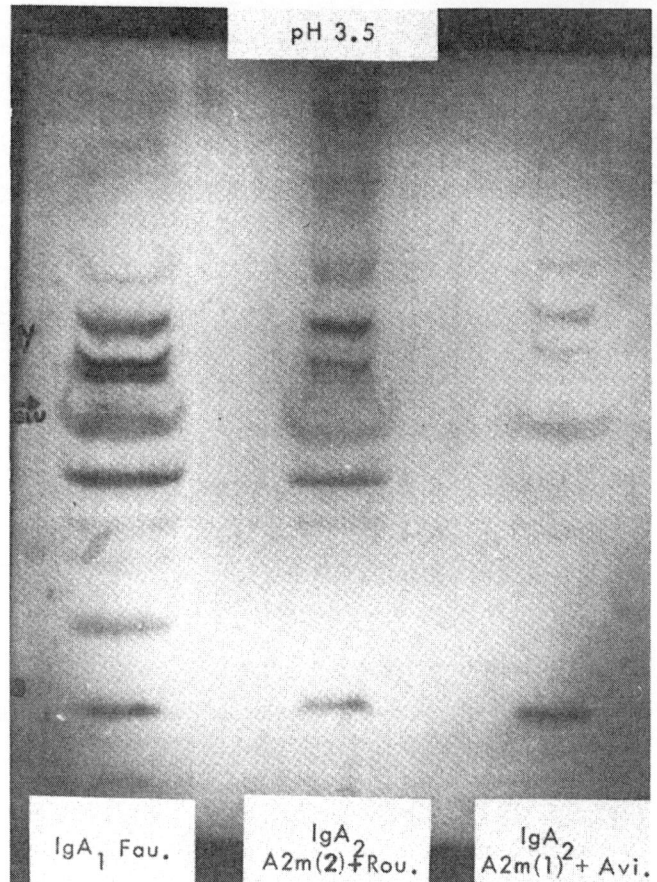

Figure 1.   Chemical typing at pH 3.5 of IgA1, IgA2m(2)+
             and IgA2m(1)+ proteins.

        Figure 2 shows the elution pattern obtained by frac-
tionation of a tryptic-peptic digest of the myeloma protein
Rou. on a column of Sephadex G-50. The hinge peptide was
localized in the first peak as for IgA1 proteins (13).

        Table I shows the amino acid composition, mobilities
and N terminal amino acids of the major radioactive peptides
isolated from the first peak (TP I, TP II, TP III, TP IV,
TP V). The peptide TP IV, which is rich in prolin, was
recognized as being the hinge peptide. Its amino acid composition was:

$Cys_{2.6}$, $Thr_{1.1}$, $Pro_{10.1}$, $Val_{3.2}$, $Leu_{1.2}$, $His_{0.99}$, $Arg_{0.91}$.

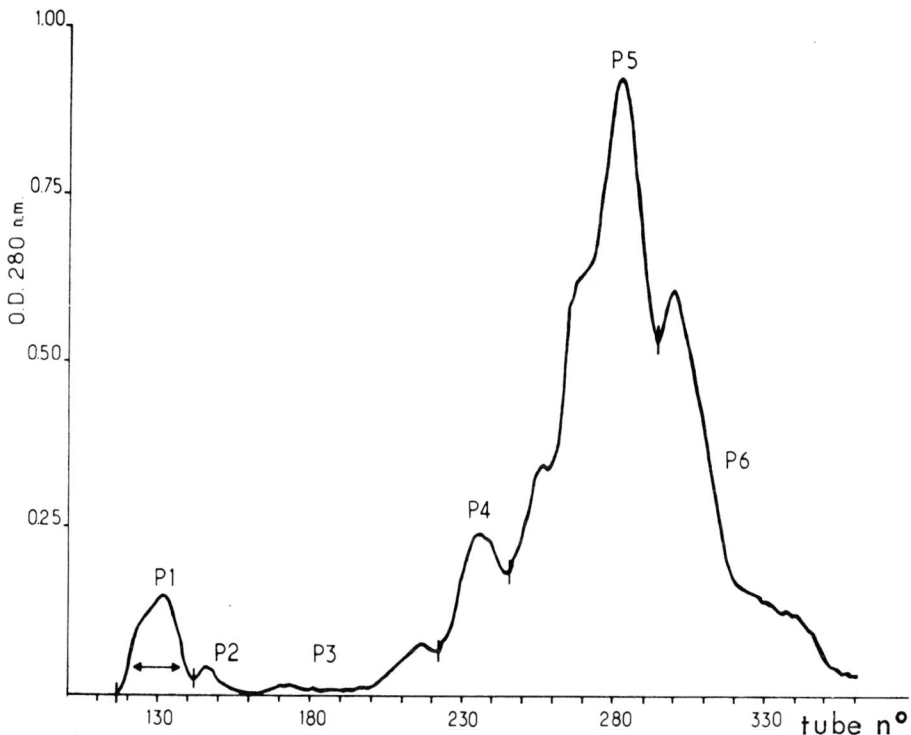

Figure 2.   Sephadex G-50, 1 M acetic acid gel filtration of
a peptic tryptic digest of protein Rou.

As the physico-chemical characteristics and the sequences of the hinge peptides of an IgA1 protein (14) and an
IgA2m(1) protein (15) are known, a comparison between these
two peptides and the hinge peptide of protein Rou. was
possible.

It was readily apparent that all these hinge peptides
contained 3 cys residues and valine as their N-terminus.
Nevertheless the hinge peptide of protein Rou. displayed the
following characteristic features. Its mobility at pH 6.5
and pH 3.5 was similar to that of the IgA1 protein and different from that of the IgA2m(1) protein which was more
anodic at pH 6.5 and more catodic at pH 3.5. In contrast
the hinge peptide of protein Rou. resembled that of the
IgA2m(1) protein since it lacked carbohydrates, 4 threonine
and 5 serine residues which were found in the IgA1 hinge
peptide.

Table 1. Amino acid composition of carboxy-methyl cysteine peptides obtained from partial reduction and alkylation of the peak 1 of Sephadex G-50 column fractionation.

Peptides[a]	TP I		TP II	TP III	TP IV	TP V
	1a	1a'	2a	3	4	5
Lys						1.00
His					0.99	
Arg			0.80		0.91	
CM Cys	present	0.40	0.40		1.70	0.11
Asp	1.00	1.00	1.00	0.53		
Thr	0.60	2.30			1.07	1.00
Ser	2.50	1.30	2.00	1.10		1.02
Glu	1.80	1.30	2.20	1.00		1.20
Pro			1.90		10.07	0.98
Gly	3.30	1.70	2.30	7.30		1.10
Ala	1.00	1.00	0.90	0.53		2.10
1/2 Cys					0.90	0.65
Val			1.80		3.20	
Leu	0.40	2.40	1.00		1.20	1.10
Tyr			0.60			
CHO		+				
mob. at pH6.5	1.34	0.28	0.54	0	0.15	0
NH term.	Asp	Leu	Asp	Gly	Val	Lys

[a]Compositions are reported as moles of amino acid per mole of peptide. Hydrolysis for 22 hours.
TP: trypsin pepsin.

     The number of proline residues in the hinge peptide Rou. was 10 as compared to 8 and 12 in the peptides of IgA2m(1) and IgA1 respectively. After digestion of the hinge peptide Rou. by subtilisin, we obtained 2 peptides, one containing 1 cysteinyl and 2 proline residues and the other containing 2 cysteinyl and 8 proline residues. The carboxyterminal amino acids of the hinge peptide Rou. were Arg-Leu whereas only Arg was found in the two other peptides. However, it should be noted that Abel and Grey (16) found also Arg-Leu at the carboxyterminal of the hinge peptide of an IgA1.

     Although these data focus only on a limited section of the IgA heavy chains and although lack of material precluded the determination of the sequence of the hinge peptide Rou., our results suggest that the hinge region of the IgA2m(2) variant is more similar to that of the A2m(1) proteins than to that of IgA1 subclass. This is in keeping with the more recent phylogenic divergence of the IgA2 subclass. The presence of the H-L bridge in the A2m(2) variant may be interpreted as the remaining corresponding ancestor to the IgA1 subclass. However, it should be emphasized that at least two features of the A2m(2) hinge peptide Rou. differ from those of the A2m(1) variant: 1) Its electrophoretic mobility which is similar to that of the IgA1 hinge peptide, precluding the chemical typing of this variant since the heavy-light bridge is also present. 2) The number of pro-line residues which seems to be unique.

These features should be carefully correlated with antigen specificity in further studies since it is well known that the control by allelic genes may be effective at multiple positions along the Ig heavy chains.

Acknowledgements: These studies were supported in part by a grant from Institut National de la Santé et de la Recherche Médicale (INSERM) (n° 73.4.033.2).

REFERENCES

1. Feinstein, D. and Franklin, E.C., Nature 212:1496, 1966.
2. Kunkel, H.G. and Prendergast, R.A., Proc. Soc. Exp. Biol. Med. 122:910, 1966.
3. Vaerman, J.P. and Heremans, J.F., Science 153:647, 1966.
4. Vyas, G.N. and Fudenberg, H.H., Proc. Nat. Acad. Sci., Wash. 64:1211, 1969.
5. Kunkel, H.G., Smith, W.K., Joslin, F.G., Natvig, J.B. and Litwin, S.D., Nature 223:1247, 1969.
6. Jerry, L.M., Kunkel, H.G. and Grey, H.M., Proc. Nat. Acad. Sci., Wash. 65:557, 1970.
7. van Loghem, E., Wang, A.C. and Shuster, J., Vox Sang. 24:481, 1973.
8. Mihaesco, E., Seligmann, M. and Frangione, B., Nature 232:220, 1971.
9. Frangione, B. and Franklin, E.C., FEBS Letters 20:321, 1972.
10. Frangione, B. and Wilstein, C., J. Mol. Biol. 33:893, 1968.
11. Offord, R.E., Nature 211:591, 1966.
12. Gray, W.P., Methods in Enzymology 11:469, 1967.
13. Wood, K.R. and Wang, K.T., Biochem. Biophys. Acta 133: 369, 1967.

14. Frangione, B. and Wolfenstein-Todel, C., Proc. Nat. Acad.
     Sci. 69:3673, 1972.
15. Wolfenstein-Todel, C., Frangione, B. and Franklin, E.C.,
     Biochemistry 11:3971, 1972.
16. Abel, C. and Grey, H., Nature New Biol. 233:29, 1971.

THE CARBOHYDRATE COMPOSITION OF GLYCOPEPTIDES ISOLATED FROM IgA2 IMMUNOGLOBULIN

M. Tomana, W. Niedermeier, J. Mestecky and
F. Skvaril*
Division of Clinical Immunology and Rheumatology,
Univeristy of Alabama in Birmingham and
*Institute for Clinical and Experimental Cancer
Research, University of Bern, Switzerland

Analyses of the carbohydrate content of eleven IgA1 and six IgA2 myeloma proteins revealed that, besides the known restriction of galactosamine to IgA1 subclass (1,2), statistically significant quantitative differences exist between the carbohydrate composition of the two subclasses. The greater amounts of fucose, mannose, and galactosamine in IgA2 immunoglobulins explain the higher total carbohydrate content of these proteins (Table 1). No statistical differences were found in the galactose and sialic acid content of the subclasses. The relatively high content of fucose in IgA2 immunoglobulins suggests that these proteins contain more highly branched oligosaccharides than proteins of the IgA1 subclass.

The glycopeptides were isolated from a polymeric IgA2 immunoglobulin (Fe1) that had a λ type of light chains and sedimentation constant of 9.5S. Polyacrylamide gel electrophoresis in 10M urea at pH 9.4 showed J chain to be present. In this protein, carbohydrates had less galactose and sialic acid than most other IgA2 immunoglobulins.

One hundred mg protein was incubated with pepsin (enzyme substrate ratio 1:100) for 16 hours at 37°C and pH 2. After neutralization with NaOH, the solution was adjusted with NaCl and with sodium phosphate buffer (pH 7) to the final concentration 0.15M and .01M respectively. The peptide mixture was applied to a 1.3 x 41 cm column containing Agarose with a covalently linked concanavalin A (Glycosilex-Miles - Yeda Ltd.,

Table 1.   Differences in Mean Carbohydrate Compositions of
IgA1 and IgA2.

| Carbohydrate | mean conc. (%)[a] | | F | P |
	IgA1[b]	IgA2[c]		
Fucose	0.13 (0.047)	0.48 (0.165)	45.26	0.0001
Mannose	1.28 (0.199)	2.44 (0.544)	41.50	0.0001
Galactose	1.49 (0.163)	1.22 (0.414)	3.69	0.0712
Glucosamine	1.36 (0.222)	2.75 (0.723)	36.46	0.0001
Galactosamine	0.46 (0.133)	0.00 (0.000)	70.78	0.0001
Sialic Acid	1.38 (0.149)	1.27 (0.663)	0.32	0.5887
Total	6.09 (0.684)	8.16 (2.04)	9.81	0.0068

[a]Figures in parentheses are standard deviations.
[b]Mean of 11 samples of IgA1.
[c]Mean of 6 samples of IgA2.

Rehovot, Israel). Peptides containing carbohydrate were
detected in peak A´ and in fractions eluted with 5% methyl-
α-D-mannoside (peak B) (Fig. 1). Fractions corresponding to
the peak A´ were lyophilized, dissolved in 1% ammonium
bicarbonate buffer (pH 7.3), and applied to the Sephadex G-25
(fine) column equilibrated in the same buffer. The first
peak from this column appeared to represent a homogeneous
glycopeptide. A single component was detected when this
glycopeptide was examined by polyacrylamide gel electrophoresis
in SDS and 9M urea (pH 7.2) and by high voltage electrophoresis
on filter paper in a pyridine-acetate buffer (pH 3.65).
Glycopeptides, eluted with methyl mannoside (peak B) from the
concanavalin A column, were partially separated from methyl
mannoside on a Sephadex G-10 column. During this process,
some glycopeptides of lower molecular weight may have been
lost in fractions that contained methyl mannoside and salt,
but no attempts were made to recover them. Fractions corresponding to the first large peak from the Sephadex G-10
column were freeze dried, redissolved in 0.1M acetic acid,
and applied to Sephadex G-50 (medium) column (Fig. 2). Peak
I was electrophoretically homogeneous. Glycopeptides in peaks
II and III were further purified by gel filtration on a
Sephadex G-25 column. Polyacrylamide gel electrophoresis of
purified fractions II and III showed the presence of one main
and several minor components. Complete resolution was
achieved by preparative high voltage electrophoresis on filter

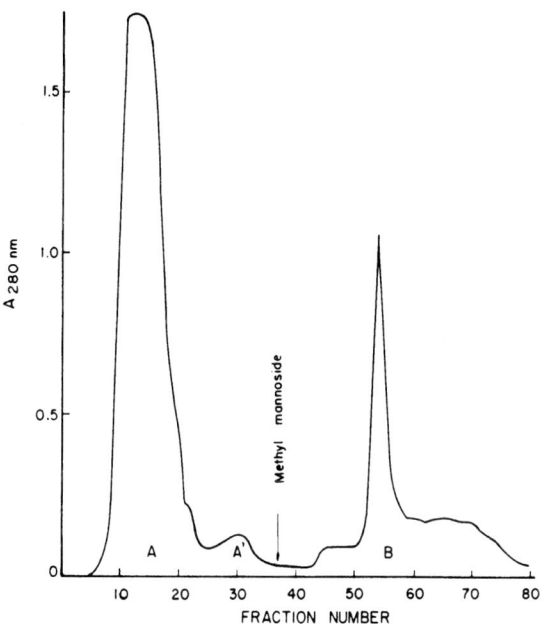

Figure 1. Separation of glycopeptides on a "Glycosilex"
column. The column 1.3 x 41 cm, was kept at room temperature
at a flow rate of 60 ml/h; 3.5 ml fractions were collected.
Initially the column was developed with a 0.01M phosphate
buffer (pH 7) containing 0.15 M NaCl. Elution was achieved
with 5% methyl α-D-mannoside in the same buffer.

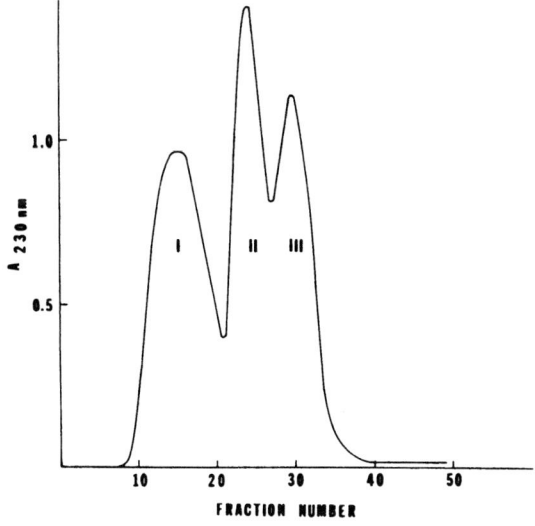

Figure 2. Separation of glycopeptides on a Sephadex G-50
(medium) column. The column 1.5 x 87 cm equilibrated in
0.1M acetic acid, was run at a flow rate of 60-70 ml/h; 3.5
ml fractions were collected.

paper. Amino acid composition, molecular weight, and further
characterization of the isolated glycopeptides will be
described elsewhere. Neutral sugars and amino hexoses were
determined by gas liquid chromatography (3), and sialic acid
was determined by the method of Warren (4). Table 2 summarizes
results of the carbohydrate analyses. The content of each
monosaccharide was expressed in relation to mannose, which
was artitrarily assigned a value of 5 residues per glycopeptide molecule.

Our results do not exclude the possibility that some
of the isolated glycopeptides contained more than one
oligosaccharide.

Table 2. The Carbohydrates in IgA2 (Fel) Glycopeptides
(Moles per 5 moles of mannose)

	Peptide A´	Peptides Eluted from Concanavalin Column		
		I	II	III
Fucose	0.8	1.0	0.8	0.4
Mannose	5.0	5.0	5.0	5.0
Galactose	1.8	2.7	2.1	0.4
Glucosamine	5.4	5.8	4.1	4.7
Sialic Acid	0.0	0.4	0.3	0.0

SUMMARY

Of four glycopeptides isolated from IgA2 immunoglobulins
by the affinity chromatography technique, two contained fucose,
mannose, galactose, glucosamine, and sialic acid, another
had this same composition except that it lacked sialic acid,
and the last appeared to contain only mannose and glucosamine.

REFERENCES

1. Wang, An-Chuan and Fudenberg, H.H., J. Immunol. 105:1286,
    1970.
2. Grey, H.M., Abel, C.A. and Zimmerman, B., Ann. N.Y. Acad.
    Sci., 190:37, 1971.
3. Tomana, M., Mestecky, J. and Niedermeier, W., J. Immunol.
    108:1631, 1972.
4. Warren, L.J., J. Biochem., 40:465, 1971.

MOUSE IgA MYELOMA PROTEINS WITH ALPHA CHAIN DELETIONS: A COMPARISON WITH HUMAN ALPHA CHAINS WITH DELETIONS

J. Frederic Mushinski
Laboratory of Cell Biology
National Cancer Institute
Bethesda, Maryland 20014

For several years our laboratory has been investigating a small group of mouse IgA myeloma proteins which have heavy chains smaller than those of most IgA myeloma proteins. Dr. Howard Grey and his colleagues have just presented interesting data characterizing a shortened human alpha chain (1), so it now seems appropriate to review the current state of knowledge about the shortened mouse alpha chains. There are striking similarities but also important differences among the properties characterizing the deleted heavy chains from man and mouse. We will discuss possible mechanisms which may produce such heavy chains in the mouse and whether the same mechanisms are responsible for the appearance of defective alpha chains in man.

Several hundred plasmacytomas have been induced in inbred strains of mice, primarily in the BALB/c and NZB strains, by intraperitoneal injections of adjuvants or mineral oils, as developed and described by Dr. Michael Potter (2). About 60% of the BALB/c plasmacytomas synthesize and secrete IgA myeloma proteins into the serum, and among a large number carefully examined, eight have been found that secrete IgA proteins with defective heavy chains. The defective IgA proteins were recognized when they were found in high concentration in the urine of the tumor-bearing mice. Subsequent studies on the nature of these urinary IgA molecules were aided by the existence of two transplantable tumor lines, Adj.PC-6A and Adj. PC-6C, both of which originated from the same adjuvant-injected BALB/c mouse. Adj.PC-6A secretes IgA molecules

which are found only in the serum or ascites while the
protein synthesized by Adj.PC-6C is also excreted into the
urine. Similarities in tryptic peptide fingerprints of the
light chains from the two proteins suggest that they are
identical. The two myeloma proteins share idiotypic antigenic
determinants, located in the Fab part of the molecule, so we
assume that the amino-terminal portion, containing V_H and
V_L, is the same in both molecules (3). Thus the antigenic
and physical differences that do exist between these closely
related prototypes of the two types of IgA myeloma proteins,
serum localized and urine excreted, may be presumed to be
located in the Fc fragment of the heavy chain.

Physicochemical studies of Adj.PC-6A protein (4,5) showed
that it exists in serum as 7,9,11, and 13 S disulfide-linked
polymers of four-chain subunits. Each subunit is made up of
two light chains, with molecular weight of about 23,000 daltons, and two heavy chains, with molecular weight of about
54,000 daltons. The 6A protein, like most polymeric mouse
IgA myeloma proteins, does not have disulfide links between
the light and heavy chains. Instead, the two light chains
are disulfide linked, and the heavy chains are disulfide bonded
only to other heavy chains (6). The carboxyl-terminal amino
acid of 6A protein and most other mouse IgA proteins is
tyrosine (6).

Adj.PC-6C protein is isolated from urine as a 3.9 S half
molecule consisting of one light chain disulfide bonded to
one heavy chain. The molecular weights of these light and
heavy chains are 23,000 and 46,000 daltons, respectively (5).
There is no tendency of this half molecule to polymerize
beyond its two chain subunit which has a molecular weight of
about 68,000 daltons. The carboxyl terminus of 6C protein
is glutamine (unpublished data). This molecular weight data
and carboxyl terminus is much the same as that reported for
another half molecule IgA myeloma protein, MOPC-47A protein
(4). The above data are summarized in Table 1 and compared
with the pertinent data available from analysis of the human
alpha chain, Vo, which has been presented in greater detail
earlier (1).

The similarities between Vo and 6C protein include their
rarity, their normal-sized light chains, the size of the
remnant of heavy chain, and the localization of the missing
polypeptide fragment to the Fc end. The differences between
them are the carboxyl-terminal amino acids, which probably

Table 1. Physicochemical Comparison of Mouse and Human IgA
Myeloma Proteins with Defective Alpha Chains

Property	Mouse (3,4,5)	Human (1)
Prevalence	Rare - Eight Cases: MOPC-4G, Adj.Pc-6C*, MOPC-47A, MOPC-88, MOPC-116, MOPC-287, McPC-844, and McPC-2185	Rare- 1Case, Vo
Purified from	Urine	Serum
Degree of assembly	Halfmolecule only (H_1L_1)	Monomer only (H_2L_2)
Interchain disulfides	H-L only	H-L and H-H
Light chain size	Intact, M.W.=23,000	Intact
Heavy chain size	M.W.= 46,000	M.W.= 40,000
Location of heavy chain deletion	Fc	Fc
Carboxyl terminus	Glutamine	Glycine

*Model protein used for data in this table.

immediately precede the deletion, and the nature of the interchain disulfide bonding. Both mouse defective alpha chains
that have been studied, 6C and 47A proteins, have glutamine
as carboxyl terminus, whereas Vo heavy chain has glycine.
Species differences in the C_H region may be responsible for
this difference. However, if the other six defective alpha
chains also prove to end in glutamine, then there will be
reason to believe that there is some termination mechanism
operating at exactly the same site in all these myelomas or
that these short alpha chains represent a new C_H subtype for
IgA molecules. The disulfide arrangement for Vo is probably
the same as for IgA molecules with undeleted alpha chains,
but the L-H disulfide bond in 6C protein is quite different
from that in 6A protein which has no L-H disulfides and
probably is the molecule from which 6C was derived. Species

differences in C_H sequence and configuration could permit
such different sequellae from a similar carboxyl-terminal
deletion if an unpaired, free cysteine residue were left in
the shortened mouse alpha chain, and if the cysteine reacted
preferentially with a light chain rather than with another
deleted alpha chain. A new mouse IgA subclass would explain
these findings, too.

The origin of the deletions in mouse and human myelomas
remains speculative but the mechanisms may be similar. Our
studies on 6A and 6C proteins may be pertinent not only to
the mouse alpha chains but also to those in man. Studies of
intracellular synthesis and assembly of 6C protein showed
only intact light chains and disulfide bonded half molecules
with a molecular weight of about 68,000 (5). This indicates
that there was no larger heavy chain which was degraded proteolytically to the deleted alpha chain either inside or
outside the cell. Translational differences may be influencing
protein synthesis in the Adj.PC-6C cells, but the transfer-RNA
patterns examined so far show a high degree of similarity
unusual for different tumors (7). Cell-free synthetic experiments are needed to completely rule out this possibility. The
eight tumors which produce short alpha chains may represent
clones of cells which are making a different and rare subclass
of IgA molecules. Using a homologous antiserum specific for
half molecule IgA proteins, we tested normal serum and other
body fluids by double diffusion looking for evidence of such
molecules in normal mice (3). No positive reactions were
found rendering this hypothesis unlikely, although it cannot
be ruled out conclusively until the test is repeated with a
more sensitive assay. The most probable explanation for the
appearance of these deleted alpha chains in mouse and human
myelomas is a DNA mutation which deleted a stretch of alpha
chain structural genome or functionally deleted the carboxyl-
terminal stretch of heavy chain by inducing premature termination of transcription or translation. Further structural
studies of these defective and intact alpha chains as well as
in vitro studies of the mutations of cloned IgA-producing mouse
myelomas cells may help to elucidate the mechanisms involved
in producing alpha chains with deletions.

REFERENCES

1. Grey, H.M., Despont, J.-P., Abel, C.A. and Penn, G.M. This
Symposium.
2. Potter, M. Physiol. Rev. 52:52, 1972.

3. Lieberman, R., Mushinski, J.F., and Potter, M. Science 159:1355, 1968.

4. Seki, T., Apella, E. and Itano, H.A. Proc. Nat. Acad. Sci., U.S. 61:1071, 1968.

5. Mushinski, J.F. J. Immunol. 106:41, 1971.

6. Abel, C.A. and Grey, H.M. Biochemistry 7:2682, 1968.

7. Mushinski, J.F. Biochemistry 10:3917, 1971.

DISCUSSION

Dr. Grey - Dr. Penn has obtained antisera specific for the Vo protein and there is no indication that there is any subclass related to this protein in normal human serum. From my understanding of the mouse half molecules studied by Dr. Apella and Dr. Mushinski there certainly are striking similarities with the Vo protein since both involve C-terminal deletions. However, it is not clear why, in the mouse situation, there is the absence of inter-heavy chain disulfide bridges, whereas in Vo they are present. Also, since the mouse protein is of the IgA_2 type, which normally lacks LH disulfide bridges, why are LH disulfide bonds present?

Dr. Cebra - I have always been intrigued by the presence of N-acetylgalactosamine in IgA_1 and in IgA molecules in general. I wonder if Dr. Putnam or some of the other speakers know enough about the glycopeptide at the hinge region to tell us whether it contains both N-acetylglucosamine and N-acetylgalactosamine. If only N-acetylgalactosamine is present in the hinge region then possibly the enzyme catalyzing attachment of this first unusual sugar recognizes some unique sequence in the hinge polypeptide. If the N-acetylgalactosamine is located more peripherally on the oligosaccharide and N-acetylglucosamine is attached directly to the peptide chain then the existence of a unique glycosyltransferase may be indicated which could be linked in expression to IgA_1 production. I wonder whether such an enzyme - the glycosyl-transferase for N-acetylgalactosamine may be linked in either expression or genetically to synthesis of an immunoglobulin chain?

Dr. Putnam - The problem with the hinge peptide in our hands is that we never get the whole hinge peptide sufficiently pure to be able to say that it does not contain glucosamine. It is a very large tryptic glycopeptide that is usually contaminated with another large tryptic glycopeptide that contains glucosamine. By use of the sequencer we get a double sequence on the hinge peptide and the glucosamine-containing peptide. We obtained the sequence of the hinge

229

peptide by thermolysin digestion and isolation of the
subpeptides and by correlating the sequence of these with
our previous studies of the hinge peptide of the Ha IgA
protein. Even in the glycopeptide fraction from the thermolysin digest two glycopeptides are present together and
are difficult to separate. The one from the hinge contains
galactosamine and has 30 amino acid residues, whereas the
other from elsewhere in the α1 chain contains glucosamine
but has only two amino acid residues. Fortunately, the
thermolysin subpeptide containing glucosamine is washed out
of the sequencer cup after the second step so we get a single
unambiguous sequence for the galactosamine glycopeptide from
the hinge. We have tried other techniques to separate the
galactosamine and the glucosamine glycopeptides but so far
without success. Although I can not give you an unambiguous
answer, we do not believe glucosamine is present in the hinge
peptide. Perhaps Dr. Frangione's laboratory can help further
on this question.

Dr. Spiegelberg - I would like to ask Dr. Putnam about the
carbohydrate attachment near the N-terminus. Was this
associated with a special variable subgroup?

Dr. Putnam - I don't think it was associated with any
particular subgroup. My belief is that it is just a consequence of having the sequence Asn-Leu-Ser. This accords with
the prototype sequence Asn-X-Thr/Ser which is not absolutely
obligatory, but which is commonly the sequence to which carbohydrate is attached. However, in our experience we have had
at least two light chains which have that kind of sequence
which do not have the carbohydrate attached. I think it is
just the chance occurrence of that sequence, which when
recognized by the transglycosidase, becomes a site for
attachment of carbohydrate.

Dr. Spiegelberg - In collaboration with Dr. Grey we have
described several IgG myeloma protein heavy chains which
also had carbohydrate on the variable region; one protein,
I recently looked at, did not fit in $VH_{1,2,3}$.

Dr. Putnam - I see. Is that carbohydrate close to the
beginning of the molecule?

Dr. Spiegelberg - It is near residue 30.

Dr. Putnam - I want to point out that we do have to he care-

ful as to whether carbohydrate is present or not when we are
using the automatic sequencer because that really doesn't
pick up the carbohydrate. When we use the sequencer, we
generally miss the residue there. We have to get it from
the small glycopeptides, which are sequenced and analyzed
for carbohydrate by conventional methods.

Dr. Capra - Just to clarify that point. In the sequencer
if you get an asparagine residue, it is asparagine; if you
have aspartic, it is aspartic. If you get nothing and have
to back-hydrolyze to find an aspartic acid, then we go and
look for carbohydrate. We have not run into an asparagine
in the first 30 residues of the five proteins we have
studied nor any other proteins. We have located carbohydrate
in IgA proteins as in other proteins by the routine procedures.
I don't see that it is a problem with the sequencer at all.

Dr. Inman - When we were at the Stockholm meeting, you will
recall that an investigator who sequenced a μ chain was
unable to designate a cysteine residue which could have been
attached to a J chain. Was the IgM whose μ chain sequenced
you reported tonight associated with J chain, and do you
have any information regarding the place of covalent attachment of the J chain to the μ chain?

Dr. Putnam - J chain is associated with all the IgM proteins
that we have tested including the one we sequenced and also
with our polymeric IgA proteins, but of course the amount
is very small. Although we have isolated J chain and have
a certain amount of data on it, we have no more data and
perhaps less data than has been reported by other workers.
We do not have specific evidence as to the site of combination
of the J chain in the IgM we sequenced. We make the
assumption that the work on the relative degree of susceptibility to reduction of the different disulfide bridges
implicated the bridge which is now called the intersubunit
bridge at Cys-414 as the point of attachment of the J chain.
However, we have no specific evidence of the kind that I
think that others have given here where by use of the
diagonal method they actually isolated the peptide which has
the J chain attachment.

EVIDENCE FOR A COMMON SYNTHETIC ORIGIN FOR SECRETORY AND SERUM IgA*

G.N. Abraham,[†] E. Santucci and R.F. Jacox

Department of Medicine and Microbiology
University of Rochester School of Medicine
Rochester, New York 14642

INTRODUCTION

Experimental evidence has been obtained which demonstrates that the synthesis of the IgA moiety of the secretory IgA molecule occurs in cells separate from those in which the secretory piece component is synthesized. The data supporting this have been described in excellent reviews and will not be reiterated here (1,2). Immunochemical evidence which establishes that the secretory and serum IgA portions may be derived from the same source in humans is lacking.

One approach to partial solution of the problem would be the isolation of serum and salivary IgA antibodies of identical specificity, and demonstration that these have equivalent active antibody site structure. Data which demonstrate structural identity of the variable region of the two antibodies would thus provide strong evidence for the concept that both serum and salivary IgA variable regions have a common synthetic origin.

The availability of monoclonal IgA anti-IgG autoantibodies (rheumatoid factors) in serum of patients with rheumatoid arthritis and knowledge that many of these persons have

*These studies supported in part by U.S.P.H.S. Grant #
 AI-11550-01 and the Monroe County Cpt. of the Arthritis Fdn.
†G.N.A. is a Post-doctoral fellow of the Arthritis Fdn.

anti-IgG activity in their saliva, allows testing of this
concept by direct and comparative immunochemical methods.

MATERIALS AND METHODS

Analytical and preparative ultracentrifugation, and
Sephadex G-200 column chromatography of serum, and isoelectric focusing techniques of the purified proteins were
performed as previously described in detail (3).

IgA anti-IgG globulin was isolated by adsorption of
serum on a bromoacetyl cellulose human IgG 1 immunoadsorbent
(3). The latex positive eluate contained IgG, IgA and IgM.
IgM was separated by Sephadex G-200 column chromatography,
and the IgA from IgG by DEAE cellulose chromatography utilizing a 0.01 M and 0.15 M pH 7.4 phosphate buffer gradient.
The IgA which eluted with the 0.15 M buffer is the serum
IgA utilized.

Secretory IgA was isolated from a 24 hour saliva specimen as follows: Saliva containing anti-IgG activity (slide
latex test) was clarified by centrifugation for 30 minutes
at 10,000 rpm and 4 C, and placed directly on a Sephadex
G-200 column. The first elution peak contained IgA by
immunodiffusion, and all the anti-IgG activity. The fractions comprising this peak were pooled, concentrated by per-
vaporation, placed on DEAE cellulose column and the IgA
purified using the 2-step phosphate gradient. The latter
procedure was abandoned since precisely the same isoelectric
focusing profile was obtained for IgA purified only by
Sephadex G-200 as by Sephadex G-200 and DEAE cellulose.

The specificity of the serum and salivary IgA for the
various IgG heavy chain subclasses, and IgG subunits was
determined by inhibition of the hemagglutination reaction
between "Ripley"-coated human O-positive erythrocytes (4),
and the purified IgA preparations. The procedure is performed as previously described (4).

Binding studies were performed utilizing the modified
micro-equilibrium molecular sieving technique (3). Sephadex
G-100 was utilized as the "semi-permeable" membrane.

Isolation of secretory piece from salivary IgA was
performed as described by Lamm and Greenberg (5). 1 mg of
I^{125} labeled preparations of serum or salivary IgA

containing 10^6 cpm were each added to 50 mg of secretory IgA
purified from human colostrum (6). The samples were extensively reduced in 8M urea by DTT and alkylated with iodoacetamide. After dialysis against H_2O and lyophilization, they
were dissolved in 70% formic acid, degraded with cyanogen
bromide for 20 hours, and applied to Sephadex G-100 columns
equilibrated with 1M acetic acid. Fractions were neutralized
with NaOH, counted for radioactivity, and tested for the
presence of secretory piece utilizing specific rabbit anti-
human secretory piece antibody.

RESULTS

The results are divided into three sections: First
are studies which demonstrate the presence and composition
of the circulating serum immune complexes. Next are the
studies which demonstrate that the salivary IgA contains
secretory piece and is thus not polymerized serum IgA.
Finally, data are provided which demonstrate identity of
the variable regions of both autoantibodies.

Serum studies: The serum and saliva utilized were obtained from a patient with severe rheumatoid arthritis who
recently developed Sjögren's syndrome. The serum IgA level
was 500 mg% by radial immunodiffusion. Figure 1 demonstrates
the schlieren patterns obtained by analytical ultracentrifugation of a 1/2 dilution of the patient's serum, and shows
prominent 9S and minor 22S complex peaks.

Sephadex G-200 chromatography (Fig. 2) demonstrates that
anti-IgG activity is associated with regions in which IgG and
IgA are present. Preparative ultracentrifugation of the
serum at pH 2.8 and pH 7.4 illustrates that prominent shifts
of IgA and IgG (and smaller amounts of IgM) occur into upper
gradient fractions suggesting that serum complexes may be
comprised of these immunoglobulins.

Studies were next performed to grossly characterize the
serum and salivary IgA anti-IgG globulins. Both IgA preparations contained only kappa type light chains by immunodiffusion. Analytical ultracentrifugation of dilute solutions
(OD 280 = 0.450-secretory and 0.520-serum), utilizing UV
scanner optics yielded $S_{20,w}$ values of 10.87 and 6.89 respectively. No evidence of aggregates was noted. Restricted
heterogeneity was confirmed by isoelectric focusing over a
pH 3-10 gradient. Figure 3 illustrates the profiles

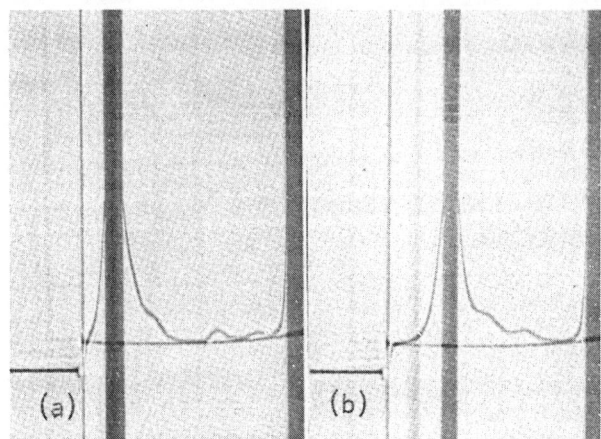

Figure 1. Schlieren pattern of patient serum in phosphate buffered saline pH 7.4. Photographs were taken at 42 (a) and 66 (b) min. after maximum speed of 56,000 rpm was reached and show 22S (a) and 9S (b) peaks.

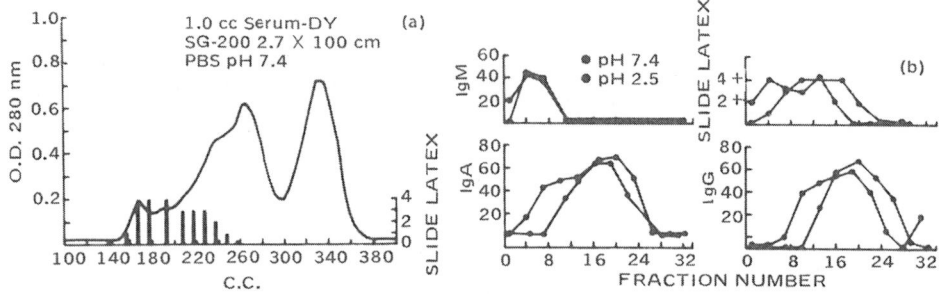

Figure 2. Sephadex G-200 chromatogram of serum (a); and (b) 10-40% sucrose density gradient ultracentrifugation at pH 7.4 and pH 2.5 of serum. IgG, IgA, and IgM in gradient fractions assayed by standard radial immunodiffusion. Scale is in mm. of precipitin ring diameter. Major shifts of IgG, IgA and slide latex activity into upper gradient fractions are noted.

obtained for the proteins. The peak of the serum IgA is at 4.50 and that of the secretory IgA at 4.75. Both have profiles as restricted as purified myeloma proteins similarly processed.

Evidence was next provided that the salivary IgA (11S) was not polymerized serum IgA by demonstrating that it contained a component immunologically identifiable as secretory piece, not present in the serum IgA preparation. First, antiserum specific for secretory IgA demonstrated spur

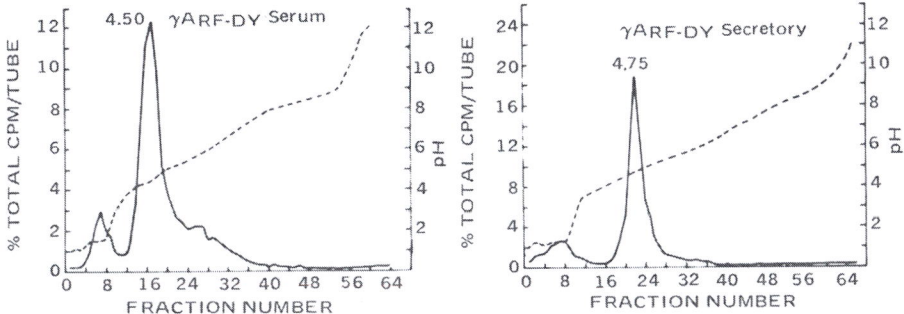

Figure 3. Isoelectric focusing profiles of secretory
and serum IgA-Dy. Conditions: 110 ml ampholine column.
pH range 3-10. 350 volts constant, for 48 hours.

formation of the salivary over the serum IgA. The same
antiserum absorbed with pooled IgA kappa and lambda myeloma
proteins reacted with the secretory but not the serum IgA
rheumatoid factor. Finally, a component reacting in a precipitin reaction with specific anti-secretory piece antibody
was identified in the salivary but not the serum IgA. This
latter experiment will be described in detail:

Radiolabeled preparations of both IgA proteins were
added to purified secretory IgA carrier, isolated from human
colostrum, extensively reduced and alkylated, and finally
cyanogen bromide degraded as described above. The samples
were placed on Sephadex G-100 columns and fractionated.
Fig. 4 illustrates that the salivary IgA contained a prominent peak of radioactivity not seen in the preparation of
serum IgA. This peak further corresponds to the position of
secretory piece demonstrated in the colostral IgA carrier by
immunodiffusion utilizing specific anti-secretory piece
antibody. No precipitation of radioactivity was attained
with rabbit anti-human IgA, IgG, IgM, kappa or anti-whole
human serum antisera in either preparation. Thus, secretory
component is identifiable only in the salivary IgA preparation.

Experiments were next performed to determine that the
active antibody site portions of these IgA proteins were
identical. Specificity of both preparations was shown by
hemagglutination inhibition. Hemagglutination of "Ripley"-
coated human 0-positive erythrocytes by the serum and salivary IgA was inhibited by varying concentrations of IgG of
the 4 major heavy chain subclasses and IgG 1 subunits. As
noted in Table 1, equal hemagglutination inhibition spectra
are noted for the IgA secretory and serum preparations.

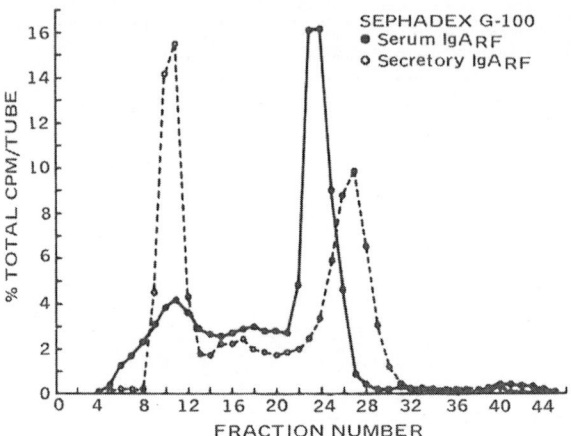

Figure 4. Sephadex G-100 chromatograms of completely reduced and alkylated I^{125} labeled serum and secretory IgA
rheumatoid factors, after degradation with cyanogen bromide.
Secretory piece from carrier colostral IgA was detected
by immunodiffusion in fractions 7-13 of both columns.

Table 1. Hemagglutination inhibition results.
          conc. IgA sec.=0.07 mg/ml; IgA ser.=.05.
          Procedure as in ref (4).

Inhibitor	Sample	Concentration of inhibitor mM/ml				
		3-4	2.0	0.8	0.4	0.2
IgG 1	IgA-sec	0	0	0	0	0
	-ser	0	0	0	0	Tr
IgG 2	IgA-sec	0	0	1+	1++	2+
	-ser	0	0	0	0	1+
IgG 3	IgA-sec	Tr	1+	2+	2+	4+
	-ser	0	Tr	1+	1+	3+
IgG 4	IgA-sec	Tr	1+	2+	3+	4+
	-ser	0	1+	1+	3+	3+
Fc	IgA-sec	0	0	0	0	2+
	-ser	0	0	0	Tr	3+
IgG 1 H	IgA-sec	0	0	Tr	2+	4+
	-ser	0	0	1+	3+	3++
IgG 1 H tryptic	IgA-sec	0	0	0	3+	4+
	-ser	0	Tr	1+	1+	4+

Strongest inhibition is shown for intact IgG 1 and IgG 2 and
Fc fragment. IgG 1 heavy chains, its tryptic digests, and
IgG 3 and IgG 4 are partially inhibitory. Fab and L chains
were non-inhibitory. Thus the specificities of the two
antibody preparations are identical.

Limited studies were performed to determine the relative binding affinities of the two anti-IgG preparations, by the micro-equilibrium molecular sieving technique. In order to conserve reactants only two points were tested. The assumption was made that the affinity of these anti-IgG proteins might be similar to that of a well-characterized (3) monoclonal IgA- anti-IgG. Thus, a 15/1 molar ratio of IgG 1 Fc piece to anti-IgG was utilized to determine the valence of these IgA proteins at antibody site saturation. At this level the serum IgA was determined to have 1.67 moles of Fc bound/mole of IgA, and the salivary IgA 3.6 moles Fc/mole of IgA. Thus, valences of 2 and 4 were assumed for calculation of a single association constant-k_a. The k_a values were determined at a 4/1 molar ratio of Fc/IgA. The k_a values found were 1.35×10^6 L/M for the salivary and 1.9×10^6 L/M for the serum IgA. Thus, within the constraints of this particular experiment, the binding constants of these autoantibodies are the same.

Studies were performed to demonstrate that the light chains of these antibodies were equivalent. Aliquots from the peak tubes of both preparations obtained from the previous isoelectric focusing experiments were added to purified IgG 1 myeloma protein carrier. Light chains were obtained after reduction and alkylation and Sephadex G-100 chromatography of the samples at acid pH. The L chains were then analyzed by isoelectric focusing over a pH range of 3-10, the peak tubes pooled and the experiment repeated over a pH range of 3-6. Figure 5 illustrates the profiles obtained. Isoelectric points of 4.12 and sharp, spiked electrofocusing patterns were found for both preparations.

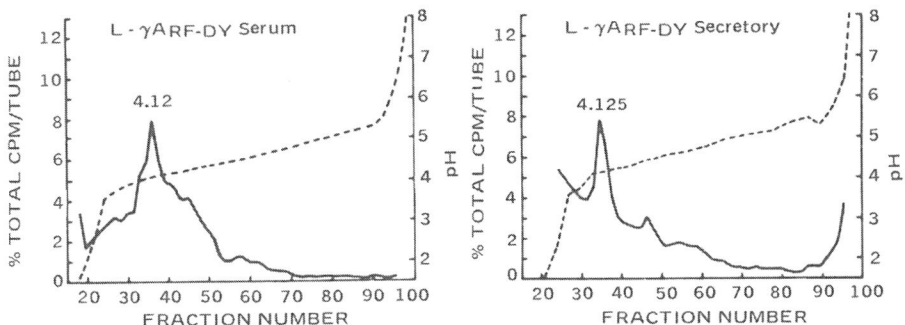

Figure 5. Isoelectric focusing profiles of L chains isolated from secretory and serum IgA-Dy. Conditions: 110 ml ampholine column; pH range 3-6; 350 volts constant for 42 hours.

Further evidence that these light chains were similar was obtained from amino acid sequence data. 1 mg of light chain from each preparation was subjected to automated Edman degradation for 4 positions. The amino terminal sequence for both proteins is Asp-Ile-Glu-Met. Thus, both light chains belong to the V_k-1 subgroup.

SUMMARY

This study was specifically directed to provide data which support the concept that the Fv or active antibody site regions of particular monoclonal serum and salivary IgA anti-IgG autoantibodies are identical. By the criteria of identical antigenic specificity, binding site avidity, light chain identity by isoelectric focusing and light chain variable region class similarity, these antibodies have identical active antibody combining sites. It is assumed that their origin is common.

Caution must, however, be exercised as to the applicability of this situation to the general state. First, the sharp isoelectric point of the salivary IgA component and its single light chain type indicates that this may be the only secretory IgA population present in this patient's saliva. Further, despite the presence of other 7S non-rheumatoid factor IgA in the patient's serum, the 7S IgA rheumatoid factor is estimated to comprise nearly all of the 500 mg% present in this patient's serum. Thus, it is possible that suppression of non-rheumatoid factor IgA synthesis is present. In short, these data may be unique and applicable only to this particular disease state. The data must be confirmed for another IgA antibody system.

REFERENCES

1. Tomasi, T.B. and Bienenstock, J., Adv. Immunol. 9:2, 1968.
2. Tomasi, T.B., Bull, D., Tourville, D., Montes, M. and Yurchak, A., in The Secretory Immunologic System, p. 3 and 41, Edited by D.H. Dayton, Jr. et al., U.S. Government Printing Office, Washington, D.C., 1971.
3. Abraham, G.N., Clarke, R.A. and Vaughan, J.H., Immunochemistry 9:301, 1972.
4. Taylor, H. and Abraham, G.N., Clin. Exp. Immunol. 13: 529, 1973.
5. Lamm, M.E. and Greenberg, J., Biochemistry 11:2744, 1972.
6. Pincus, C.S., Lamm, M.E. and Nussenzweig, V., J. Exp. Med. 133:987, 1971.

STUDIES ON THE PRIMARY STRUCTURE OF HUMAN SECRETORY COMPONENT

Charlotte Cunningham-Rundles, Michael E. Lamm,
and Edward C. Franklin
New York University Medical Center
New York, New York 10016

INTRODUCTION

Secretory component occurs in external secretions in two forms, bound and free. The former is an integral part of the secretory IgA molecule, the attachment being covalent in the human. Free secretory component, on the other hand, is present in secretions unattached to other protein. The bound and free forms of secretory component, in both human (1,2) and rabbit (3) have been previously compared in terms of size, amino acid composition, and antigenic determinants and found to be similar, and possibly identical. In order to extend the comparison of the bound vs. free secretory component we have done peptide mapping studies and determined their N-terminal amino acid sequences.

MATERIALS AND METHODS

Free and bound secretory components were isolated from human colostrum as described in references 1 and 2 respectively. For amino acid sequence and tryptic peptide mapping studies, secretory component was completely reduced and alkylated. In some instances easily reduced cystines were first alkylated with ^{14}C-iodoacetic acid and then dialyzed before complete reduction and alkylation with cold iodoacetamide. Amino acid sequences were determined (4) with a Spinco Model 890 automated sequencer. The N-terminal amino acid was also determined by thin layer chromatography after dansylation (5,6).

RESULTS

The tryptic peptide maps of bound and free secretory components were similar, the only definite differences being two extra peptides in the map of bound secretory component. Some 45-50 ninhydrin-positive peptides were observed, a number consistent with the lysine and arginine content of secretory component (1,2). By autoradiography, 4 peptides in each map were significantly radioactive (as a result of ^{14}C-alkylation after partial reduction), and these were the same in both bound and free secretory component.

The first 16 residues of free secretory component are: Lys-Ser-Pro-Ile-Phe-Gly-Pro-Glu-Glu-Val-Asp-Ser-Val-Glu-Gly-Gly-. Only the first 14 residues of bound secretory component were identified with certainty and these were identical.

A comparison between the sequence of the first 16 residues of human secretory component and the known sequences of other proteins was made by computer (National Biomedical Research Foundation, Washington, D.C.). No significant homologies were found.

DISCUSSION

These studies on the primary structure of secretory component emphasize further the close relationship between the bound and free forms. The tryptic peptide maps, which reflect the amino acid sequence of the entire protein, were similar after staining with ninhydrin. The easily reduced half-cystines in bound secretory component include those which join it to the remainder of the secretory IgA molecule. The homologous (as revealed by the autoradiographs of the peptide maps) easily reduced half-cystines in free secretory component, on the other hand, most likely are part of an intrachain disulfide bridge since free secretory component is known to be a single chain and we have been unable to demonstrate any free sulfhydryl groups in it.

Direct evidence for identity of sequence at the N-terminus was obtained. However, the stretches which were sequenced represent only small portions of large proteins. The lack of homology of sequence between secretory component on the one hand, and H and L chains on the other, is not unexpected since secretory component is synthesized in epithelial cells (7) whereas H and L chains are made by plasma cells. Although from the information available it is not yet possible to speculate on its evolutionary origin, it is likely that secretory component is a unique protein species which functions in an immunological role as part of secretory IgA and also in other ways by itself.

SUMMARY

From previous work the two forms of secretory component, bound and free, are known to be similar and possibly identical. In the present studies the tryptic peptide maps of bound and free human secretory component are shown to be similar, including the easily reduced cystine peptides, and the amino acid sequences for the first 14 residues from the N-terminus are identical. There are no homologous stretches of sequence in other proteins.

Acknowledgements: Supported by Grants AI-09738, AM-02594 and AM-01431 from the NIH.

REFERENCES

1. Kobayashi, K., Immunochemistry, 8:785, 1971.
2. Lamm, M.E. and Greenberg, J., Biochemistry, 11:2744, 1972.
3. O'Daly, J.A. and Cebra, J.J., Biochemistry, 10:3843, 1971.
4. Edman, P. and Begg, G., Europ. J. Biochem., 1:80, 1967.
5. Gray, W.R., Methods Enzymol., 11:;39, 1967.
6. Woods, K.R. and Wang, K.T., Biochim, Biophys. Acta, 133: 369, 1967.
7. Tomasi, T.B., Jr., Tan, E.M., Solomon, A. and Prendergast, R.A., J. Exp. Med., 121:101, 1965.

PRODUCTION OF AN Fc FRAGMENT FROM HUMAN IMMUNOGLOBULIN A BY AN IgA-SPECIFIC BACTERIAL PROTEASE

Andrew G. Plaut, Robert J. Genco,
and Thomas B. Tomasi, Jr.

Tufts-New England Medical Center Hospital,
Boston, Massachusetts, and the Schools of
Dentistry and Medicine, State University of
New York at Buffalo, Buffalo, New York

INTRODUCTION

Enzymatic proteolysis of human immunoglobulin A yields Fab_α fragments but the Fc_α is degraded to small peptides. The unavailability of Fc_α has hampered to some extent certain studies of IgA, e.g., its primary structure and the attachment site of secretory component and J chain. Recently, while studying human intestinal immunoglobulins, it was observed by Mehta et al. (1) that normal feces contain an IgA fragment which was shown to be Fc_α, and that feces contain a proteolytic enzyme which cleaves both serum and secretory IgA to yield Fab_α and Fc_α. Of considerable interest is that the enzyme is produced by bacteria in those regions of the alimentary tract heavily populated by bacteria, principally the mouth and the colon. We have termed the enzyme IgA protease because enzymatic activity has thus far been found only against IgA.

METHODS AND RESULTS

IgA protease activity is detected by incubating purified serum myeloma IgA (at a concentration of 5.0 mgm/ml in Tris-HCl buffer, .05 M, pH 8.1) with an equal volume of enzyme (prepared as outlined below) at 37° C for periods of 30 minutes to 20 hours. Highly active enzyme gives discernible

proteolysis after 30 minutes. Digests are studied by immunoelectrophoresis (Figure 1) which reveal Fab$_\alpha$ and Fc$_\alpha$ fragments and variable amounts of undigested IgA. The Fab$_\alpha$

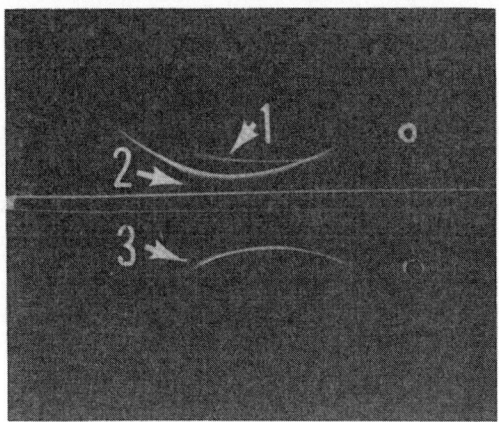

Fig. 1. Immunoelectrophoresis showing Fc$_\alpha$ (1) and Fab$_\alpha$ (2)
fragments produced by IgA protease. The antiserum is unab-
sorbed rabbit anti-human IgA. The fragments show a reaction
of immunologic non-identity and have an electrophoretic migration similar to that of starting IgA substrate (3).
Anode is to the right.

fragment is immunologically identical to that derived by
trypsin proteolysis. The identification of the Fc$_\alpha$ fragment
rests on these criteria: 1) it reacts with alpha chain-
specific antisera; 2) it is devoid of immunologically detectable light chain antigenic determinants; 3) it shows
a reaction of non-identity with the Fab$_\alpha$ fragment; 4) it
is partially identical, but antigenically deficient, to the
initial IgA; and 5) it has a faster (more anodal) electrophoretic mobility than Fab$_\alpha$ and intact IgA by immunoelectrophoresis and polyacrylamide disc gel electrophoresis. Fc$_\alpha$
enzymatically derived from myeloma IgA protein and purified
by Biogel P- 200 molecular sieve chromatography is heterogeneous in size as shown by its multiple banding pattern on
5% polyacrylamide disc gel electrophoresis and analytical
ultracentrifugation. Mild reduction of such preparations
using 10 mM dithiothreitol (DTT) yields a homogenous 3.0 S
Fc$_\alpha$ fragment which has a molecular weight of 41,500 as determined in 6 M guanadine hydrochloride by the meniscus deple-

tion method (2). It migrates as a single band in disc gel electrophoresis. The size heterogeneity of unreduced Fc_α is thought to be due to the monomer-polymer mixture of the starting IgA myeloma.

IgA protease activity as defined by the ability to release intact Fc_α from myeloma IgA protein is found in cell-free filtrates of normal human feces, mixed human saliva, and suspensions of dental plaque in buffer at pH 8.1. These fluids are all exposed to a large bacterial population. Activity is negligible or absent in fasting human small intestinal fluid, secretin-stimulated pancreatic fluid, bile, and saliva obtained directly from the parotid duct. Homogenates of normal human rectal mucosa in Tris buffer pH 8.1 are also negative and remain so following physical and chemical treatments which rupture subcellular particles. The enzyme is found in the medium following aerobic culture of whole feces, saliva, and several oral bacterial isolates, predominately streptococcal species.

IgA protease can be partially purified from culture fluid of Streptococcus sanguis (American Type Culture Collection #10556) grown in a variety of nutrient media. Todd-Hewitt medium and a modification of a published synthetic medium (3) suitable for streptococcal cultivation give the best enzyme yield. Two liters of a 48-hour, non-gassed, aerobic culture at 37° C are centrifuged and solid ammonium sulfate is slowly added to the supernatant to a final concentration of 60%. The resultant precipitate is dissolved in normal saline, dialyzed exhaustively against saline at 4° C and the final volume adjusted to approximately 5% of the starting volume of culture supernatant. Acetone is slowly added to a volume of 70% (final v/v) at 4° C. The gummy precipitate is evacuated to remove traces of acetone and dissolved in Tris buffer, 0.5 M, pH 8.1. This crude preparation has potent IgA protease activity, and work is now in progress to further purify the enzyme.

Naturally occurring IgA protease can be obtained from centrifuged suspensions of feces in buffer. The clear, cell-free supernatant is applied to a DE-52 cellulose column equilibrated in Tris-HCl buffer (.05 M, pH 8.1 containing .25 M NaCl) and eluted with the same buffer. The single step eluate is then treated with ammonium sulfate and acetone as outlined above for bacterial culture fluids.

The molecular weight of fecal IgA protease is approximately 40-60,000 based on centrifugation in sucrose density

gradient using appropriate marker proteins of known molecular weight. The enzyme is active in the pH range 6.5-8.5
and is irreversibly inactivated when heated to 55° C for 30
minutes at pH 8.1. Enzyme activity is fully inhibited in
5 mM ethylendiaminetetraacetic acid (EDTA), indicating that
activity is metal dependent. Following removal of EDTA by
dialysis, activity can be restored by Zn^{2+}, Co^{2+}, or Mn^{2+};
Ca^{2+} and Mg^{2+} are less effective, and other bivalent cations
are difficult to evaluate because they appear to alter the
IgA substrate. 10 mM diisopropylfluorophosphate (DFP) has
no effect on IgA protease activity, indicating that it is
not a serine endopeptidase. No formal comparison of fecal
enzyme with that elaborated by S. sanguis has as yet been
undertaken, but both exhibit resistance to DFP inhibition
and are EDTA sensitive.

The specificity of the enzyme is quite restricted.
Partially purified naturally occurring (fecal) preparations
having potent IgA cleaving activity also act on human colostral IgA to produce Fab_α and Fc_α fragments. IgA protease
does not appear to cleave human IgG or IgM, but a complete
absence of such activity has not been established with certainty. Active enzyme does not significantly cleave
classical protease substrates, e.g. casein, gelatin, or Azo-
coll. Using the ninhydrin reaction (4) to detect exposure
of newly exposed α-amino groups, IgA protease does not cleave
the synthetic peptides $CBZ-gly-L-phe-NH_2$ or $hip-L-leu-NH_2$,
dipeptides selected because they are suitable substrates for
other metal-dependent extracellular bacterial proteases. The
present lack of a suitable substrate for the rapid, quantitative assay of IgA protease is hampering attempts to isolate
and characterize the enzyme.

                              DISCUSSION

Although characterization of IgA protease is still incomplete, it functions in catalytic amounts to cleave IgA at
the hinge region and thus may be regarded as an endopeptidase.
Its inhibition by metal chelating agents but not DFP and its
optimal function at neutral pH are characteristics of certain
other bacterial endopeptidases (5), among which are thermolysin
(from B. thermolyticus), neutral proteases of B. subtilis and
B. megaterium, proteases produced by certain fungi of the
genera Aspergillus and Streptomyces, and collagenases elaborated by several microbial species. In our hands, commer-

cial preparations of thermolysin and B. subtilis neutral
protease readily cleave IgA, but do not produce an Fc_α fragment. Most bacterial neutral proteases require Ca^{2+} for
stability (but probably not for catalytic action) and can
hydrolyze casein and certain dipeptide substrates. The
markedly restricted specificity of IgA protease suggests
that it may be more akin to collagenase-type enzymes.

The location of IgA protease in human alimentary tract
fluids correlates with high bacteria populations in dental
plaque, saliva, and feces, and activity is absent in fluids
less exposed to bacteria. The presence of Fc_α fragments in
normal feces and the capacity of unconcentrated saliva or
fecal fluid to cleave secretory IgA suggests a potential
role for this enzyme in the secretory immune system. At
this time, the nature of this role is unknown.

Supported by USPHS (NIH) Grants AM AI 16607, DE 02814,
and AM 10419 and Research Career Development Award AI 70420
(to Dr. Plaut).

REFERENCES

1. Mehta, S. K., Plaut, A. G., Calvanico, N. J. and Tomasi,
      T. B., Jr., J. Immunol., in press.
2. Edelstein, S. J. and Schachman, H. K., J. Biol. Chem.,
      242: 306, 1967.
3. Carlsson, J., Caries Res., 4: 305, 1970.
4. Williams, C. A. and Chase, M. W. (editors), in Methods
      in Immunology and Immunochemistry, Vol. II, p. 275,
      Academic Press, New York, 1968.
5. Matsubara, H. and Feder, J., in The Enzymes. Edited
      by P. D. Boyer, Vol. III, p. 765, Academic Press, New
      York, 1971.

PRECIPITIN CROSS-REACITONS BETWEEN HUMAN AND ANIMAL J-CHAINS

J.P. Vaerman,* K. Kobayashi,** and J.F. Heremans*

Dept. of Experimental Medicine,* Univ. Catholique
de Louvain, Brussels, Belgium, Dept of Biochemistry,** Hokkaido University, Sapporo, Hokkaido,
Japan

INTRODUCTION

The J-polypeptide chain of polymeric IgA, secretory IgA
and/or IgM has been identified in the human (1,2), dog (3),
rabbit (1), mouse (4), pig (5), bovine (6), sheep (7), phea-
sant, toad, catfish (8), shark (9), chicken, rat, but not in
tortoise (10) by means of gel electrophoresis in alkaline urea
of the reduced-alkylated or S-sulfonated immunoglobulins.
The finding of J-chain in such phylogenetically distant species as catfish and shark, points to the primitive character
of this polypeptide (8,9).

The close similarity in amino acid composition of
J-chains from human (2), rabbit (11), canine (3) and porcine
(5) origin, as well as the reported serological cross-
reaction between human and canine J-chains (3), has led us
to investigate whether J-chains from many animal species
would cross-react with human J-chains.

MATERIALS AND METHODS

<u>Antisera</u>. Two rabbits were repeatedly (more than 10-
times) injected with 0.25-0.5 mg of purified J-chains from
S-sulfonated human secretory IgA (12). The antisera were
absorbed by means of glutaraldehyde insolubilized human
serum and L-chains. Specificity was checked by the absence
of reaction with human serum, milk, L-chains and α-chains,
and by the presence of a single and strong precipitin line

upon diffusion against human J-chains obtained by S-sulfona-
tion (12) and complete reduction-alkylation (13) of polymeric
immunoglobulins (Fig. 1,1).

Isolation or Partial Purification of Polymeric Animal Igs

Dog. SIgA was isolated from canine milk (14) and monoclonal IgA from a myeloma serum (3); polyclonal IgM was
partially purified from normal serum by euglobulin precipitation followed by gel-filtration on Sepharose 6B.
  Cat and hedgehog. DEAE and Sephadex G 200-fractions of
serum containing polyclonal IgM and polymeric IgA (15) were
used after concentration by salting-out.
  Bovine, goat, sheep, pig and horse. Polyclonal serum IgM
was obtained by salting-out (35% saturated ammonium sulfate)
DEAE-fractions eluted at high ionic strengths (15); S-IgAwas
provided by Sephadex G 200-fractions of colostrum or milk
(15).
  Guinea-pig. SIgA was isolated from milk (16) and IgM was
partially purified from normal serum as for the dog.
  Rat. Monoclonal IgA and IgM were isolated from the sera
and ascites of LOU/Ws1 rats bearing transplantable immunocy-
tomas (17). Polyclonal IgM was partially purified from the
sera of rats parasitized with Trypanosoma brucei, by gel
filtration and euglobulin precipitation.
  Mouse. Polyclonal IgM was obtained as for rats and monoclonal polymeric MOPC-315 IgA was partially purified from
serum by Sephadex G 200 and removal of euglobulins.
  Chicken. IgM and SIgA were isolated from normal serum and
bile, respectively (18).
  Tortoise IgM was purified from serum (19).

    All the samples were analyzed by agarose-gel electro-
phoresis and immunoelectrophoreses, using specific antisera
(14), to verify the presence of large amounts of IgM, IgA
or both, and to evaluate the relative proportions of IgA
and/or IgM, as compared to other proteins.

Preparation of Animal J-Chains

    The purified and enriched immunoglobulin solutions were
dialyzed against 5M guanidine-HCl buffered at pH 8.0 with
solid Tris. After reduction (0.03 M dithiothreitol) and
alkylation (.10 M iodoacetamide), the samples were further
dialyzed against saline, centrifuged at high speed, and the
supernatants were concentrated by lyophilisation.

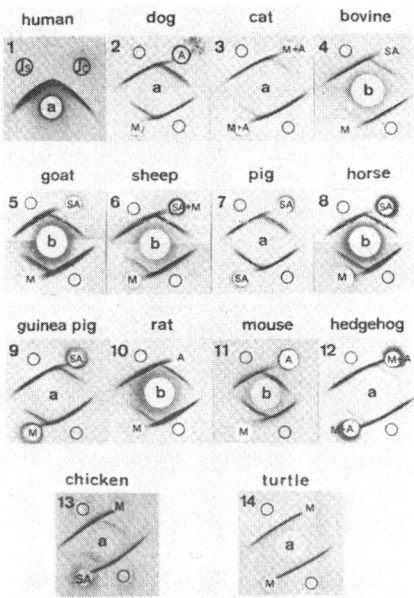

Fig. 1 - Ouchterlony analyses of human and animal J-chains
with anti J-chain (a) or (b). Js, Jc: human J-chains obtained
from S-sulfonated and completely reduced-alkylated polymeric
immunoglobulins, respectively; A: polymeric serum IgA;
M: IgM; SA: secretory IgA.
Unmarked wells received human J-chains.

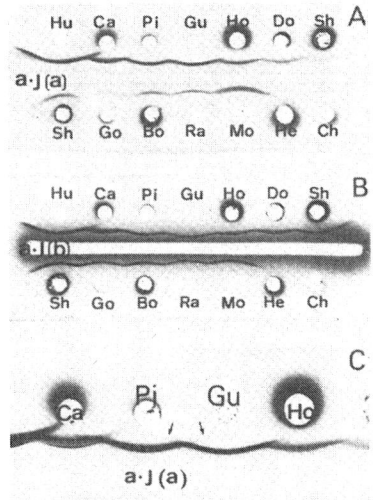

Fig. 2 - Cross-reactions given by anti J-chain antisera.
Hu: Human; Ca: Cat; Pi: Pig; Gu: Guinea-pig; Ho: Horse;
Do: Dog; Sh: Sheep, Go: Goat; Bo: Bovine; Ra: Rat;
Mo: Mouse; He: Hedgehog; Ch: Chicken. C is an enlargement
of a part of A, to emphasize spurs and double spurs (arrows).

RESULTS

Typical cross-reactions between human and animal J-chains including dog, cat, bovine, goat, sheep, pig, horse, hedgehog, guinea-pig, rat, mouse and chicken, are illustrated in Figure 1, 2-13. The specificity of these cross-reactions was confirmed by the patterns of partial identity with human J-chains and by the disappearance of all reactions after absorption of the antisera with purified human J-chains. No reactions were observed with any of the unreduced animal immunoglobulins.

One of the antisera failed to precipitate with the chicken and hedgehog J-chains (Fig. 2B), whereas both failed to react with the tortoise J-chains (Fig.1,14). Surprisingly, all cross-reactions obtained with antiserum anti-J (b) displayed apparent reactions of identity among each other (Fig. 2,B), whereas cross-reactions with anti-J (a) gave rise to distinct spurs (Fig.2, A and C).

DISCUSSION

The wide cross-reactions observed between human and animal J-chains confirm the chemical similarities already reported and suggest that large homologies will be found between the amino acid sequences of these J-chains. The fact that even fowl J-chain cross-reacted with human J-chain is noteworthy. A cross-reaction between fowl and human μ-chains, but not γ-chains has been detected suggesting that μ-chain genes may have been preserved during evolution (20). Similarly, our data support the hypothesis that the J-chain may be a polypeptide of great evolutionary stability. Whether or not this is related to the putative biological function of stabilizing polymeric immunoglobulins remains a matter of speculation.

REFERENCES

1. Halpern, M.S. and Koshland, M.E., Nature 228:1276, 1970.
2. Mestecky, J., Zikan, J. and Butler, W.T., Science 171: 1163, 1971.
3. Kehoe, J.M., Tomasi, T.B., Ellouz, F. and Capra, D., J. Immunol. 109:59, 1972.
4. Parkhouse, R.M.E., Nature-New Biology 236:9, 1972.
5. Zikan, J., Immunochemistry 10:351, 1973.
6. Butler, J.E., Biochim, Biophys. Acta 251:435, 1971.

7.   Heimer, R., Jones, D.W. and Maurer, P.H., Biochemistry
     8:3937, 1969.
8.   Weinheimer, P.F., Mestecky, J. and Acton, R.T.,
     J. Immunol. 107:1211, 1971.
9.   Klaus, G.G.B., Halpern, M.S., Koshland, M.E. and
     Goodman, J.W., J. Immunol. 107:1785, 1971.
10. Vaerman, J.P., Lebacq-Verheyden, A.M., Bazin, H. and
     Heremans, J.F., Unpublished results.
11. O'Daly, J.A. and Cebra, J.J., Biochemistry 10:3843, 1971.
12. Kobayashi, K., Vaerman, J.P. and Heremans, J.F., Biochim.
     Biophys. Acta 303:105, 1973.
13. Kobayashi, K., Vaerman, J.P. and Heremans, J.F.,
     Immunochemistry (In press).
14. Reynolds, H.Y. and Johnson, J.S., Biochemistry 10:2821,
     1971.
15. Vaerman, J.P., Studies on IgA Immunoglobulins in Man
     and Animals, Sintal, Louvain, 1970.
16. Vaerman, J.P. and Heremans, J.F., J. Immunol. 108:637,
     1972.
17. Bazin, H., Deckers, C., Beckers, A. and Heremans, J.F.,
     Int. J. Cancer 10:568, 1972.
18. Lebacq-Verheyden, A.M., Vaerman, J.P. and Heremans, J.F.,
     Immunology 22:165, 1972.
19. Acton, R.T., Weinheimer, P.F., Shelton, E., Niedermeier,
     W. and Bennett, J.C., Immunochemistry 9:421, 1972.
20. Mehta, P.D., Reichlin, M. and Tomasi, T.B., J. Immunol.
     109:1272, 1972.

Acknowledgement: Fig. 1 and 2 are published with the permission from The Williams & Wilkins Co., Baltimore (10/12/73).

DISULFIDE BRIDGES OF HUMAN IMMUNOGLOBULINS A$_1$ AND A$_2$

C. Wolfenstein-Todel, E. Mendez, F. Prelli,
B. Frangione and E.C. Franklin

New York University School of Medicine
550 First Avenue, New York, N.Y.   10016

We have previously reported the sequences of the peptides containing the labile disulfide bridges of IgA1 (1) and IgA2, Am2(+) (2). In order to further characterize the similarities and differences between these subclasses, we have now extended our studies to an examination of all the disulfide bridges of these molecules.

The partially reduced and alkylated heavy chains were completely reduced and carboxymethylated with (^{14}C) iodoacetic acid, and subjected to trypsin digestions. The soluble tryptic peptides were fractionated on Sephadex G-50 and purified. The insoluble material was further digested with pepsin and the radioactive peptides were isolated. Table I shows a comparison of the sequences obtained from the constant region. The peptides clearly belonging to the variable region have not been included. Five of the peptides (T1, T2, T3, TP4 and TP5) appear to be present in both subclasses besides the previously reported C-terminal peptide (2,3).

Three additional peptides (T6, T7, and T8) showed a high degree of homology. Peptides T2, T3 and T7 were also obtained by Moore and Putnam (4) from another IgA1 protein. Hence, all of these probably belong to the constant region of the α1 and α2 chain respectively, and account for a total of 13 cysteines. Peptide T9, which contains the heavy-light disulfide bridge (1) was identified in two different IgA1 myeloma proteins, and thus it too can be located in the constant region of the human α1 chain.

Peptide T9 from IgA2 does not show any apparent homology with any of the peptides reported for IgA1. Its complete sequence has not been established, but it probably contains the previously reported peptide Pro(Asp,Cys,Thr, Glu_2,Pro,Gly_2,Ala,His). The peptide T10 obtained from IgA2 does not show any homology either, but it could contain peptide TP5, isolated from both IgA1 and IgA2.

Peptide T8 includes the previously described "Hinge" region (1,2,5), but its sequence has now been extended at its N-terminal end, where the homology is maintained. The "hinge" peptide of IgA2, Am2(+) differs from that of IgA1 since it lacks carbohydrate and has a gap of about 13 residues, just in the place where duplication of a small fragment was identified in A1 molecules.

Because of the presence of 3 cysteines in such close proximity and of the clustering of interchain disulfide bridges of the hinge in the subclasses of IgG, the arrangement of disulfide bridges in this region of the molecule was studied by diagonal electrophoresis. For this purpose, an IgA1 myeloma protein was digested with pepsin followed by trypsin, and fractionated on Sephadex G-50. The first peak was further digested with subtilisin and studied by diagonal electrophoresis at pH 3.5. Two sets of cysteic acid-containing peptides were obtained.

Two peptides were present in the same region of the paper: TPS 1a: Val-Thr-Val-Pro-Cys-Pro-Val-Pro-Ser-Thr-Pro-Pro-Thr-Pro-Ser-Pro-Ser-Thr-Pro-Pro-Thr-Pro(Ser,Pro,Ser) and TPS 1b: Cys-Leu-Ala. Since they run together in the first dimension on electrophoresis, and only separate after oxidation, they must have been originally bound to each other by a disulfide bridge:

Val-Thr-Val-Pro-Cys-Pro-Val-Pro-Ser-Thr-Pro-Pro-Thr-Pro...
                    |
                    Cys-Leu-Ala

The sequence Cys-Leu-Ala is included in the peptide: Pro-Ala-Thr-Gln-Cys-Leu-Ala-Gly-Ser-Lys, which represents a portion of peptide T6 (Table I) and was isolated from the same first peak eluted from Sephadex G-50. This peptide is probably derived from the Fd region since it is absent from an α chain disease protein.

The other set of cysteic acid peptides also contained two main ones: Cys-Cys-His-Pro-Arg and Asp-Leu-Cys-Gly-Cys. In addition two other peptides derived from these were isolated from the same region of the paper, but in low yield: These are (Cys,His,Pro)Arg and (Asp,Leu,Cys,Gly). Based on the different yield of the peptides, it seems likely that the last two are bound to each other by a disulfide bridge:

$$
\begin{array}{c}
\text{Cys-His-Pro-Arg} \\
| \\
\text{Asp-Leu-Cys-Gly}
\end{array}
$$

This intrachain bridge is probably located in the Fc fragment since the peptide Asp-Leu-Cys-Gly-Cys can be recovered from an α chain disease protein.

In the absence of definitive data, the following models can be proposed for the carboxy terminal end of the hinge of IgA1:

1) Two symmetric interchain and 1 intrachain bridge per α chain

```
    ┌──────────────┐
 -Cys-Cys-His-Pro-Arg    Asp-Leu-Cys-Gly-Cys
    |      ┌──────────────────────────┐  |
 -Cys-Cys-His-Pro-Arg    Asp-Leu-Cys-Gly-Cys
```

2) Two labile intrachain bridges per α chain

```
    ┌──────────────────────────┐
 -Cys-Cys-His-Pro-Arg    Asp-Leu-Cys-Gly-Cys
    └──────────────────────────────────────┘
```

3) Four asymmetrical interchain bridges:

```
 ─►Cys-Cys-His-Pro-Arg    Asp-Leu-Cys-Gly-Cys─►
      |       ＼               ＼         |
 ◄─Cys-Gly-Cys-Leu-Asp    Arg-Pro-His-Cys-Cys◄─
```

Since Abel and Grey (6) isolated the "hinge" peptide both as monomer and dimer, we can discard model 2, leaving models 1 and 3. Model 3 is unlikely since it would require an anti-parallel arrangement which has not been noted in any immunoglobulin to date. Taking the total hinge and associated peptides there would appear to be 2 interchain bridges and 2 intrachain disulfide bridges per α chain (Fig. 1) (Model 1). Model 3 which is less likely would yield 4 asymmetric interchain bridges and 1 intrachain disulfide bridge per α chain.

TABLE I

Comparison of Sequences around the Disulfide Bridges of IgA1 and IgA2,Am2(+)

Subclass	Peptide	Sequence[a]
A1 – A2	T1	K G N T F S C M V G H E A L P L A F T E K
A1 – A2	T2	L S L(H.R)P A L(Z.D.L.L.L.G.S.E.A.B.L.T.C.T.L.T.G.L.)R
A1 – A2	T3	S V T C H V K
A1 – A2	TP4	A C L
A1 – A2	TP5	T C L A R
A1 – A2	b	A E V D G T C Y
A1	T6	D L C G C Y S V S S V L P G C A E P H G B K
A2	T6	(Z.P.H,T,T,Z,A,F)K
A1	T7	N F P P S E D A S G D L Y T T S S Z L T L P A T Q C L A G S K
A2	T7	(—)— P D G K
A1	T8	(H)P T N P S E D V T V P C P V P S T P P T S P S T P P T P(S,P,S)C C H P R
A2	T8	H Y ——— GAP ——— P P P P C C H P R
A1	b	T F T C T A A Y P E S K
A2	b	T(C.T.A.A.H.P.E.L)K
A1	T9	S L C S T Z P B G B(C,B,T,Z,P,P,P,G,G,A,A,V,L,L,L,F,F,I,Y.)K
A2	T9	L A G D P(B,C,T,T,S,S,Z,Z,G,G,A,A,V,M,L,L,L,H,K,R)
A2	T10	G Z B(C,B,T,T,S,Z,A,A,V,L,)R

a – Identical sequences are indicated with solid lines.

b – Previously reported (1-3)

```
  ┌──────────┐   ┌─────┐
Cys-Leu-Ala...—Cys—...—Cys-Cys—...Asp-Leu-Cys-Gly-Cys
                            │                  │
Cys-Leu-Ala...—Cys—...—Cys-Cys—...Asp-Leu-Cys-Gly-Cys
  └──────────────────┘   └───────────────────┘
```

Figure 1:   Model of the Hinge Region of IgA1

In the case of IgA2, Am2(+), the "hinge" peptide was resistant to further proteolysis and could not be split by subtilisin digestion. After diagonal electrophoresis at pH 3.5, two other peptides were found in the same region of the paper (2); Glx-Cys-Pro-Asp-Gly-Lys and Asp-Leu-Cys-Gly-Cys. The carboxy terminal sequence of the hinge peptide of IgA1 and of IgA2, Am2(+) is the same. Thus it seems probable that the structure proposed for IgA1 applies also to IgA2. The peptide Glx-Cys-Pro-Asp-Gly-Lys is located in a region with striking homology (peptide T7, Table I) to the one con- taining the sequence Cys-Leu-Ala which was found to be bound to the first cysteine of the "hinge" in IgA1. Hence it seems likely that it too forms an intrachain disulfide bridge with the corresponding cysteine in the "hinge" of IgA2, Am2(+).

In conclusion, in spite of some differences in the amino acid sequence of the hinge of the α1 and α2 chains, their 3 dimensional arrangement appears to be similar and to involve an unusual degree of folding not yet noted in other classes of immunoglobulins.

REFERENCES

1. Wolfenstein, C., Frangione, B., Mihaesco, E. and Franklin, E.C., Biochemistry 10:4140, 1971.
2. Wolfenstein-Todel, C., Frangione, B. and Franklin, E.C., Biochemistry 11:3971, 1972.
3. Prahl, J.W., Abel, C.A. and Grey, H.M., Biochemistry 10:1808, 1971.
4. Moore, V. and Putnam, F.W., Biochemistry 12:2361, 1973.
5. Frangione, B. and Wolfenstein-Todel, C., Proc. Natl. Acad. Sci. USA 69:3673, 1972.
6. Abel, C.A. and Grey, H.M., Nature (London) 223:29, 1971.

DISCUSSION

Dr. Mestecky - The partial primary sequence of bovine secretory component was presented several years ago. Is there any sequence homology between human and bovine secretory components?

Dr. Tomasi - Data obtained by Dr. Capra and myself on the primary structure of bovine secretory component (A) isolated in its free form from bovine colostrum were compared with the data obtained by Cunningham-Rundles et al. on the human secretory component (B).

	1	2	3	4	5	6	7	8	9	10	11	12	13	14	15
A.	Lys	Ser	Pro	Ile	Phe	Gly	—	—	—	Asp	Val	Asp	Ser	Val	Asp	Gly
B.	Lys	Ser	Pro	Ile	Phe	Gly	Pro	Glu	Glu	Val	Asp	Ser	Val	Glu	Gly

Important points in this comparison are as follows: There appears to be a deletion at position 7 and 8 in the bovine protein. The proteins are aligned in order to maximize homology. Eleven of the 13 residues in the two proteins are identical. The two differences at positions 9 and 14 are one base changes involving a glutamate - aspartate. There appears to be considerable homology in the N-terminal region of these two proteins. This finding is consistent with recent studies in our laboratory showing that immunological cross reactions exist between these two proteins using an antibovine secretory component antiserum.

Dr. Kunkel - I want to ask Dr. Vaerman whether he tested rabbit J chain. He immunized the rabbit, and if you are going to interpret this in an evolutionary sense, you have to think that the rabbit J chain would also be very similar. Then the question comes up, how did you get antibodies? Do you have any data on that, Dr. Vaerman?

Dr. Vaerman - We tested the rabbit J chain obtained from IgM preparations and treated similarly, but we could find no reaction with the rabbit J chain.

Dr. Kunkel - This also suggests that the homology is not as great as you might think.

Dr. Good - I just think we must not let Dr. Vaerman sit
down with such an extraordinary finding before we really
understand it. If I understood him correctly, this is
really unique. He mentioned that the cross reaction to an
IgM had extended far down in phylogeny. I wonder whether
or not that was really a cross reaction to a J chain in that
IgM. We have looked over the phylogenetic range for relationships to all of the other immunoglobulins, one to another, and when you get down as far as the fishes, you see
just no cross reactivity with human immunoglobulins. Here
research tells us that cross reactions to J chains go all
down the phylogenetic scale. This kind of cross reactivity
one sees only with histones and DNA. This brings up a clinical question. Have you looked, for example, in lupus
patients for antibodies to the J chain? Such might be a
fruitful search.

Dr. Vaerman - The answer is no.

Dr. Wang - I have a comment in regard to Dr. Capra's report.
Dr. Capra mentioned that he found specific high percentage
of the VHIII heavy chains among IgA myeloma proteins he examined. Actually, we pointed out the preferential association between VHIII subgroup and alpha chains two years ago
in a paper in Proceedings of the National Academy of Science
in 1971. Since then, we have analyzed heavy chains of IgA
isolated from normal individuals using two different methods
for isolation. One is the conventional method, that is, to
use sodium sulfate precipitation followed by ion exchange
chromatography and followed by gel filtration. The normal
IgA heavy chain prepared this way had a figure of about 33%
VHIII versus about 20% for IgG heavy chains. The second
isolation method is by immunoabsorption,using a column of
conjugated anti-IgA. The IgA heavy chain from normal persons isolated in the manner have about 40-45% VHIII which is
approximately twice as high as that found in IgG.

Dr. Hanson - I was very interested in the communication of
Dr. Plaut since we have in cooperation with Dr. Motas from
Romania been using a reductase described by Tietze and isolated from rabbit liver to degrade secretory IgA. That
reductase causes secretory IgA to fall apart into 7S IgA and
some free secretory component. Now, similar reductases are
produced by many E. coli strains. I wonder if it could be
poooiblc that in the maLerial that Dr. Plaut worked with
such reductases could be present as well, and start the

reaction by having the secretory IgA turn into 7S IgA
which would be more prone to be degraded by the proteolytic
enzyme that he describes. Also, I would like to ask him
whether he knows what kind of microorganism produces this
enzyme and whether it is commonly found.

Dr. Plaut - The point raised in the first instance as to
whether this possibly is two enzymes is one that we have
not rigorously excluded although all the evidence at the
moment, while purification is going on, suggests that there
is one. I might also add that I don't know whether your
reductase is a metal dependent enzyme. Do you know?

Dr. Hanson - Not that I know.

Dr. Plaut - Our enzyme, if treated with EDTA, entirely loses
its activity. Whether there are two enzymes there or not,
I cannot say for sure. Secondly, the type of organism that
produces this enzyme is something that Dr. Genco and I are
now studying in great detail. At the moment I can tell you
that Streptococcus sanguis is catalog #10556 from the
American Type Culture Collection. Streptococcus sanguis,
10557 from A.T.C.C., does not definitely elaborate the enzyme as far as we can tell, and so there is a considerable
amount of variability involved in which species do so.
S. mutans is negative.

Dr. Butler - I would add to Dr. Tomasi's comment concerning
the similarity of secretory components. We have obtained
cross reactivity among secretory components of different
species. Antiserum to bovine secretory component cross
reacts most strongly with that from the sheep and goat, and
cross reacts to a lesser extent with human and porcine secretory components. At present, we have not obtained cross
reactivities with any of the rodent secretory components,
particularly rat secretory component which has been isolated
in my laboratory.

Dr. Dawes - I would like to ask Dr. Abraham how he collected
the saliva from this one patient—whether in fact, the saliva
was collected directly from one or another salivary gland
or whether it was whole saliva.

Dr. Abraham - We need a stimulatory procedure in a patient
with Sjögren's disease. We simply admitted the patient to
our clinical research center and just asked her to spit

for 24 hours, and we obtained a total of approximately 10
or 11 ml of saliva.

Dr. Dawes - There is one possibility which I would like to
ask Dr. Abraham about. These patients with Sjögren's
disease, as he mentioned, have very low flow rates particularly from the parotid glands. They usually have a very
poor state of oral health, inflamed gingivae, and high flow
rate of gingival crevice fluid. Is it possible that in
this patient there was a flow of plasma IgA from the gingival
crevice into the mixed saliva that perhaps combined with
some free secretory component?

Dr. Abraham - The answer to that is no. The experiment
showed that the IgA was combined with secretory component.
It would be highly unlikely, if it were a serum transudate,
that there would be no IgG contaminating it, especially since
the patient was hyper-IgG-globulinemic to about 2,500 mg%.

Dr. Dawes - Thank you. Could I ask Dr. Plaut one question,
please? If one collects a mixed sample of saliva, what will
be the half-life of IgA in that saliva in view of your finding of the proteolytic enzyme? Normally, of course, the
saliva is continually replaced in the mouth and swallowed and
we need to know this to assess whether the proteolytic enzyme
could have importance in the oral cavity.

Dr. Plaut - At the moment I cannot recall if the half-life
of IgA in saliva has been studied. It is a continuously
flowing system, which would make its study difficult and
half-life hard to interpret.

Dr. Dawes - The implication from your talk as I perceived it
was that it was possible that the secreted IgA that comes
into the oral cavity could be broken down quite quickly by
this proteolytic enzyme.

Dr. Plaut - Unconcentrated saliva takes time to split IgA;
in other words, it takes 10 to 12 hours to give a significant
split of IgA in our standard system which contains IgA at
4 milligrams per ml. I don't know if that helps to answer
your question or not. Dr. Mestecky, I wonder if I could
take this opportunity to point out something that I should
have emphasized, and that is the difficulty of detecting
proteolysis of IgA on immunoelectrophoresis. I mentioned
that this can be circumvented to some extent by using IgAs

of slow electrophoretic mobility because the Fc fragment, as
has been shown years ago for IgG, is of the same mobility
in all the IgAs we've studied. So an electrophoretically
slow IgA is the best substrate since the mobility of the
released Fc is much faster relative to unsplit substrate.

Dr. Fudenberg - I make this comment only because I assume
the Proceedings here will be published. Upon listening
to the J-chain data presented today, I think there is one
reference which should be included in the volume. Eight
or nine years ago, Suzuki and Deutsch published a paper
saying that the molecular weight of subunits of IgM did
not add up to the total molecular weight of the parent
molecule, and pointed out that something else must also be
present. Because of the erroneous molecular weight of light
chains in the literature at that time, they felt it represented extra L-chains. "At that point in time," (pardon
the expression) everyone scoffed at this and said it could
not be so as it went against the prevailing dogma; therefore,
Deutsch did not publish similar data regarding the polymer
IgA. Their molecular weights corresponded approximately to
several J-pieces per IgM molecule. Therefore, if these
Proceedings are going to be published, I think the Suzuki
and Deutsch reference should be included with new interpretations of their data (Suzuki, T. and Deutsch, H.F., J. biol.
Chem. 242:2725, 1967).

SESSION D

FUNCTION

CHAIRMAN: FREDERICK W. KRAUS

IMPLICATIONS OF SECRETORY IMMUNE SYSTEM IN VIRAL INFECTIONS

P.L. Ogra, R.B. Wallace, G. Umana, S.S. Ogra,
D. Kerr Grant and A. Morag

Departments of Pediatrics and Microbiology,
State University of New York at Buffalo and
University of Iowa, Iowa City
Division of Virology, Children's Hospital, 219
Bryant Street, Buffalo, New York 14222

Considerable evidence is available to suggest that secretory immunoglobulins play an important role in protection
against certain viral diseases (1). The extent of the secretory immune response elicited at an external mucosal surface
and its relative contribution in the mechanisms of antiviral
immunity seems to be intimately related to pathogenesis and
course of the viral infection (2). The development and biologic function of various secretory immunoglobulins, particularly secretory γA has been studied extensively after naturally acquired infections or after immunization with live attenuated or inactivated viral vaccines. Antibody activity against
viral antigens has been demonstrated in several organs and
external mucosal tissues (1-6). The development of specific
secretory immunity in different tissues after infection with
some of these viruses is discussed below.

DEVELOPMENT OF VIRAL SPECIFIC SECRETORY ANTIBODY

Poliovirus. After immunization with live attenuated
poliovaccine (Sabin) administered orally, and inactivated vaccine (Salk) inoculated parenterally, it was demonstrated that
serum γM, γG and γA responses were strikingly similar with
either type and route of immunization (7). However, secretory antibody response to poliovirus appeared in the nasopharynx and alimentary tract following oral immunization with the
live vaccine. The antibody was first detected 2-3 weeks after
immunization and persisted, in stable titers, for as long as

5 years to date (7). Although no secretory antibody response
was observed in the nasopharynx and alimentary tract after
parenteral immunization with inactivated vaccine, intranasal
instillation of this vaccine resulted in prompt induction of
secretory γA response in the nasopharynx, with little or no
response in serum immunoglobulins (8). The secretory response
after intranasal immunization with inactivated vaccine was
transient. Detectable antibody levels persisted in the nasopharynx for 3-4 months, and no evidence of anamestic response
was observed after reimmunization. In another series of experiments in infants with double barrelled surgical colostomy,
local immunization of distal colon with live poliovaccine
resulted in a specific γA poliovirus antibody response largely
confined to the immunized distal colon. Lesser titers of γA
antibody were observed in the non-immunized proximal segments
of colon, and no antibody activity was found in the non-
immunized nasopharynx. Despite these differences in the
antibody response in different segments of alimentary tract,
all patients manifested an antibody response in serum γG, γA,
and γM immunoglobulin which was comparable to the response
obtained after oral feeding of poliovaccine in normal children
(9). Immunization of distal colon with inactivated poliovaccine resulted in the appearance of poliovirus specific
secretory antibody response confined to the immunized segment
without any response in the non-immunized areas of colon,
nasopharynx or in the serum (9).

In similar studies local antibody response to poliovirus
was observed in the human female genital tract following local
immunization with inactivated poliovaccine (5). The response
after intravaginal immunization was characterized by the
appearance of γA and infrequently γG poliovirus antibody in
the vagina within 7 days of local immunization. Intrauterine
immunization resulted in the appearance of antibody response
in the uterus, which was essentially limited to γG immunoglobulin, with little or no γA antibody response. No antibody
response was observed in the nasopharynx and serum after
genital immunization. Intramuscular immunization with inactivated vaccine resulted in the appearance of γG response
in the genital tract, 2-5 weeks after immunization, and the
response was correlated with the height of γG response in
the serum (5).

Other investigations have provided evidence for the existence of secretory immune system and local antibody production

in the mucosa of middle ear in patients with secretory otitis
media (6). Paired specimens of serum and middle ear fluid
obtained from children with secretory otitis media were tested
for the distribution and proportions of antibody activity
against polio and other viruses in the major classes of immunoglobulins. These children had been previously immunized
with live poliovaccine or infected or immunized against mumps,
measles or rubella virus. The predominant viral specific
antibody activity in the serum was associated with γG,
although low levels of γA antibody were also found frequently.
On the other hand, antibody activity in the middle ear against
the viruses listed above, was predominantly associated with
γA immunoglobulin. The ratios of γG:γA antibody in the middle
ear ranged from 1:1 to 1:6, while their ratios in the serum
ranged from 10:1 to 10:3 respectively (Table 1).

TABLE 1

The ratio of γG:γA antibody activity against poliovirus type
I, mumps, measles and rubella viruses in human serum and
middle ear fluids.

	Mean Ratio of γG:γA Antibody	
	Serum	Middle Ear
Poliovirus type I	10:2	1:4
Mumps	10:1	1:2
Measles	10:1	1:1
Rubella	10:3	1:6

In order to define the nature of local antibody production in the central nervous system, groups of rhesus monkeys
were immunized with live virulent (Mahoney) type I poliovirus,
Sabin or Salk vaccine administered intrathalamically, orally
or intranasally. Intrathalamic immunization with live virulent virus resulted in the appearance of γG specific poliovirus
antibody in the central nervous system with little or no antibody response in the serum. Highest antibody activity was
found in those areas of brain and spinal cord which were char-
acteristically affected by poliomyelitis infection (Table 2).
In addition, mononuclear cells staining specifically for γG
immunoglobulin were regularly observed in those areas of brain
which contained γG poliovirus antibody. No γM or γA poliovirus
antibody or immunoglobulin containing cells were observed in
the brains of infected monkeys. No immunoglobulins or immuno-

competent lymphoid tissue could be detected in the brains of
normal or sham immunized monkeys (10).

These observations suggest that many internal organs and
external mucosal surfaces have the capacity to display local
immunologic responses, which when elicited by local application
of the antigen, are quite independent of the systemic antibody
responses. The evidence presented strongly suggests that the
secretory antibody response to poliovirus in the nasopharynx
and alimentary tract is of γA type and is produced locally as
a result of availability of the viral antigen to the mucosal
immunocompetent cells. The induction of poliovirus specific
secretory antibody in local sites is determined to a large
extent by the route of immunization (parenteral or local),
type of viral antigen (live virulent, attenuated or inactivated) employed, and the type of immunocompetent tissue
available at the secretory sites.

TABLE 2

Distribution of poliovirus antibody and γG containing cellular
element in the central nervous system following intrathalamic
inoculation of live virulent (Mahoney) type I poliovirus.

	Poliovirus Antibody Titer[a]	γG Containing Cells
Nasopharynx	4	NT[b]
Serum	< 1	NT
Spinal Fluid	32	+[c]
Cervical Cord	64	+
Vermis	128	+
Thalamus	128	+
Occipital Cortex	< 1	0[d]

a   Expressed as reciprocal of dilution
b   Not Tested
c   Present
d   Absent

Hepatitis B Antigen (HB Ag). In addition to the parenteral route of transmission, acute viral hepatitis associated
with HB Ag can be acquired by non-parenteral or oral routes.
HB Ag was detected frequently in the serum, feces, nasopharynx and urine of patients with a naturally acquired HB Ag

infection. The amount of antigen detected in the secretions
was variable, although in many patients the antigen was found
in the feces for as long as 4 months after its initial detection. Anti-HB Ag antibody response in the serum was characterized by infrequent appearance of γG antibody which persisted for as long as 7 months. The antibody response in nasopharynx and feces was characterized by the development of γA
anti-HB Ag antibody activity 2-3 months after the detection
of antigen (11). The development of secretory antibody was
observed only in the secretions of those subjected who manifested high level of HB Ag in the secretions. Patients in whom
little or no HB Ag was detectable in secretions failed to manifest any secretory antibody response (Table 3). These observations further support the concept of local antibody production in the alimentary tract. Furthermore, these data suggest
that optimal concentrations of locally available antigen are
required for induction of detectable secretory antibody
responses.

TABLE 3

Relationship of the HB Ag titer in the feces to the subsequent
development of secretory antibody to HB Ag in feces.

Highest Titers of HB Ag in Feces	No. Patients Tested	No. Patients with Antibody Response to HB Ag in Feces
1:2[a]	4	0
1:4	3	1
1:8	2	1
1:32	3	3

a Expressed as reciprocal of dilution of fecal extract with
an initial immunoglobulin concentration of 80 mg/100 ml.

   Rubella Virus. In recent years, several types of live
attenuated rubella virus vaccines have been developed. Of
these, HPV-77 and Cendehill strains of rubella vaccine have
been licensed for routine use in this country, and RA27/3
strain has been extensively used in Europe. Careful analysis
of recent immunization data have revealed that although high
levels of serum antibody to rubella are regularly elicited
after parenteral immunization with HPV-77 or Cendehill vaccine,
approximately 80-85% of such vaccinees are susceptible to naso-

TABLE 4

Effect of re-infection challenge with wild (Brown) or live attenuated rubella vaccine (HPV-77, RA27) in subjects previously immunized with HPV-77 or RA27 live rubella vaccine.

Total No. Subjects Studied	Antigen and Route	Percent Subjects with Antibody Response		Antigen and Route	Percent Subjects with >4 fold Booster Effect		% of Subjects With Virus Shedding in Nasopharynx
		Serum γG	Nasopharynx γA		Serum γG	Nasopharynx γA	
16	HPV-77 S.C.[a]	100	6	Brown I.N.	93	100	75
15	HPV-77 S.C.	100	0	RA27 S.C.	6	20	0
15	HPV-77 S.C.	93	13	RA27 I.N.	21	66	13
25	RA27 S.C.	100	50	Brown I.N.	44	40	24
21	RA27 I.N.[b]	95	85	Brown I.N.	25	24	30
10	Natural	100	100	Brown I.N.	10	10	0

a HPV-77/DK-12 rubella vaccine administered subcutaneously
b RA27/3 rubella vaccine administered intranasally

pharyngeal reinfection with naturally occurring wild rubella
virus.   The incidence of such reinfection after natural disease is in the range of 1-2% (12-14). The implication of
secretory immune system in nasopharyngeal immunity to rubella
virus was studied in children after natural infection or immunization with HPV-77 or RA27/3 rubella virus vaccines (15).
Although the serum immunoglobulin response following naturally
acquired infection or immunization (regardless of its type or
route) was generally similar, the secretory response following
natural infection or intranasal immunization with RA27/3 was
characterized by the regular appearance of γA rubella antibody
in the nasopharynx.   However, little or on nasopharyngeal antibody activity was observed after subcutaneous immunization with
HPV-77 live rubella vaccine. Subsequent natural reinfection
in HPV-77 vaccinated subjects regularly resulted in booster
effect on pre-existing serum antibody levels, detectable
shedding of rubella virus from the nasopharynx or development
of significant nasopharyngeal γA antibody response as shown
in Table 4. Despite the lack of secretory response after
parenteral immunization with HPV-77 rubella vaccine,
subcutaneous immunization with RA27/3 rubella vaccine resulted
in the appearance of secretory γA antibody in at least 40-50%
of such vaccinees. It should be pointed out that intranasal
immunization with RA27/3 resulted in secretory antibody
response in approximately 75-80% of subjects (16). These
differences may indicate that in addition to the replicating
nature of immunizing vaccine and the route of administration,
certain other inherent properties of live attenuated virus
vaccines may enable them to preferentially distribute the
antigen to mucosal immunocompetent tissues and elicit specific
secretory antibody responses, particularly when the vaccines
are administered by a parenteral route of inoculation.

ANTIVIRAL FUNCTION OF SECRETORY γA

There is evidence to suggest that γA immunoglobulins
have viral neutralizing capacity (1) (2). Studies carried
out in man after natural or vaccine induced viral infections
and subsequent reinfection challenge, have provided indirect
evidence of in-vivo viral neutralizing activity for secretory
immunoglobulins at the external mucosal surfaces. Nasopharyngeal antibody induced as a result of intranasal immunization with inactivated poliovaccine prevents nasopharyngeal
colonization of poliovirus after oral reinfection with live
attenuated poliovaccine. Such inhibitory effect of nasopharyngeal antibody was demonstrated in the absence of a detect-

able poliovirus antibody activity in the serum (8). Similar
effects after nasopharyngeal reinfection with live attenuated
poliovirus were observed in infants with double barrelled
colostomy described earlier. Following initial immunization
in the distal colon, high levels of poliovirus γA antibody
were detectable in the immunized colon, but no antibody
activity was observed in the non-immunized nasopharynx. After
the closure of the colostomy, these infants were fed with live
poliovaccine administered orally. Virus excretion studies
after nasopharyngeal reinfection showed that non-immune nasopharynx became infected, but the immunized distal colon
manifested little or no shedding of the virus (9). These
observations suggest that locally immunized segments of
respiratory and alimentary tracts develop resistence to
colonization and replication of poliovirus. The locally
induced immunity appears to be associated with the development
of specific secretory γA antibody to poliovirus.

A relationship between nasopharyngeal immunity and
tonsils and adenoids was demonstrated in a study of poliovirus
antibody levels in serum and nasopharynx before and after
tonsilloadenoidectomy (T&A) in children immunized with live
poliovaccine. Secretory γA poliovirus antibody response was
present in all children before T&A. Following T&A pre-
existing nasopharyngeal antibody levels fell sharply with
mean antibody titers decreasing 3-4 fold. In some younger
children, the secretory antibody levels dropped 6-8 fold.
In addition, the nasopharyngeal antibody response in children
after T&A was found to be 2-4 fold lower than in children
with intact tonsils (17). The mechanism for the lowered
nasopharyngeal γA activity after T&A is not clear. It is
probable that removal of significant mass of lymphoid tissue,
particularly in younger children, may be a contributing factor.
These observations may partly explain the increased evidence
of paralytic polio following T&A (17).

The role of nasopharyngeal antibody in respiratory
immunity to rubella was studied in children after primary
immunization with HPV-77 or RA27 live attenuated rubella
virus vaccines or after prior natural infection. As discussed
earlier, the serum antibody response following either
immunization or infection were generally similar. However,
the nasopharyngeal γA antibody response was regularly observed after natural infection, intranasal immunization with
RA27 vaccine and frequently after subcutaneous RA27 immunization. Nasopharyngeal antibody rarely appeared after

immunization with HPV-77 vaccine (Table 4).   3-4 months after
primary immunization or infection, many subjects were re-
challenged with live virulent (Brown) or RA27 live attenuated
rubella virus administered intranasally or subcutaneously.
The incidence of reinfection, as evidenced by a four fold or
greater rise of pre-existing serum and nasopharyngeal antibody levels, and the detection or rubella virus in the nasopharyngeal secretions is presented in Table 4.   Highest
incidence (93%) of reinfection with live virulent (Brown)
rubella virus was observed in HPV-77 vaccinees. On the other
hand, only about 44% of subcutaneously immunized and 25% of
intranasally immunized RA27 vaccinees could be successfully
reinfected with virulent virus (Table 4).   The ability to
resist nasopharyngeal reinfection appeared to be closely
associated with the presence and the level of pre-existing
nasopharyngeal γA antibody.   These results suggest a role of
nasopharyngeal γA antobody in preventing or limiting the outcome of nasopharyngeal reinfection with rubella virus.   In
addition, nasopharyngeal and rarely subcutaneous reinfection
with RA27 live rubella virus in HPV-77 vaccines resulted in
a booster serum antibody response, and the development of
nasopharyngeal antibody.   Since successful booster immunization has not been observed after reinfection with HPV-77
rubella vaccine, these data suggest a potentially beneficial
use of intranasal reimmunization with RA27 rubella vaccine in
patients previously immunized with HPV-77 vaccine.

MUCOSAL IMMUNITY IN γA DEFICIENCY

The observations related in the preceeding sections
suggest a protective role of secretory γA antibody in viral
immunity.   However, it is well known that a small proportion
of normal human population is either markedly deficient or
totally lacking the γA immunoglobulins.   Such apparently
healthy subjects and other patients with γA deficiency syndrome do not seem to be unduly susceptible to recurrent viral
infections (18).   Several investigators have demonstrated
that γA deficient mucosal tissues are quantitatively replaced
by cells containing γM and γG immunoglobulins, particularly
in the alimentary tract (19).

Antibody responses to polio and rubella virus was studied
in the serum and nasopharyngeal secretions of several γA
deficient patients after intranasal inoculation with inactivated poliovaccine or natural rubella infection.   Nasopharyngeal
antibody response to poliovirus in patients with total absence

or selective deficiency of γA was characterized by the appearance of γG and occassionally γM class of poliovirus antibody
4-6 days after immunization. The response persisted for 3-4
months. During the course of these studies, few patients
developed natural rubella infection with development of γM
and subsequently γG rubella antibody in the serum. The secretory antibody response in these patients was characterized
by the appearance of γG rubella antibody in the nasopharynx,
which persisted in stable titers for as long as 12 months.
The outcome of intranasal reinfection challenge with RA27/3
live rubella vaccine in these patients was significantly
influenced by the level of pre-existing nasopharyngeal antibody, regardless of the antibody titer in the serum. Patients
with lowest nasopharyngeal γG rubella antibody level were
successfully reinfected with rubella vaccine, with nasopharyngeal virus shedding, while those with high nasopharyngeal
titers successfully resisted intranasal reinfection (20).
These data suggest that a deficient or absent serum and
secretory γA system may be effictively compensated by local
mucosal production of γG and to a small extent by γM viral
specific antibodies. Thus, these observations provide an
explanation for the apparent immunity to induced viral
infection in γA deficient patients.

GENERAL DISCUSSION

Extensive studies of the secretory immune system indicate
that secretory immunoglobulins particularly γA, serve an
important function at mucosal surfaces in antiviral immunity.
However, little information is available regarding the role
of cell-mediated immunity, interferon, and other factors in
the mechanism of defense at external mucosal surfaces.
Recent studies of Waldman (21) have suggested induction of
local cellular immunity in the respiratory tract of guinea
pigs after local immunization. This immunity appeared to be
independent of any systemic cellular response.

In an attempt to characterize the human cellular immune
responses to rubella virus, a number of rubella seronegative
children were immunized with HPV-77 rubella vaccine administered subcutaneously or with RA27/3 rubella vaccine administered intranasally. 1-2 months later, the children underwent
T&A for other medical reasons. The tonsilar and adenoidal
lymphoid cells, and lymphocytes from peripheral blood were
subsequently tested for the development of specific cellular
immunity to rubella virus, employing in-vitro assay of migra-
tory inhibitory factor, and in-vitro lymphocyte transformation

TABLE 5

Patterns of migration of tonsillar and adenoidal lymphoid cells
obtained after subcutaneous immunization with HPV-77 or
intranasal immunization with RA27/3 rubella vaccine.

Immunization	No. Patient	Mean Migration Index[a] Tonsil & Adenoid Cells	p Value
None	3	1.1	
HPV-77 S.C.	8	0.95	>0.01
RA27/3 I.N.	6	0.41	<0.001

a   Migration Index = $\dfrac{\text{migration in presence of killed rubella antigen}}{\text{migration without killed rubella antigen}}$

in the presence of heat killed rubella virus antigen. Cellular immune responses were regularly demonstrated by tonsilar
and adenoidal lymphoid cells obtained after intranasal immunization with RA27/3 vaccine. On the other hand, tonsilar and
adenoidal lymphocytes obtained after subcutaneous immunization with HPV-77 conspicuously failed to elicit any evidence
of cellular immunity (Table 5). These data provide further
support to the existence of cellular immune responses in the
secretory immune system. The significance of these observations in local immunity to virus infections remains to be
defined. However, the implications of local cellular immunity
may be applicable to the mechanisms of resistence in certain
clinical and experimental situations. For example it has
been recently shown that immunization with a temperature
sensitive mutant of respiratory syncytial virus, when administered by respiratory route failed, to induce detectable secretory antibody response. However, a significant number of
such vaccines resisted a subsequent reinfection challenge
with respiratory syncytial virus (22). It is possible that
the development of local cellular immunity in the respiratory
tract may be a mechanism of protection in such individuals.

ACKNOWLEDGMENT

These studies were supported in part by grants from the
National Institute of Allergy and Infectious Disease (AI09769),
National Institute of Child Health and Human Development

(HD06321), Clinical Research Center Program of the National Institute of Health (RR-628), Wellcome Research Foundation, and Henry C. and Bertha R. Buswell Foundation.

REFERENCES

1. Tomasi, T.B. and Grey, H.M., Prog. Allergy 16:81, 1972.
2. Ogra, P.L. and Karzon, D.T., Ped. Clin. N. Amer. 17:385, 1970.
3. Ogra, P.L., in Secretory Immunologic System, eds. Dayton, D., et al., U.S. Government Printing Office, Washington, D.C., 1971, p. 259.
4. Ogra, P.L., in Comparative Immunology of Oral Cavity, eds. Mergenhagen, et al., U.S. Government Printing Office, Washington, D.C. (in press).
5. Ogra, P.L. and Ogra, S.S. J. Immunol. 110:1307, 1973.
6. Ogra, P.L., Bernstein, J.M. and Tomasi, T.B., Ped. Res. 7:293, 1973.
7. Ogra, P.L., Karzon, D.T., Righthand, F. and MacGillivray, M., New Eng. J. Med. 279:893, 1968.
8. Ogra, P.L. and Karzon, D.T., J. Immunol. 102:15, 1969.
9. Ogra, P.L. and Karzon, D.T., J. Immunol. 102:1423, 1969.
10. Ogra, P.L., Ogra, S.S., Al-Nabeeb, S., Fed. Proc. 31:759, 1972.
11. Ogra, P.L., J. Immunol. 110:1197, 1973.
12. Horstman, D.M., Liebhaber, H., LeBouvier, G.L., Rosenberg, D.A. and Halstead, S.B. New Eng. J. Med. 283:771, 1970.
13. Meyer, H.M. and Parkman, P.D., J.A.M.A. 215:613, 1971.
14. Wilkins, J., Leedom, J.M., Portnoy, B. and Salvatore, M.A., Amer. J. Dis. Child. 118:275, 1969.
15. Ogra, P.L., Kerr-Grant, D., Umana, G., Dzierba, J. and Weintraub, D., New Eng. J. Med. 285:1333, 1971.
16. Plotkin, S.A., Farquhar, J.D. and Ogra, P.L., J.A.M.A. (in press).
17. Ogra, P.L., New Eng. J. Med. 284:59, 1971.
18. Heremans, J.F. and Vaerman, J.P., in Progress in Immunology (First International Congress of Immunology), ed. Amos, B., Academic Press, N.Y., p. 875, 1971.
19. Savilhati, E., Clin. Exp. Immunol. 13:395, 1973.
20. Ogra, P.L. and MacGillivray, M., Ped. Res. 6:379, 1972.
21. Waldman, R.H. and Henry, C.S., J. Exp. Med. 134:482, 1971.
22. Wright, P.F., Mills, J. and Chanock, R.M., J. Inf. Dis. 124:505, 1971.

THE ROLE OF THE SECRETORY IMMUNE SYSTEM IN PROTECTION AGAINST AGENTS WHICH INFECT THE RESPIRATORY TRACT

R. H. Waldman   and R. Ganguly

University of Florida, College of Medicine
Departments of Medicine and Immunology and
Medical Microbiology, Gainesville, Florida

The field of immunology developed in an attempt to understand the observed phenomenon that, following many infectious diseases, people become immune to that disease for some time, and often this immunity is permanent. As a natural corollary of this, there developed attempts to somehow induce this immune state without causing the illness, or at least, to acceptably reduce the severity of the illness. Over the past 200 years, the corollary aim has probably proven more successful than attempts to understand the phenomenon, and the development of the several immunization practices now widely used has been the most successful aspect of the disciplines of immunology and infectious diseases (with the possible exception of the role of the latter in the generally improved state of public hygiene). In addition, we feel that this contribution from the combined efforts of the fields of infectious diseases and immunology will continue to be great, for example, in the development of vaccines against caries, herpesvirus and streptococcal infections, the hepatitides, gonorrhea and syphilis; and in improved vaccines against cholera and influenza, to name a few.

Most infectious diseases occur either wholly on secretory surfaces, or enter the body through a secretory surface. Many of these infections involve the gastrointestinal tract; this is covered elsewhere in this book.

We shall review the data on the relationship of respiratory
tract immunology and infectious diseases.

ANTIVIRAL ANTIBODY

Artenstein et al (1) demonstrated "natural" antibody
against a number of viruses in nasal secretions of normal
individuals, and showed that the antiviral substance of
normal nasal secretions belongs predominatly to the IgA
class antibody. Neutralizing activity against 2 or more
of the 8 viruses tested was found in each of the 10 normal
nasal washings.

Of greater practical importance, however, have been
recent attempts to stimulate secretory antibody, i. e., the
development of vaccines. It is generally felt that live
attenuated organisms elicit better immunity than do killed
organisms. This seems to be supported by the common observation that immunity following recovery from natural infection
is more effective and enduring than that resulting from killed
vaccines. Several live vaccines in practice, like those of
small pox and yellow fever, are very effective, and protection against these diseases is almost complete. However, it
should be noted that there have been no controlled studies
in which a live attenuated vaccine has been compared with
the comparable killed vaccine. By replicating, live infectious
agents tend to persist longer, possibly resulting in the
development of more solid immunity. This might involve a
greater antigenic mass and/or longer contact with the immunocompetent cells. Theoretically, the same result would be
obtained by administering the inactivated (but not denatured)
organisms repeatedly and in larger doses, which, however,
may be impractical. Thus the real advantage of a live vaccine
may be easier immunization procedures for wider application.
However, there are certain disadvantages of live vaccines:
(a) they necessitate more careful handling, since if the
organisms die from lack of refrigerated conditions (as is
possible in underdeveloped countries) or if a lyophilized
vaccine becomes moist, the result is a killed vaccine with
very little antigenic mass: (b) the ever present danger of
administration of an adventitious agent along with the live
organism: this is especially important with respect to viral
vaccines which are grown in a living cellular milieu, and it
is virtually impossible to rule out the presence of another
agent; (c) they are subject to the risk of mutation to
virulence.

Since secretory antibody may be important in protection, and the evidence for this will be covered below, a knowledge of the optimal method of stimulating such antibodies on mucosal surfaces is essential in determining the best immunizing procedures. It is known that parenterally administered vac= cines can elicit a secretory antibody response (2), probably by transportation of the antigen to the secretory lymphoid tissue. But it has been noted that such levels of local antibodies are usually low and result only in partial pro- tection (3). On the other hand, much more pronounced antigenic stimulation of the secretory mucosal surface has been achieved using directly applied live and/or inactivated vaccines. Following aerosol-spray immunization with an inactivated parainfluenza vaccine, higher levels of secretory antibody have been obtained, predominatly of the IgA class, as well as IgG type serum antibodies (4). Local respiratory anti- body has further been found to correlate with protection against the disease (5). Intranasal instillation of in- activated polio vaccine led to the production of nasal anti- bodies, but very little or no serum antibodies (6). No significant titers of secretory antibody developed following parenteral immunization.

Waldman et al (7) and Kasel et al (8), found that persons developed antibody in respiratory secretions more frequently and to a greater magnitude when immunized intranasally with an inactivated influenza virus vaccine than when given the vaccine by the subcutaneous route. Conversely, they also observed that a better systemic response could be elicited by subcutaneous vaccine administration than following immuniz- ation via the respiratory route. The changes in nasal wash protein, IgA, hemagglutination inhibition (HI) activity and virus neutralizing activity in persons experiencing infection with influenza virus has been reported by Alford et al (9). A rise in titer of neutralizing activity occurred around 10-14 days after inoculation in both serum and nasal secretions The rate of appearance of neutralizing activities in nasal wash specimens was further studied by Rossen et al (10). Their results indicate that nasal antibody activity tends to be detected earlier in those individuals with higher base- line IgA concentration in nasal wash specimens and the authors suggested that this phenomenon may be important in control- ling infection and preventing illness. None of the men with high base-line IgA levels in this study developed illness after challenge, whereas 3/4 of the men with low base-lines did. In this group of men, the early detection of neutralizing activity was not related to the level of serum antibody.

Thus it appears that optimal mucosal antibody response for viral neutralizing activity may be induced by either natural infection, or by direct application of killed or live attenuated virus to the mucosal surface.

It should be mentioned in this context that the secretory immune system is probably not a unitary system, i.e., stimulation of one component probably does not lead to antibody production in another. Studies conducted by Mann et al (11) and Waldman et al (12), using live and inactivated influenza virus vaccines, applied subcutaneously and/or locally, showed that a significant amount of neutralizing antibody activity in saliva, an external secretion that contains the same order of magnitude of secretory IgA as nasal secretions or sputum, could not be induced. This lends support to the local production and stimulation hypothesis, since the salivary glands are stimulated directly by antigen neither during influenza infection nor following aerosol or subcutaneous immunization. Ogra and his co-workers immunized humans with "double-barrel" colostomies into one limb of the large intestine with polio-virus antigens and found production of antibody against polio-virus only in the limb of the colostomy into which the antigen was placed, and not in the other limb nor in nasal secretions (13). In studies with influenza and rubella vaccines administered into the respiratory tract of human volunteers, it was observed that better antibody production was related to the area of the respiratory system where the immunogen droplets landed, depending on the particle size and method of administration. In other words, antigen delivered into the nose by nose drops stimulated antibody only in the nasal secretions and not in the bronchial secretions.

With respect to the localization of the secretory immune system in the respiratory tract, mention should be made of recent studies of lower respiratory secretions, i. e., material obtained by bronchoaveolar lavage (14). The immunoglobulin content of this fluid was intermediate between that of serum and upper respiratory secretions, i. e., the IgG:IgA ratio was about 3:1. Evidence was presented suggesting that the antibody found in the lavage fluid was locally produced, and that it was found in both the IgA and IgG classes.

In view of the local nature of secretory antibody production, the route and selection of particle size aimed at stimulating specific areas of the respiratory mucosa might become an important feature in immunizing procedures.

When the particle size was varied in order to study the
stimulation of antibody in the respiratory tract, it was
found that particles with a mean diameter of 1.5µ were not
retained in the nasal passage and therefore, did not give
rise to nasal antibody, but were very effective in stimulating
lower respiratory tract antibody, as analyse on sputum
from the vaccinees. On the other hand, large particle aerosol
(100µ) more effectively stimulated nasal antibody, probably
because the immunogen deposited primarily on the upper
respiratory passage. In studies with rubella vaccine, in
young adult human volunteers, the efficacy of different
particle-sizes was assessed. The volunteers who received
the vaccine by nose drops showed the highest mean nasal
antibody response while the small-particle aerosol (5 µ
average) inhaled through the mouth produced the least nasal
antibody (Table 1).

Table 1 - Nasal Secretion Antibody in Volunteers Immunized
          With Rubella Vaccine by Various Routes

Vaccine Groups	# With Antibody Rise / # Tested	Geometic Mean Titer
Aerosol	9/11	1:3
Spray	5/6	1:4
Nose Drops	9/9	1:7
Subcutaneous	4/8	1:2

Administration of vaccines by aerosol may be better
as a mass immunizing procedure, as indicated from a number of
field trials. It is more pleasant for the vaccinees to
receive, as compared to the subcutaneously administrated
immunogen. Vaccinees receiving local immunization presumably will face more local side-effects (usually mild) of
the vaccine as compared to those receiving parenteral
immunization, who experience more systemic reactions (usually
more severe).

It is possible that secretory IgA antibody is less
specific than is serum IgG antibody. Dowdle and co-workers
(15) demonstrated significant rises in nasal secretion antibody to a previous influenza A strain following A2/Hong Kong
virus immunization, while there was little or no rise in
serum antibody to the heterologous strain. In another study,
volunteers were immunized by aerosol with an Asian strain

of inactivated influenza virus vaccine prior to the appearance of the A2/Hong Kong variant. An antibody rise was
demonstrated against the vaccine strain in both respiratory
secretions and serum. Whereas there was no rise in serum
antibody to the heterologous strains A/PR8 and A2 Hong Kong
influenza, there was a significant rise in IgA antibody to
these heterologous strains (16).

PROTECTION AGAINST INFECTION AND DISEASE

The presence of secretion antibody and protection against
viral infection have been found to be correlated in several
recent studies carried out in volunteers. Perkins et al
(17) administered an inactivated rhinovirus type 13 vaccine
to adult male volunteers by the intramuscular (IM) or intranasal (IN) route.   Upon challenge with 100 TCD_{50} of
the same virus in the volunteers, the IN-group demonstrated
a significant protective effect, whereas the IM-group
developed illness with an equal frequency as the seronegative
controls. The volunteers who received the vaccine IN
developed both serum and nasal secretion antibodies, while
the volunteers who were vaccinated IM developed primarily
a serum antibody response. When the response to challenge
of the vaccinees was evaluated with the antibody levels,
only the nasal secretory antibody was found to be correlated
with protection against the disease. The correlation between secretory antibody and protection was also indicated
with rhinovirus by Cate et al (18).

In another study using type 1 parainfluenza virus for
vaccination and challenge, Smith et al (5) demonstrated
the protective role of secretory antibody against infection.
They showed that despite the fact that all the adult vaccinees possessed serum neutralizing antibody to type 1
parainfluenza virus, 50% of those challenged became infected
and contracted mild upper respiratory tract illness. It
appeared that those with higher serum antibody titers were
less likely to become infected. Subsequent analysis, however, indicated that this protective effect was associated
primarily with the level of neutralizing activity in nasal
secretions and not the serum antibody titer. Presence of
neutralizing activity in the nasal secretions was found to
be associated with a statistically significant protection
against type 1 virus infection and illness.

To test the ability of local antibody to protect against influenza virus infection, field trials have been carried out testing the efficacy of aerosol immunization before naturally occurring influenza epidemics. In several field trials, the aerosol route of immunization rendered protection rates between 70 to 80% (19-21). There were differences in the studies, primarily in the protection rates afforded by the subcutaneous groups. It is conceivable that pre-existing systemic antibody binding the injected antigen interferes with the antigen reaching the secretory mucosa resulting in a reduced secretory antibody response to parenteral antigen. Whatever may be the underlying mechanisms, it appears from these field trials that secretory IgA antibody correlated with protection against viral infection.

It is known that respiratory syncytial (RS) virus is the most frequent cause of serious respiratory disease in infancy and that lack of protection to the infection early in life occurs in spite of passively acquired maternal IgG neutralizing antibodies. This implies that serum antibodies are not protective in this infection. Furthermore, studies by Mills et al indicated that parenteral immunization with an inactivated vaccine elicited high serum antibody levels, but these were not associated with protection (22). They also showed that, in natural infection, nasal wash antibody appeared associated with inhibition of colonization and multiplication of the virus in the respiratory tract. Parrot et al (23) further demonstrated a rise in nasal fluid neutralizing activity both following natural infection with RS virus and local immunization with attenuated (cold adapted) vaccine. Moreover in this infection, the absence of local immunity in the presence of high serum antibody levels has been suggested to frequently involve a severe Arthus-like hypersensitivity reaction. If this hypothesis is borne-out by further studies, the importance of secretory antibody in protection against the pathogenesis of viral infection, is emphasized. Similar reactions have also been encountered with measles in infants previously immunized systemically with the killed vaccine. Whether such unwanted reactions in the presence of high levels of circulating antibodies are a result of imbalance between local and serum antibodies and/or is due to some other immune phenomenon, remains to be defined.

Studies indicate that local nasopharyngeal immune mechanisms are importantly related to immunity against rubella infection (24), and this is covered in the chapter by Ogra elsewhere in this volume.

In recent studies by Brunner et al (25), antibody to
Mycoplasma pneumoniae was measured in respiratory secretions
of volunteers who were challenged with the wild-type organism.
Analysis of the clinical response to challenge showed that
the respiratory tract IgA antibody was more closely related
to host resistance than was serum antibody. This corroborates
the observations of Fernald and Clyde in hamsters, in
which local immunity was also suggested to be more important
(26). Brunner et al have also carried out studies with
temperature-sensitive mutants of M. Pneumoniae, administered
via the respiratory tract. Although the tested strains
thus far reported were too virulent to be generally used,
this approach appears to offer hope for the eventual control
of illness due to M. Pneumoniae.

In experiments using aerosol challenge of animals with
Proteus sp. and Staphylococcus aureus, Jakab and Green (27)
showed that animals immunized by aerosol had markedly enhanced
pulmonary bactericidal activity against the homologous, but
not the heterologous bacterial strain. Animals immunized
intraperitoneally had slightly increased pulmonary resistance
to challenge, but significantly less than the aerosol-immunized
animals. The mechanism of this increased resistance has not
been elucidated, but it appears to be independent of serum
antibody, or at least not significantly dependent on it,
since animals immunized by aerosol had no detectable serum
antibody.

Pharyngitis caused by group A, β-hemolytic streptococci
is a mucosal infection, and might be influenced by local
immune mechanisms. In a series of recent studies, volunteers
were immunized with a purified type 1 M-protein vaccine,
either subcutaneously or by spray onto the naso-and oro-
pharynx (28, 29). The parenterally-immunized group developed
high levels of serum antibody. The aerosol-spray group
developed only low levels of serum antibody, but did develop
respiratory secretion antibody. Following challenge with
virulent homologous streptococci, there was significant reduction in illness in both groups, as compared to placebo-
immunized volunteers (Table 2). Of interest is the observation that colonization of the pharynx was not significantly
decreased in the parentally-immunized group, but was in the
locally-immunized group. Further studies are underway, but
the data suggest that both local and systemic immune mechanisms
are related to protection against illness, but that colonization is inhibited better by local immunity.

TABLE 2:   Streptococcal M-Protein Vaccine
Study: Response to Challenge

Vaccine Group (#)	Positive Culture	Illness
Placebo (41)	78%	75%
Subcutaneous (19)	42%	26%
Nasopharyngeal Spray (22)	27%	23%

CELL MEDIATED IMMUNITY ON SECRETORY SURFACES

During the last decade, there has been an upsurge of
interest in the field of cell-mediated immunity (CMI), an
area previously less well understood, as compared to the
immunoglobulin system. As a result of these studies, it
has been established that sensitized cells are important in
protection against certain infections, as much as they are
essential for the rejection of organ homografts and in tumor
immunity. Despite the fact that specifically sensitized
lymphocytes which are active in CMI constitute a distinct
mode of immune response, apparently independent of humoral
antibodies, CMI on secretory surfaces has not been studied
to any significant degree.

Recent studies suggest that the local induction of CMI
on a mucosal surface is feasible. The appearance of
sensitized lymphocytes in the respiratory tract was compared
with that present in the spleen of guinea pigs after
administration of DNP-HGG either locally (nose drops) or by
injection. The results indicated that CMI, as evidenced by
inhibition of macrophage migration in the presence of antigen,
was associated with lymphocytes obtained from the respiratory
tract of guinea pigs immunized by DNP-HGG in nose drops, but
not those immunized parenterally. However, splenic
lymphocytes from parenterally immunized animals inhibited
macrophage migration while those from locally immunized
animals did not. Thus, this immunity might be considered as
part of the secretory immune system, previously described only
in terms of humoral immunity (30).

It is obvious, therefore, that, in addition to the
secretory immunoglobulin system, CMI might also play an
important role in protection and immunity on mucosal surfaces.

Galindo and Myrvik (31) demonstrated in rabbits immunized with BCG vaccine that pulmonary CMI exists independently from that found systemically, depending upon the route of immunization. Following intravenous immunization CMI by lungs of mice correlated with protection against infection with M. tuberculosis, while the presence of sensitized lymphocytes obtained from the peritoneal cavity did not. In a study of humans, bronchoalveolar cells were obtained from PPD positive and negative individuals. Jurgensen et al demonstrated CMI by pulmonary lymphocytes from the former, but not the latter (33). However, in these studies, the stimulation of lymphocytes by local immunization was not examined. Recently Barclay et al (34) reported on their observations regarding protection of monkeys against air-borne tuberculosis by aerosol vaccination with BCG. They demonstrated that the vaccine administered intravenously or by aerosol to rhesus monkeys induced a much greater degree of protection against aerosol challenge with virulent M. tuberculosis than intracutaneous BCG vaccination. The aerosol route of vaccination was not associated with any obvious adverse side effects, such as the draining abcesses often seen following intracutaneous administration, and might have potential application in humans.

Regarding local immunization with viral antigens and the development of CMI on mucosal surfaces, guinea pigs were immunized systemically or locally with influenza vaccine into the respiratory tract and the humoral and cellular immunities were evaluated in serum and splenic lymphocytes (systemically) and in bronchial washings (local immunity). It was observed that local cellular and humoral immunity developed following immunization with nose drops but there was little systemic immune response (35). On the other hand, parenteral immunization led to the development of circulating antibody and to CMI, as determined by the inhibition of macrophage migration in splenic lymphocytes. Jurgensen et al found similar results in studies of humans (33). Thus it seems that CMI to influenza virus in the respiratory tract or in the spleen is also dependent on the route of immunization.

REFERENCES

1.   Artenstein, M.S., Bellanti, J.A. and Buescher, E.L., Proc. Soc. Exp. Biol. Med. 117:558, 1964.
2.   Rosen, R.D., Wolff, S.M. and Butler, W.T., J. Immunol. 99:246, 1967.

3. Ganguly, R., Ogra, P.L., Regas, S. and Waldman, R.H.,
    Inf. Immun. 1973 (in press).
4. Wigley, F.M., Fruchtman, M.H. and Waldman, R.H., New
    Eng. J. Med. 283:1250, 1970.
5. Smith, C.B., Purcell, R.H., Bellanti, J.A. and Chanock,
    R.M., New Eng. J. Med. 275:1145, 1966.
6. Ogra, P.L., Karzon, D.T., J. Immunol. 102:15, 1969.
7. Waldman, R.H., Wood, S.H., Torres, E.J. and Small, P.A.,
    Jr., Am. J. Epid. 91:575, 1970.
8. Kasel, J.A., Hume, E.B., Fulk, R.V., Togo, Y., Huber, M.
    and Hornick, R.B., J. Immunol. 102:555, 1969.
9. Alford, R.H., Rossen, R.D., Butler, W.T. and Kasel, J.A.,
    J. Immunol. 98:724, 1967.
10. Rossen, R.D., Butler, W.T., Waldman, R.H., Alford, R.H.,
    Hornick, R.B., Togo, Y. and Kasel, J.A. J. Am. Med.
    Assoc. 211:1157, 1970.
11. Mann, J.J., Waldman, R.H., Togo, Y., Heiner, G.G.,
    Dawkins, A.T. and Kasel, J.A., J. Immunol. 100:726, 1968.
12. Waldman, R.H., Kasel, J.A., Fulk, R.V., Mann, J.J.,
    Togo, Y., Hornick, R.B., Heiner, G.T., Dawkins, A.T.,
    Nature 218:594, 1968.
13. Ogra, P.L., Karzon, D.T., J. Immunol. 102:1423, 1969.
14. Waldman, R.H., Jurgensen, P.F., Olsen, G.N., Ganguly, R.
    and Johnson, J.E. III, J. Immunol. 111:38, 1973.
15. Dowdle, W., Coleman, M.T., Schoenbaum, S.C., Kaye, H.S.
    and Hieholzer, J.C., in The Secretory Immunologic System,
    Edited by D.H. Dayton, Jr., P.A. Small, Jr., R.M. Chanock,
    H.E. Kaufman, T.B. Tomasi, Jr., U.S. Government Printing
    Office, Washington, 1971.
16. Waldman, R.H., Wigley, F.M. and Small, P.A., J. Immunol.
    105:1477, 1970.
17. Perkins, J.X., Tucker, D.N., Knopf, H.L.S., Wenzel, R.P.,
    Kapikian, A.Z. and Chanock, R.M., Am. J. Epid. 90:519,
    1969.
18. Cate, T.R., Rossen, R.D., Douglas, R.G., Jr., Butler,
    W.T. and Couch, R.B., Am. J. Epid. 84:352, 1966.
19. Waldman, R.H., Mann, J.J. and Small, P.A., Jr., J. Am.
    Med. Assoc. 207:520, 1969.
20. Waldman, R.H. and Coggins, W.J., J. Inf. Dis. 126:242,
    1972.
21a. Liem, K.S., Marcus, E.A., Jacobs, J. and Van Strik, R.,
    Postgrad, Med. Jour. 49:175, 1973.
21b. Waldman, R.H., Bond, J.O., Levitt, L.P., Hartwig, E.C.,
    Prather, E.C., Baratta, R.L., Neill, J.S. and Small,
    P.A., Jr., Bull WHO 41:543, 1969.

22. Mills, J., Knopf, H.L.S., Kirk, J.V. and Chanock, R.M.,
     in The Secretory Immunologic System, Edited by D.H.
     Dayton, P.A. Small, Jr., R.M. Chanock, H.E. Kaufman and
     T.B. Tomasi, Jr., U.S. Government Printing Office,
     Washington, 1971.

23. Parrott, R.H., Kim, H.W., Bellanti, J.A., Arrobio, J.A.,
     Mills, J., Brandl, C.O. and Chanock, R.M., in The Secre-
     tory Immunologic System, Edited by D.H. Dayton, P.A.
     Small, Jr., R.M. Chanock, H.E. Kaufman and T.B. Tomasi,
     U.S. Government Printing Office, Washington, 1971.

24. Ogra, P.L., Kerr-Grant, D., Umana, G., Dzierba, J.
     and Weintraub, D., New Eng. J. Med. 285:1333, 1971.

25. Brunner, H., Greenburg, H., Couch, R.B. and Chanock,
     R.M., Inf. Immun. (in press).

26. Fernald, G.W. and Clyde, W.A., Jr., Inf. Immun. 1:559,
     1970.

27. Jakab, G. and Green, G., J. Clin. Invest. (in press).

28. Fox, E.N., Waldman, R.H., Wittner, M.K., Mauceri, A.A.
     and Dorfman, A., J. Clin. Invest. 52:1885, 1973.

29. Waldman, R.H., Fox, E.N., Dorfman, A., Wittner, M.K.
     and Polly, S.M., (in preparation).

30. Henney, C.S. and Waldman, R.H., Science 169:696, 1970.

31. Galindo, B. and Myrvik, Q.N., J. Immunol. 105:227, 1970.

32. Yamamoto, K., Anacker, R.L. and Ribi, E., Inf. Immun.
     1:595, 1970.

33. Jurgensen, P.F., Olsen, G.N., Johnson, J.E. III,
     Swenson, E.W., Ayoub, E.M., Henney, C.S. and Waldman,
     R.H., J. Inf. Dis. (in press).

34. Barclay, W.R., Busey, W.M., Dalgard, D.W., Good, R.C.,
     Jamicki, B.W., Kasin, J.E., Ribi, E., Ulrich, C.E. and
     Wolinsky, E., Am. Rev. Resp. Dis. 107:351, 1973.

35. Waldman, R.H., Spencer, C.S. and Johnson, J.E., Cell.
     Immun. 3:294, 1972.

THE ROLE OF IMMUNIZATION IN CONTROLLING ANTIGEN UPTAKE FROM
THE SMALL INTESTINE

W. Allan Walker, Kurt J. Isselbacher and
Kurt J. Bloch
Departments of Medicine and Pediatrics
Harvard Medical School and the Pediatric Gastro-
intestinal, Gastrointestinal, Arthritis and
Clinical Immunology Units of Massachusetts
General Hospital, Boston, Massachusetts 02114

INTRODUCTION

The intestinal absorption of intact macromolecules (1-2),
and the ability of such molecules to induce both a local and
systemic immune response has been demonstrated under natural
and experimental conditions (2-4). Patients lacking secretory
IgA frequently display elevated levels of serum antibodies
to ingested antigens suggesting that in the absence of
secretory IgA, excessive absorption of antigen has occurred
giving rise to the greater serum antibody response (5). We
have been concerned for several years with the mechanism of
uptake of antigen from the intestine and with the role of
immunization in controlling such uptake.

In an earlier morphologic study (2), a tracer protein-
enzyme, horseradish peroxidase (HRP, M.W. 40,000) introduced
into intestinal loops, was noted to be transported through
the mucosa of adult rats by a pinocytotic mechanism similar
to that described for the uptake of gamma globulins by the
intestine of neonatal rats (6). In a parallel physiologic
study, it was shown that following instillation into the
duodenum of adult rats, HRP was transported into both
intestinal lymph and portal blood. In addition, in vitro
experiments demonstrated that transport of HRP was an energy-
dependent process (8). Recently, the physiologic studies have
extended to a second protein antigen, bovine serum albumin
(BSA) (9).

To determine the effect of immunization on the intestinal uptake of macromolecules, rats were orally immunized
with HRP or BSA, and absorption of these antigens by everted
jejunal and ileal gut sacs was studies (10). In comparison
with controls, a consistent decrease in HRP uptake was noted
in both germ-free and conventional rats immunized with that
antigen (Figure 1); a similar decrease in BSA uptake was
noted in rats immunized with BSA. These observations suggested that local immunization interferes with intestinal
uptake of antigens. In subsequent studies, the effect of
parenteral immunization on uptake of antigen was examined
(11). Again it was found that immunization led to inhibition
of antigen uptake; however, intense parenteral immunization
was required to reveal this effect.

Having demonstrated that immunization inhibited the
absorption of antigens, we next attempted to determine the
mechanism of inhibition.

MATERIALS AND METHODS

Adult female rats weighing approximately 175 gms
(Holtzman Co., Madison, Wisc.) were used in these experiments.
Rats were injected intramuscularly (IM) with BSA as previously described (11). Other rats were injected intraperitoneally
(IP) with 0.5 ml of BSA (4.0 mg/ml) mixed with equal volumes
of incomplete Freund's adjuvant (Difco Laboratories, Detroit,
Mich.) on four occasions during a two month period. Animals
were studied ten or more days after the last injection. In
keeping with previous observations on gut sacs from orally
and IM immunized rats, gut sacs obtained from rats immunized
by the IP route were **also** shown to absorb significantly less
antigen than gut sacs obtained from untreated controls. (W.A.
Walker, unpublished observation)

Bovine serum albumin was labelled with $Na^{125}I$ using a
modification of the method of Greenwood et al. (12). Gut
sacs from immunized and control rats were incubated in 30 ml
of Krebs-Ringer-bicarbonate solution containing either 1 ug/ml
or 10 ug/ml of ^{125}I-BSA ($2x10^3$ cpm/ml incubation media) for
a period of 3 hrs under conditions previously described (8).
One ml samples were removed from the incubation medium
after 5,15,30,60,120 and 180 minutes. The total radioactivity in the sample was determined (8) before and after precipitation of protein with 10% trichloroacetic acid (TCA); a
constant amount of BSA was added to each sample prior to

precipitation. It was assumed that ^{125}I remaining in the
supernatant was present as free iodine or as iodine associated with small peptides (13), and that the percent of total
radioactivity remaining in the supernatant after TCA precipitation reflected the breakdown of ^{125}I-BSA.

In order to determine binding of ^{125}I-BSA, gut sacs
were removed from the media after 3 hrs and the serosal
contents drained. The sacs were then rinsed by sequential
dipping into three separate beakers containing saline. It
was assumed that antigen loosely bound to the intestinal
musosa would be eluted by the initial dipping and that
more tightly bound antigen would remain adherent to the
gut sac. After dipping, the mucosa of the gut sacs was
removed by scraping and the scrapings were homogenized. The
total concentration of ^{125}I-BSA in each beaker and extract
was determined. In some experiments involving gut sacs from
rats immunized IM, the rinsing fluid contained in the first
beaker was concentrated by negative pressure dialysis and
the concentrated fluid applied to a sucrose density gradient
and subjected to ultracentrifugation as previously described
(14).

RESULTS

Gut sacs obtained from controls and rats immunized
with BSA by either the IM or IP route were incubated with
^{125}I-BSA for 3 hrs. Thereafter the incubation media was
examined for total radioactivity before and after precipitation of protein with 10% TCA. With one exception, the
amount of radioactivity remaining in the supernatant was
greater in the immunized compared to the control groups
(Table 1). These results suggest that gut sacs from immunized rats degrade more antigen than gut sacs from controls.

In some experiments, samples of the incubation fluid
were examined at intervals. At five minutes of incubation,
gut sacs from rats immunized IP were found to bind a greater amount of labelled protein than the controls; however,
the extent of breakdown of ^{125}I-BSA was minimal at this
time. On further incubation, the extent of breakdown by
gut sacs from immunized rats increased; the difference
compared to controls was greatest at 3 hrs.

Following 3 hrs incubation, the gut sacs were dipped
sequentially in saline and the radioactivity released was

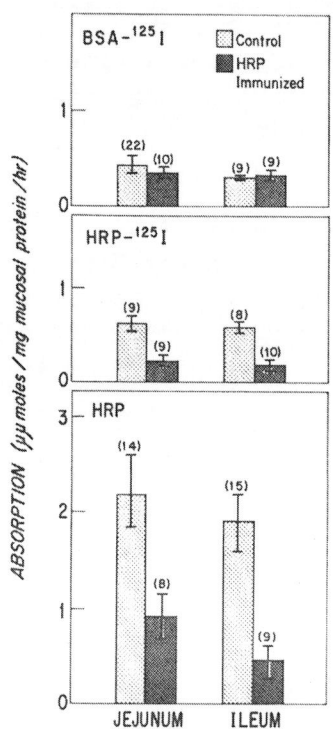

Figure 1: Absorption of antigens into the serosal fluid of rats orally immunized with enzyme horseradish perodidase (HRP) and of control rats. Number of observations per group of animals is expressed in parentheses. Uptake of HRP as measured by enzymatic assay in 12 orally immunized conventional rats was significantly less than in control animals (C). The average absorption ± S.E., per hour, in jejunum of immunized animals was 0.92 ± 0.22 pmole/mg and 2.18 ± 0.37 pmole/mg in control animals (P < .005); in the ileum, 0.45 ± 0.15 pmole/mg was abosrbed, compared with 1.89 ± 0.30 pmole/mg in controls (P < .001). Uptake of HRP as measured by radioactivity techniques was also significantly less in immunized animals than in controls (B). Average absorption ± S.E. of ^{125}I-HRP, per hour, in jejunum of immunized animals was 0.23 ± 0.04 pmole/mg and 0.61 ± 0.06 pmole/mg in controls (P < .01); in the ileum, 0.19 ± 0.06 pmole/mg was absorbed compared with 0.58 ± 0.05 pmole/mg in controls (P < .01). However, no significance difference in absorption of ^{125}I-BSA in jejunum (0.35 ± 0.04 pmole/mg versus controls 0.45 ± 0.07 pmole/mg) or ileum of immunized rats (0.32 ± 0.04) pmole/mg versus controls 0.29 ± 0.02 pmole/mg) was noted (A). (From Walker, W.A., Isselbacher, K.J. and Bloch, K.J.: Intestinal Uptake of Macromolecules: Effect of oral immunization, Science 177:608, 1972.

determined.   Considerable radioactivity was released by
rinsing the gut sacs of rats immunized IM (group A); most
of the radioactivity removed was found in the first rinse.
With one exception, this phenomenon was not observed with
gut sacs obtained from rats immunized IP (group B).   We
suspect that this difference is related to the smaller dose
of ^{125}I-BSA in the incubation medium, 10 ug per ml in the
former compared to 1 ug per ml in the latter group.   Following
prolonged incubation, there may have been insufficient
antigen available in the latter group to consistently demonstrate greater binding to gut sacs of immunized rats
compared to controls.

    The first rinsing fluid obtained from gut sacs in group
A was concentrated and applied to a sucrose density gradient.
Following ultracentrifugation, ^{125}I was detected in fractions
collected from the bottom of the gradient (Figure 2); in

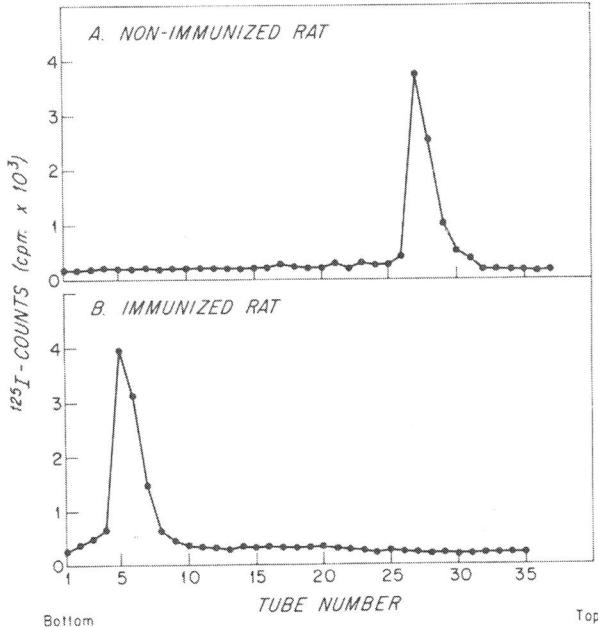

Figure 2:   Localization of ^{125}I-BSA on sucrose density
gradients.   Following 3 hr incubation of gut sacs from a
control (A) and an immunized rat (B) with ^{125}I-BSA, sacs
were rinsed and the first rinsing fluid concentrated and
applied to the gradient.   Radioactivity appeared in the upper
zone of the gradient in the control and in a zone near the
bottom of the gradient in the sample from the immunized
rat.

TABLE I

Fate of $125I$-BSA after exposure to gut sacs from immunized rats and control rats

Animals	Route of Immunization	Dose of 125I-BSA in incubation medium	Breakdown[a]		First rinsing fluid[b]		Residual mucosal binding[c]	
			Jejunum	Ileum	Jejunum	Ileum	Jejunum	Ileum
Group A								
1	IM	10 ug/ml	342	260	150	200	123	135
2			58	156	1100	900	69	110
3			356	200	167	185	84	97
4			187	455	154	145	142	105
Group B								
1	IP	1 ug/ml	1680	215	167	142	132	105
2			390	316	120	115	39	110
3			233	240	105	109	117	116
4			416	375	118	103	110	111

a Refers to the amount of BSA degraded by gut sacs during 3 hr incubation. Since gut sacs of slightly different sizes were used, calculations were based on the number of mg of mucosal protein obtained by scraping. Degradation is expressed as a per cent of breakdown observed with sacs from control rats.

b Total radioactivity of solution in which gut sacs were initially rinsed after incubation for 3 hrs with 125I-BSA. Counts were related to the number of mg of mucosal protein obtained by scraping and expressed as a per cent of control.

c Total radioactivity remaining in extracts of mucosal scrapings after sequential dipping. Counts were related to the number of mg of mucosal protein and expressed as a per cent of control.

contrast, rinsing fluid obtained from controls and treated
similarly, showed radioactivity at the top of the gradient.
The location of the label in the latter experiments is similar
to the location of intact ^{125}I-BSA applied to the sucrose
density gradients. It seems likely that gut sacs from these
immunized animals released ^{125}I-BSA still bound to antibody,
while presumably free ^{125}I-BSA was released from the controls.

Following sequential dipping, mucosal extracts were
prepared from gut sacs of control and immunized rats and
the amount of radioactivity associated with the extracts
were determined. Considerable variation in results was seen
in group A; in group B immunized rats, with one exception,
showed slightly greater residual binding than controls.

DISCUSSION

Previous studies have shown that oral immunization
or intensive parenteral immunization specifically inhibit
the uptake of the immunizing protein antigen, but not that
of an unrelated antigen. The present study suggests that
enhanced degradation of the antigen may account for the
decrease in uptake observed. From the information available,
the following sequence may be tentatively suggested. Initial
exposure of gut sacs from immunized rats to soluble antigen
in vitro leads to the rapid association of antigen with
the mucosal surface. At this site, antigen-antibody complexes may be degraded by local proteases. The exact site
of antigen binding and degradation remains to be determined;
either the glycocalyx (15) or the cell surface itself may
serve these functions.

Residual binding of labelled antigen to the mucosa
of gut sacs from immunized rats, may reflect labelled protein which has escaped degradation and has become tightly
adherent to epithelial cells or incorporated within such
cells or others in submucosal structures. In the majority
of experiments, mucosal scrapings from immunized rats show
slightly greater antigen binding than did controls. Whether
the radioisotope was actually within epithelial or other
cells of the lamina propria was not determined. It is possible that such binding reflects the presence of antibody
in or on the tissue rather than intra- or inter-cellular
uptake. In group A, rat #3 is of special interest. This rat
showed enhanced destruction of antigen during prolonged
incubation of gut sac with BSA. On subsequent rinsing of

the gut sac in saline, considerable weakly bound ^{125}I-BSA
was released in the first rinse. After rinsing, the radioactivity detected in the mucosal extract was less than that
of the control. These results suggest that in this animal,
antigen did not become firmly associated with the mucosa
of the gut. One would predict that in this animal, uptake
of antigen would be markedly inhibited. According to our
view, secretory antibody prevents uptake of soluble antigen
by combining with antigen, at some distance from the immediate surface of the cell. This concept is analogous to one
proposed by Williams and Gibbons (16) to explain the
inhibition by secretory antibody of the colonization of
epithelial cells by bacteria.

It should be stressed that we are reporting preliminary
observations. The nature of the high molecular weight
substance responsible for binding antigen in the density
gradient experiments remains to be identified as antibody.
Furthermore, the exact site of antigen breakdown in relation
to the epithelial cell surface and the specificity of the
enhanced breakdown of antigen remain to be determined.

Acknowledgements: Miss Pamela Gleason, a student at
Connecticut College for Women, New London, Connecticut
worked on this study as part of a student summer project.
This work was supported in part by a contract from the United
States Army Medical Research and Development Command
(Contract DADA-17-70-C-0113), U.S.P.H.S. grants (AM-5067,AM-
3564, AI-10129, and AM-16269) and grants from the Massachusetts
Chapter of Arthritis Foundation and L.H. Bendit Foundation.

REFERENCES

1. Bernstein, I.D. and Ovary, Z., Int. Arch. Allergy 33:521,
    1968.
2. Cornell, R., Walker, W.A. and Isselbacher, K.J., Lab.
    Invest. 25:42, 1971.
3. Korenblat, R.E., Rothberg, R.M., Minden, P. and Farr, R.S.,
    J. Allergy 41:226, 1968.
4. Crabbé, P.A., Nash, D.R., Bazin, H. et al., Lab Invest.
    22:448, 1970.
5. Buckley, R.H. and Dees, S.C., N. Eng. J. Med. 281:465, 1969,
6. Clark, S.L., J. Biophys. Biochem. Cytol. 5:41, 1959.
7. Warshaw, A.L., Walker, W.A., Cornell, R. and Isselbacher,
    K.J., Lab. Invest. 25:675, 1971.

8. Walker, W.A., Cornell, R., Davenport, L.M. and Isselbacher, K.J., J. Cell Biol. 54:195, 1972.

9. Warshaw, A.L., Walker, W.A. and Isselbacher, K.J., Gastroenterology 64:188, 1973.

10. Walker, W.A., Isselbacher, K.J. and Bloch, K.J., Science 177:608, 1972.

11. Walker, W.A., Isselbacher, K.J. and Bloch, K.J., J. Immunol 111:221, 1973.

12. Greenwood, F.C., Hunter, W.M. and Glover, J.S., Biochem. J. 89:114, 1963.

13. Steinman, R.M. and Cohn, Z.A. J. Cell. Biol. 55:616, 1972.

14. Walker, W.A., Field, M., Davenport, L.M. and Isselbacher, K.J., Proc. Nat. Acad. Sci. (in press) 1973.

15. Ugolev, A.M., Gut 13:735, 1972.

16. Williams, R.C. and Gibbons, R.J., Science 177:697, 1972.

LACK OF C3 ACTIVATION THROUGH CLASSICAL OR ALTERNATE PATHWAYS BY HUMAN SECRETORY IGA ANTI BLOOD GROUP A ANTIBODY

H.R. Colten and J. Bienenstock

Children's Hospital Medical Center, Boston, Mass., and McMaster University, Hamilton, Ontario, Canada

There have been several reports showing that serum IgA antibody does not fix Cl or activate the complement sequence as judged by the classical hemolytic assay following aggregation of the molecule either by heat or bisdiazobenzidine (BDB) (1 - 7). Similar attempts with secretory IgA have led to the same conclusions (8).

The biological function of secretory IgA is at best poorly understood and since aggregated myeloma IgA will activate the alternate pathway we have investigated the ability of pure 11S secretory IgA anti blood group A antibody prepared by the methods of Moreno and Kabat (9) to bind Cl or activate the alternate pathway when combined with antigen on the human red cell surface. We have also looked at the activity in this system of BDB treated non-specific secretory IgA.

Human blood group A red cells (1.5×10^8 per ml) were sensitized with sub-agglutinating doses of pure 11S secretory IgA anti A. Autologous fresh serum was added as a source of complement. The mixtures were incubated at $37^{\circ}C$ for 1 hr and the residual C3 activity was measured with a functional hemolytic assay. Preparations of reagents used and details of the assay system are as described by Rapp and Borsos (10). In order to look for possible inhibitors of the alternate pathway, assays were also performed in autologous serum diluted 1 : 3. BDB aggregation of secretory IgA was performed as reported

elsewhere (11).   C4 deficient guinea pig serum was
obtained from Dr. M. Frank.   Agarose electrophoresis and
immunofixation of Properdin factor B (GBG) was done by the
method of Alper (12).

Table 1

Cells	Antibody (µg)		Serum	C3 activity *
Human A	#1 anti A	4.3	Human	1800
Human A	#2 anti A	8.8	Human	2040
Human A	–		Human	1850
–	BDB agg. sec. IgA	0.1	Human	880
–	–		Human	1220
Human A	#3 anti A	12	C4 Def.gp	780
–	#3 anti A	12	C4 Def.gp	789
Human A	–		C4 Def.gp	830
–	–		C4 Def.gp	760

*   Detection of serum yielding 63% lysis in standard C3
      hemolytic assay (1 effective C3 molecule/cell)

As seen in Table 1, C3 was not utilized by secretory
IgA anti A bound to the red cell surface either in
autologous or C4 deficient serum.   Figure 1 shows that no
cleavage of GBG occurred in these systems, demonstrating
the lack of ability under these conditions of secretory
IgA to activate the alternate pathway.   Three separate
preparations of secretory IgA have given the same results.

BDB treated secretory IgA showed activation of C3 at
0.1 µg of sensitizing IgA at 1/120 of the dose at which no
activation occurred on the cell surface.   Similar results
were obtained with a second IgA preparation.

Thus, 11S secretory IgA antibody on the red cell
surface appears unable to activate the complement system
by either route.   These results are supported by several
reports on the inability of secretory IgA antibody to
cause opsonization of bacteria or red cells (13-17) in the
presence of complement, although some conflicting
evidence exists (18-20).

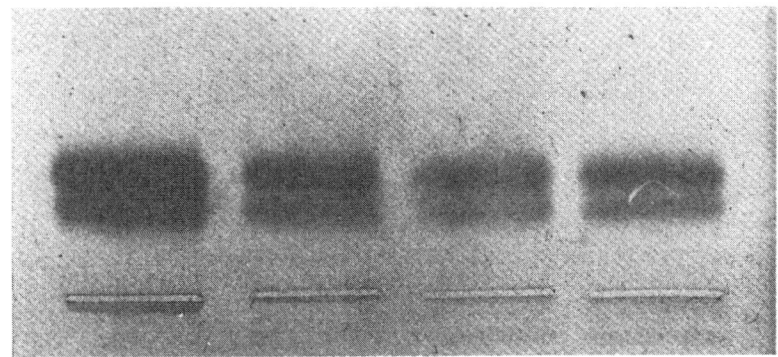

Sec IgA   o   +   +   o

  A rbc   o   +   +   +

A serum   +   +   +   +

Agarose gel electrophoresis showing lack of conversion of
C3 after incubation of secretory IgA antibody and red
cells

     It should be noted that secretory IgA of only one
specificity was studied, therefore more general
conclusions should be deferred.

REFERENCES

1. Ishizaka, T., Ishizaka, K., Borsos, T., and Rapp, H.
   J. Immunol. 97: 716, 1966.
2. Adinolfi, M., Mollison, P.L., Polley, M.J., and Rose,
   J.M., J. Exp. Med. 123: 951, 1966.
3. Heremans, J.F., Vaerman, J.P., and Vaerman, C., J.
   Immunol. 91: 11, 1963.
4. Rawson, A.J., and Abelson, N.M., J. Immunol. 93: 192,
   1964.
5. Vaerman, J.P., and Heremans, J.F., Int. Arch. Allergy
   Appl. Immunol. 34: 49, 1968.
6. Frommhagen, L.H., and Fudenberg, H.H., J. Immunol. 89:
   336, 1962.
7. Ishizaka, T., Ishizaka, K., Salmon, S., and Fudenberg,
   H.H., J. Immunol. 99: 82, 1967.
8. South, M.A., Cooper, M.D., Wollheim, F.A., Hong, R., and
   Good, R.A., J. Exp. Med. 123: 615, 1966.

9. Moreno, C., and Kabat, E.A., J. Exp. Med. 129: 871, 1969.

10. Rapp, H.J., and Borsos, T., in The molecular basis of Complement Action, Appleton, Century, Crofts, N.Y., 1970.

11. Ishizaka, K., Ishizaka, T., and Lee, E.H., J. Immunol. 95: 771, 1965.

12. Alper, C.A., and Propp, R.P., J. Clin. Invest. 47: 2181, 1968.

13. Huber, H., Douglas, S.D., Huber, C., and Goldberg, L.S. Int. Arch. Allergy Appl. Immunol. 41: 262, 1971.

14. Eddie, D.S., Schulkind, M.L., and Robbins, J.B. J. Immunol. 106: 181, 1971.

15. Wilson, I.D., J. Immunol. 108: 726, 1972.

16. Quie, P.G., Messner, R.P., and Williams, R.C., J. Exp. Med. 128: 553, 1968.

17. Zipursky, A., Brown, E.J., and Bienenstock, J., Proc. Soc. Exp. Biol. Med., 142: 181, 1973.

18. Kaplan, M.E., Dalmasso, A.P., and Woodson, M., J. Immunol. 108: 275, 1972.

19. Reynolds, H.Y., and Thompson, R.E., J. Immunol. 111: 369, 1973.

20. Knop, J., Breu, H., Wernet, P., and Rowley, D., Aust. J. Exp. Biol. Med. Sci. 49: 405, 1971.

DISCUSSION

Dr. Montgomery - I have two questions, one for Dr. Ogra
and the other one I guess is a more general question. Let's
take the specific one first. Dr. Ogra, did you ever put
dead polio or any other type of viral vaccine in the gut and
look at a remote secretory site such as mammary tissue? You
looked at a distal mucosal surface, if I understood your data
correctly, and didn't see an antibody response. Did you
ever look at a site such as mammary tissue?

Dr. Ogra - We have looked at a number of sera-negative
pregnant women who were immunized with inactivated polio
vaccine given intranasally or parenterally and live Sabin
vaccine given orally, and what we have found so far is that
inactivated vaccine when given intranasally, does not induce
a serum response or a mammary response. When inactivated
vaccine is given intramuscularly, a very profound mammary
response and a very good serum response is obtained. When
live vaccine was given orally, an appreciable mammary response
and a fairly decent serum response was obtained.

Dr. Montgomery - Thank you. That takes care of that question. The other question concerns Dr. Walker's presentation.
The pinocytotic mechanism -- I need a clarification for my
own mind -- it works for HRP and BSA. Do you have any idea
concerning such a mechanism operative in a bacterial situation? Would the bacteria be absorbed in that way? The
second part of the question is that if such bacterial
antigens would be absorbed in that way, would you envision an
antibody to block such an absorption in a bacterial system?
I may be pre-empting someone else's talk, but I was curious
if you had any comments on that.

Dr. Walker - What we were presenting is primarily related
to soluble antigens; we have not specifically worked with
bacteria although there have been reports of bacteria being
taken up by the intestine by other investigators. I would
assume that this would take place through an altered mucosal
barrier, most likely on ingestion of the cell itself.

Dr. Kunkel - I wanted to ask Dr. Walker whether he did any
measurements of antibody at the mucosal surface. If there

is antibody there, I would think you'd expect your results.
Perhaps your technique is a very indirect way of measuring
local antibody.

Dr. Walker - Both pertain; first of all, we did measure
quantitative antibody activity using a modification of the
Farr technique on secretions, extracts of mucosa as well
as serum. Using a radioautography immunodiffusion technique
and to determine specific antibody, we were able to demonstrate the class specific antibodies in secretions as well
as in mucosal extracts from the animals immunized. We
could not look specifically at gut sacs after they had been
exposed to antigen because the antibodies were probably
complexed with antigen and could not be identified. We
looked at the serum from these animals however, and they
had the same levels of antibody activity as those in which we
looked for secretions and extracts. We looked at animals
handled in a similar fashion for secretions. This is what
we based our immunization data on.

Dr. Dawe - Just a comment on the first two papers from, you
might say a divergent field, i.e. veterinary medicine.
There is an intranasally administered vaccine, available
commercially in veterinary medicine which contains two
modified live viruses: infectious bovine rhinotracheitis and
parainfluenzae 3 plus Pasteurella. The interesting thing
about this is that the modified live parenterally administered
IBR vaccine cannot be used in pregnant females and that it
induces abortions in large numbers of them, but when you use
the intranasally administered vaccine, it gives extremely
good protection and does not have the problem of abortion
that they see. This is now available and massive doses are
being used in the Midwest in large populations of cattle, and
I think here's a model that we might be considering where we
can get larger numbers to study some of these problems, rather
than having the problem of dealing with humans -- back to the
idea of comparative medicine.

Dr. Good - I'm very glad that the issue of the local immunity
system pertaining to cell-mediated immunity was raised, and
the very fine work that has been done by Henney and Waldman
brought to the front. Dr. Mueller and I have been very much
interested in this issue vis-a-vis the gastrointestinal tract
as well as the respiratory tract. Mueller has been doing
experiments very parallel to the early experiments of Henney
and Waldman in our laboratories but using stimulation via the

GI tract. He has found clear evidence that local immunity
related to cell-mediated functions can be induced without
initiating very many cell-mediated functions in the systemic
domain. We think this might have important implications
with respect to the local defense against certain virus,
fungus and bacterial infections. The vaccine strain polio
infections that occur in children with severe combined
immunodeficiency disease are a case in point as Drs. Lopez,
Biggar, Park and I found. Children just do not eliminate
these viruses no matter how much antibody we give them
parenterally or enterally. Upon reconstitution of cellular
immunity, and in some instances we have reconstituted
vis-a-vis the cellular mechanism, they will promptly eliminate
the virus from their secretions. I really think this all
needs much more study but I can go this far at present. I
really think that cell-mediated immunity is a very important
component of the local immunity system. I was a little
confused by what Dr. Bienenstock said. He gave us clear
evidence that antibody of the IgA system on red blood cells
directed against a particular antigen on the red blood cells
does not activate the complement system. However I did
understand him to say that, as others have found, aggregated
IgA will activate the complement system. Wouldn't a more
relevant analysis be whether antigen-antibody complexes
alleviate IgA rather than whether antibodies against red blood
cells do so? Crucial quantitative issues may be involved
in the latter that require precise analysis which has not
yet been presented.

Dr. Bienenstock - The problem is, Dr. Good that Harvey
Colton tried to do that, but there are extreme technical
problems relating to the use of blood group A substance in
this particular system. All I was trying to point out was
that a biological system with antigen-antibody complexes was
more relevant to this question than potentially BDB treated
immunoglobulin.

Dr. Freter - I have a question for Dr. Walker. There is a
recurrent idea popping up in work of various people that
local immunity may be based, at least in part, on leukocytes
"crawling out" of the mucosa and phagocytizing bacteria. Did
you notice in your preparations in the fluids of your cells
any kind of leukocytes that might have explained the increased
breakdown of your antigens?

Dr. Walker - No, Dr. Freter, we did not.

Dr. Newcomb - I've got a question for Dr. Waldman. In the
guinea pig, you and Chris Henney have shown that you did
not get MIF produced by cells from bronchial washings unless
preceded by local immunization. Recenlty Kaltreider and
Salmon demonstrated that T cells did not appear in canine
bronchial washings unless preceded by non-sepcific
irritation or antigens. I wonder if there might be some
connection.

Dr. Waldman - I think the data on the canine cells suggest
that there are no T-cells as measured by PHA stimulation.
I think one might question whether or not this is an
adequate assay for the presence of T-cells. Certainly in
other systems one can find evidence for T-lymphocytes present
all the time. Of course, most animals are constantly under
some sort of stimulation; they are not in antigen-free
circumstances, so I can't answer. I don't know whether or
not there needs to be some sort of prior antigenic stimulation.

Dr. Bockman - Some years ago Dr. Winborn and I studied the
intestinal absorption of ferritin in hamsters in the normal
condition and after previous immunization. Although it was
not quanitative we got the distinct impression that after
immunization there was a distinct increase in the amount of
absorbed ferritin within the epithelial cells. I'll be
looking forward to Dr. Walker's second hypothesis: the
absorption of more of the material into the cells and the
breakdown of lysozomal mechanisms. With respect to the
question of absorption of bacteria, we didn't find absorption
of bacteria in these types of cells but there is a location
where bacteria seem to be absorbed as a normal process and
that's in the specialized, what we refer to as follicle
associated, epithelium which is demonstrated, for instance,
in the rabbit appendix. Later on I hope to show some of the
fine structure of that follicle associated epithelium in
the appendix of experimental animals as well as in the human.

Dr. Butler - I would like to make a comment on Dr. Walker's
paper which relates to the interpretation of antibodies that
occur in the sera of patients with IgA deficiencies. We
have been studying these antibodies for the last few years
and similar to other investigators, have found the presence
of anti-ruminant antibodies. Many of these antibodies are
directed against ruminant immunoglobulins and in our hands,
and in agreement with reports in the literature, are directed
particularly against bovine IgM. However, we found another

antigen which is part of the epithelial cell glycocalyx of
the bovine mammary gland (which we call BAMP) that is also
an antigen against which we find antibodies in patients with
IgA deficiencies. Following Dr. Fudenberg's paper which
showed that patients with anti-ruminant IgM antibodies could
also have antibodies to human IgM, we decided to look for
the presence of antibodies in IgA deficient patients to human
epithelial cell mucoproteins. Rabbit or human antibodies
to BAMP failed to react, by indirect fluorescence, with 300
normal human biopsies, but we did find something quite
interesting. Human epithelial-cell-derived neoplasms have
this antigen or something which has antigenic determinants in
common with BAMP on their surface and the sera of patients
with these neoplasms contain antibodies to BAMP. Hence,
antibodies to BAMP occur either in individuals with IgA
deficiencies and without known tumors, or patients with
epithelial cell neoplasms. At this point we are wondering
whether there is some correlation between IgA deficiency
and a deficiency of the thymus which effects immune surveil-
lance. Hence, serum antibodies to the bovine proteins may
not necessarily indicate the intestinal absorption of food
antigens, but may in some cases represent antibodies to
tumor antigens.

BACTERIAL ADHERENCE TO MUCOSAL SURFACES AND ITS INHIBITION BY SECRETORY ANTIBODIES

R. J. Gibbons

Forsyth Dental Center
Boston, Massachusetts

INTRODUCTION

To understand how antibodies in secretions can protect against bacterial infection, it is necessary to understand the requirements for microbial colonization of mucosal surfaces. It is obvious that bacteria must proliferate on these surfaces, and consequently antibodies have been studied for their ability to kill bacteria in association with the complement and phagocytic systems. However complement-dependent bactericidal reactions and opsonization appear to be of lesser importance on mucosal surfaces than in systemic environments. This is because the secretions which bathe man's mucous surfaces lack at least several components of the complement system, and the mucinous glycoproteins present possess anti-complementary activity. Moreover, active leukocytes are not common on most mucosal surfaces. Finally, secretory immunoglobulin A (S-IgA), the predominant antibody type in secretions, has not been generally found to mediate such bactericidal activities (1).

It may be that IgA and other antibodies in secretions can kill bacteria by mechanisms yet to be discovered. However, recent studies of indigenous streptococci in the mouth have elucidated another parameter which is essential for bacterial colonization of mucosal surfaces and is independent of those factors which affect microbial growth or death. It has been shown that bacteria selectively adhere to these surfaces, and the degree to which they adhere influences the extent to which they colonize (2-7).

This simple ecological concept appears to be of
fundamental importance for understanding the ecology of
indigenous and pathogenic bacteria, and it offers an
explanation as to how antibodies in secretions, including
S-IgA, may influence bacterial colonization.

ADHERENCE AND COLONIZATION OF INDIGENOUS BACTERIA

It has been known for several years that certain
bacterial species selectively colonize different sites within
the human oral cavity. For example, Streptococcus sanguis,
S. mitis and frequently S. mutans comprise high proportions
of the streptococcal populations on teeth; yet S. salivarius
does not (5,6,8). Rather S. salivarius is the predominating
Streptococcus species found on the tongue, while S. mitis
predominates on buccal mucosa (6,8-10). The reasons for this
selective bacterial colonization in various oral niches have
never been clear. They were presumed to be due to differences
in the growth of these species as a result of postulated
differences in nutrient availability between sites. However,
few convincing data are available to support these possibilities. Our laboratories have found that these streptococci
and other oral species exhibit surprising differences in their
abilities to attach to the surfaces of the tongue, cheek, or
teeth. The relative ability of all species thus far studied
to attach to a given surface in the mouth has been found to
correlate directly with the proportions of that species found
indigenously (2-7). Thus the ability of these indigenous
organisms to attach to surfaces appears to determine both the
location and extent to which they may colonize.

One can theorize that in environments which contain
surfaces exposed to a fluid flow, bacteria must either adhere
to a surface or else multiply at a rate which exceeds the
dilution rate caused by the fluid flow if they are to
colonize. Otherwise the organisms are simply washed away.
Most of man's mucous membranes, as well as the eye, heart,
bladder, etc. represent examples of such environments. It
has long been recognized that most of the bacteria found in
the oral cavity and in the intestinal canal of man and animals
are firmly attached to the surfaces present (7, 10,11).
Microbial growth in most of these environments appears to be
occurring at a slow overall rate (12, 13), and it is likely
slower than the dilution rate resulting from the flow of
secretions. Under these conditions, the ability of an
organism to adhere to an exposed surface or become mechanical-

ly entrapped in a protected niche would be essential for it's colonization.

Because epithetial surfaces desquamate continuously, a bacterial clone is not likely to have the opportunity to proliferate for an extended period of time on a given epithelial cell. This situation, together with a relatively slow overall rate of growth, would have the effect of minimizing shifts in bacterial populations due to differences in growth rates between species. In addition, organisms which become dislodged must reattach to the constantly renewing mucosa for colonization to continue. The net effect of a small difference in the ability of two species to attach to a mucosal surface therefore becomes compounded with time. Consequently, the extent to which a given species may colonize such an environment would be largely influenced by its innate capacity to adhere, and by the number of bacterial cells available for attachment.

ADHERENCE OF PATHOGENIC BACTERIA

The importance of adherence in determining if and where indigenous bacteria may colonize implies that adherence should also be important for the colonization of pathogenic organisms. It seems likely that the extent to which a pathogen can attach to a surface should influence the extent to which it may colonize, and thus be related to its virulence. Many pathogens have been observed to adhere to mucosal epithelium. Moreover, direct correlations have been reported between the ability of strains of gonococci (14), S. pyogenes (15), Shigella flexneri (16), enteropathogenic E. coli (17,18) and Mycoplasma species (19) to adsorb to mucosal surfaces and their ability to initiate infections.

The relationship between the adherence and the virulence of Streptococcus pyogenes has been studied in our laboratories. S. pyogenes possesses an array of antigens, but the most important appears to be the M protein. The presence of this type specific antigen is well documented to be essential for virulence (20,21). It is also known that naturally acquired immunity to infection by S. pyogenes is directed against this surface antigen. We have found that virulent strains of S. pyogenes possessing M protein attached well to human buccal and pharyngeal cells, whereas an avirulent mutant lacking M protein adsorbed poorly (15,22). Tryptic removal of M protein from virulent strains greatly reduced their ability to adsorb.

It was also found that treatment of virulent strains with
type specific anti-M serum inhibited their ability to attach
to epithelial surfaces. These and other data indicate that
the virulence related M protein surface antigen of S. pyogenes
participated in its adherence to mucosal surfaces, thereby
fostering its colonization (15,22).

Jones and Rutter (18), subsequently reported that the
virulence-related K88 surface antigen of enteropathogenic
strains of E. coli associated with piglet diarrhea promoted
attachment of the organism to the small intestine. Antiserum
to the K88 antigen also inhibited the adherence of virulent
strains. Similar findings have recently been reported for
pili antigens involved in the adherence of virulent gonococci
(14). On the basis of these and other examples, it seems
likely that surface antigens of many pathogenic bacteria
influence their adherence to mucosal surfaces. These would
be expected to affect colonization of the pathogen, and hence
relate to its virulence.

ANTIBODY MEDIATED INHIBITION OF BACTERIAL ADHERENCE

Several investigators have shown that when various
bacteria are introduced into the mouth, the nasopharyngeal
area, or the intestinal canal, the organisms are generally
rapidly cleared (23-25). Thus the cleansing action existant
on mucosal surfaces is apparent. The mucous secretions,
aided by cilial beating of epithelial cells in the trachea,
or by forces imposed by the tongue and mastication in the
oral cavity, or intestinal motility and peristalsis in the
upper bowel appear to be major cleansing forces. Their
collective actions, along with epithelial cell desquamation,
nonspecifically limit bacterial colonization on mucosal
surfaces.

Several lines of evidence led us to recently propose
that antibodies, and particularly S-IgA, may augment the
cleansing action of secretions and provide protective
immunity by inhibiting the adherence and colonization of
bacteria (26,13). S-IgA antibodies are capable of specifically binding to antigenic components on the surfaces of
bacteria, and of causing their agglutination (1). In light
of the participation of antigenic bacterial surface components
in their adherence, this property of S -IgA per se could
interfere with microbial colonization, thereby providing
protective immunity. This possibility seemed likely

because antisera directed against surface antigens of V. cholerae (27), S. pyogenes (15,22), E. coli (18) and S. salivarius (26) have been shown to inhibit the attachment of these species to mucosal surfaces. Serum antibodies also inhibit the formation of adherent deposits of S. mutans (28) in vitro.

The studies of Freter with experimental cholera also provided evidence which enabled us to formulate this hypothesis (27,29,30). Freter observed that induced coproantibodies were protective against experimental infection by V. cholerae. He further observed that when live vibrios were introduced into intestinal loops of immunized animals, or animals to which hyperimmune antiserum had been administered, the vibrios tended to remain free in the lumen, whereas greater numbers of vibrios could be cultured from the mucosal lining of non-immune animals. Freter therefore recognized that there was an inverse relationship between the number of viable vibrios recoverable from intestinal linings and immunity. He hypothesized that either the antibodies were directly inhibiting the adsorption of the vibrios, or that there was an antibody-dependent antibacterial reaction occurring on the mucosal surface (27,29,30). In subsequent investigations data were obtained which supported the latter possibility, but it was pointed out that a direct effect upon bacterial adsorption could not be ignored (29). These experiments were conducted before data were available concerning the selective nature of bacterial adherence and its influence on bacterial colonization.

We have recently found that S-IgA isolated from human parotid saliva contained agglutinating antibody against some strains of S. salivarius and S. mitis, but not other serotypes of these species (26). The S-IgA preparation was found to inhibit attachment to human buccal epithelial cells of those strains against which it exhibited antibody activity, but it had no detectable effect on the adherence of other strains (26). S-IgA antibodies evidently react with bacterial surface antigens and sterically hinder attachment of the organisms to epithelial cells. The antibody-bacterial reaction could occur as the organisms are growing on the mucosal surface so that dislodged cells have an impaired ability to reattach, or it could occur with bacteria transiently present in the secretions (Fig. 1)

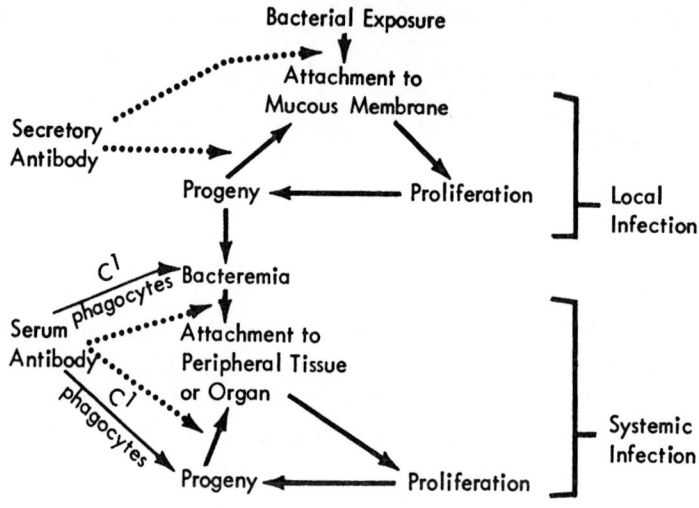

POSSIBLE ROLE OF ANTIBODY MEDIATED INHIBITION OF BACTERIAL
ADHERENCE IN LOCAL AND SYSTEMIC IMMUNITY

It should be noted that a small degree of inhibition of
adherence becomes multiplied by the constant need for bacterial reattachment occurring on desquamating mucosal surfaces.
Thus, immunoglobulin-mediated inhibition of adherence of one
serotype relative to another would lead to the elimination of
the affected strain in a highly efficient manner. Teleologi-
cally, this may account for the low titres of S-IgA and other
immunoglobulins which are generally detected in secretions.

In systemic infections, the pathogen must gain entrance
to the bloodstream, and then a similar sequence of events
involving attachment, multiplication, and reattachment to
either the same or a distant tissue may occur (Fig. 1). Serum
antibodies typified by IgG and IgM may facilitate killing of
the pathogen at any of these stages with mediation of the
complement and phagocytic systems. However, it is clear that
immune sera also inhibit bacterial attachment. Consequently
it is reasonable to postulate that serum antibodies may also
contribute to systemic immunity by interfering with the
adherence and colonization of the agent at peripheral sites,
thereby reducing dissemination of the infection.

ADHERENCE INHIBITION IN LOCAL IMMUNITY

There are a variety of data which directly support, or
are consistent with the concepts advanced. For example,
Fubara and Freter (31) have recently reported that purified

S-IgA obtained from gut washings of orally vaccinated germ-
free mice passively protected against experimental cholera
infection. This protection was associated with a reduction
of the vibrio populations which adsorbed to the intestinal
mucosa. Similarly, in a preliminary report, Griffen and
Paulissen (32) observed that intestinal washings of orally
immunized mice contained motility-inhibiting antibodies to
Salmonella enteriditis. The appearance of antibody in
intestinal secretions was related to a more rapid clearance
of S. enteriditis following oral challenge.

Certain examples of naturally acquired immunity provide
other supportive data. A state of immunity commonly exists
following recovery from an infectious bacterial agent whereby
the host is protected from re-infection. This immunity to
re-infection has been observed for beta hemolytic streptococci, staphylococci, pneumococci, Mycoplasma species and
Corynebacterium diphtheriae. Immunity following these natural
infections is frequently type specific, and in many cases it
appears to affect the ability of the pathogen to colonize
locally on mucosal surfaces. One of the best examples stems
from the studies of Watson and coworkers (33). They observed
that when monkeys were inoculated intranasally with virulent
strains of S. pyogenes, the organisms colonized the mucosal
surfaces of the animals for weeks before being eliminated.
A state of immunity developed, for when these animals were subsequently challenged with the same M type of S. pyogenes, the
inoculated organisms were not generally detected after 24
hours. However different M types of the organism could successfully colonize such animals. These observations indicate
that a type specific immunity to S. pyogenes can be induced
following natural infection in primates. This immunity acted
by preventing colonization of the challenge organism on the
mucosal surface, and it was associated with a rapid clearance
of the pathogen. That this entailed an inhibition of adherence is further suggested by the fact that the immunity was
directed against the type-specific M protein surface antigen
which is involved in the attachment of this pathogen to mucosal surfaces (15,22).

POTENTIAL ECOLOGICAL EFFECTS OF SECRETORY ANTIBODIES

Other data are available which suggest the existance of
an immunological selection pressure imposed upon bacteria
colonizing mucosal surfaces. Several investigators have shown
that over time, there is a continual changeover of the sero-

types of E. coli which colonize the intestinal canal of man
(34,35). The conversion and selection of bacterial serotypes
has been most intensively studied by Miller and co-workers
(36,37). These investigators observed that when germfree
animals were monoinfected with a specific serotype of V.
cholerae, the inoculated serotype prevailed for approximately
2 weeks and then was replaced by a different serotype which
had arisen by mutation. This changeover of serotype was
accelerated if the animals were previously immunized with the
strain inoculated. Conversely, almost complete inhibition of
serotype conversion occurred when the animals were treated
with the immunosuppressant agent, cyclophosphamide. Thus
these investigators concluded that a potent immunologic
selection pressure can be imposed upon bacteria colonizing
mucosal surfaces. Although it was not demonstrated, it seems
likely that immunoglobulins present in the secretions bathing
these surfaces were involved.

It is clear that man's mucous secretions contain low
titres of antibodies against indigenous bacteria (1). Hence
these antibodies should influence the colonization of indigenous organisms. Data are available which suggest that the
adherence of many indigenous bacteria is suppressed in the
oral cavity, and this is seemingly mediated in part by
secretory antibodies (26). For example, epithelial cells
scraped directly from human buccal surfaces average only 10 to
15 bacteria per epithelial cell, even though these cells are
continuously exposed to concentrations of S. salivarius, S.
mitis and other indigenous bacteria approaching 10^8 organisms/
ml of saliva. If the epithelial cells are washed and incubated with suspensions of these streptococci grown in vitro,
hundreds of organisms attach to each epithelial cell in less
than an hour. Thus it is clear that these streptococci, as
they exist in saliva, possess a reduced capacity to attach to
mucosal surfaces. Brandtzaeg and coworkers (38) have shown
that salivary bacteria are coated with IgA. Similarly, the
bacterial deposits on human teeth have been found to contain
significant quantities of IgA and IgG (39). The demonstrated
ability of immunoglobulins to inhibit the attachment of bacteria to epithelial surfaces therefore seems to be at least
partially responsible for the suppressed adherence of salivary
organisms.

The apparent existance of an immunologic selection
pressure imposed upon bacteria colonizing mucosal surfaces has
important implications for understanding the aggressive ecolo-

gical behavior of infectious agents (26). It has generally been assumed that once small numbers of a pathogen are introduced on a mucosal surface, the organisms somehow overgrow indigenous bacteria and attain numerical prominence. But there are few data which suggest that either the nutritional requirements or the potential growth rates of pathogens are sufficiently different from those of indigenous bacteria to achieve this effect. However, in a non-immune individual, a pathogen represents a serotypically novel organism in the environment. Thus, unlike most other bacteria present, it would possess a temporary immunologic selective advantage whereby it could adhere and colonize unimpeded by secretory antibodies. This would enable small numbers of a pathogen to attach prominance within a relatively short period of time in a manner quite analogous to the selection pressure which enables small numbers of a mutant serotype to emerge during the process of serotype conversion. Once the pathogen has colonized in high numbers, it would stimulate an antibody response. Because this may be augmented by tissue dammage produced by toxins or lytic enzymes, the antibody response would likely be greater than that to most indigenous bacteria. Consequently the adherence of the pathogen would become inhibited to a greater extent than most of the indigenous flora, and the pathogen would become selectively eliminated. An immune state would now exist whereby the individual would be protected against re-infection by the same serotype. However, should colonization of the pathogen progress slowly and elicit a comparable secretory antibody response to that imposed against indigenous bacteria, the pathogen would exist in a transient balanced or "carrier state" in which its adherence and colonization would be similar to that of indigenous bacteria. In this state of partial suppression, the pathogen would colonize for weeks or months as serotypes of indigenous bacteria appear to do before being eliminated or undergoing serotype conversion. It is apparent from these discussions that the selective nature of bacteria adherence and its role in colonization has broad applicability to many problems related to infection and immunity.

REFERENCES

1. Tomasi, T.B., and Grey, H.M. Prog. Allergy 16:81, 1972.
2. Gibbons, R.J., and van Houte, J. Infect. & Immun. 3:567, 1971.
3. van Houte, J., Gibbons, R.J., and Banghart, S. Archs Oral Biol. 15:1025, 1970.

4.   Liljemark, W.F., and Gibbons, R.J.   Infect. & Immun. 4:
     264, 1971.
5.   van Houte, J., Gibbons, R.J., and Pulkkinen, A.J.   Archs.
     Oral Biol. 16:1131, 1971.
6.   Liljemark, W.F., and Gibbons, R.J. Infect. & Immun. 6:852,
     1972.
7.   Gibbons, R.J. "Ecology and Cariogenic Potential of Oral
     Streptococci", Streptococci and Streptococcal Diseases.
     L. W. Wannamaker & J. Matsen, eds., pgs. 381-385, Academic
     Press, N.Y., 1972.
8.   Carlsson, J. Odont. Revy 18:55, 1967.
9.   Krasse, B. Odont. Revy 5:203, 1954.
10. Gibbons, R.J., Kapsimalis, B., and Socransky, S.S.   Archs.
     Oral Biol. 9:101, 1964.
11. Savage, D.C. Microbial Pathogenicity in Man and Animals.
     Cambridge University Press, 1972.
12. Gibbons, R.J.   J. Dent. Res. 43:1021, 1964.
13. Gibbons, R.J., and Kapsimalis, B. J. Bacteriol. 93:510,
     1967.
14. Punsalang, A.P., and Sawyer, W.D.   Infect. & Immun. 8:255,
     1973.
15. Ellen, R.P., and Gibbons, R.J.   Infect. & Immun. 5:826,
     1972.
16. Labrec, E.H., Schneider, H., Magnani, T.J., and Formal,
     S.B.   J. Bacteriol. 88:1503, 1964.
17. Bertschinger, H.V., Moon, H.W., and Whipp, S.C.   Infect. &
     Immun. 5:606, 1972.
18. Jones, G.W., and Rutter, J.M.   Infect. & Immun. 6:918, 1972
19. Sobeslansky, O., Prescott, B., and Chanock, R.M.   J. Bact-
     eriol. 96:695, 1970.
20. Lancefield, R.C.   J. Immunol. 89:307, 1962.
21. Maxted, W.R., and Widdowson, J.P. "The Protein Antigens of
     Group A Streptococci", Streptococci and Streptococcal
     Diseases.   L. W. Wannamaker & J. Matsen, eds., pgs. 251-
     266, Academic Press, N.Y., 1972.
22. Ellen, R.P., and Gibbons, R.J.   Ab. 284, IADR, 1973.
23. Bloomfield, A.L. Johns Hopkins Hosp. Bull. 13:14, 1920.
24. Dixon, J.M.S.   J. Path. Bact. 79:131, 1960.
25. Cooke, E.M., Hettiaratchy, I.G.T., and Buck, A.C.   J. Med.
     Microbiol. 5:361, 1972.
26. Williams, R.C., and Gibbons, R.J.   Science 177:697, 1972.
27. Freter, R.   Texas Rpts. on Biol. and Med.   27:299, 1969.
28. Evans, R.T., and Genco, R.J.   Infect. & Immun. 7:237, 1973.
29. Freter, R.   Infect. & Immun. 6:134, 1972.
30. Freter, R.   Infect. & Immun. 2:556, 1970.
31. Fubara, E.S., and Freter, R.   J. Immunol. 111:395, 1973.

32. Griffen, B.R., and Paulissen, L.J. Abstract M25, 73rd
     Meeting, Amer. Soc. Microbiol., 1973.
33. Watson, R.F., Rothbard, S., and Swift, H.F. J. Exp. Med.
     84:127, 1946.
34. Robinet, H.G. J. Bacteriol. 84:896, 1962.
35. Cooke, E.M., Ewins, S., and Shooter, R.A. Brit. Med. J.
     4:593, 1969.
36. Sack, R.B., and Miller, C.E. J. Bacteriol. 99:688, 1969.
37. Miller, C.E., Wong, K.H., Feeley, J.C., and Forbines, M.E.
     Infect. & Immun. 6:739, 1972.
38. Brandtzaeg, P., Fjellanger, J., and Gjeruldsen, S.T. J.
     Bacteriol. 96:242, 1968.
39. Taubman, M.A. Abst. 881, IADR, 1972.

SPECIFICITY OF ANTIBODIES TO STREPTOCOCCUS MUTANS; SIGNIFICANCE IN INHIBITION OF ADHERENCE

Robert J. Genco, Richard T. Evans, and
Martin A. Taubman
School of Dentistry, State University of New
York and Forsyth Dental Center
Buffalo, N. Y. and Boston, Mass.

INTRODUCTION

Shortly after strains of Streptococcus mutans were shown to be cariogenic, they were found to produce dextran and levan polymers from sucrose. These polymers are responsible for the ability of S. mutans to adhere to, and colonize smooth surfaces of teeth (1-3; cf. reviews 4,5). The large molecular weight dextrans and levans are necessary for the formation of plaques on teeth which in turn, appears to be a requirement for cariogenicity. This is supported by the finding that a mutant of S. mutans, lacking the ability to produce these polymers, is no longer cariogenic (6). We have shown the adherence of S. mutans to wires can be inhibited by antiserum to whole S. mutans cells (7). In the same experiments we found that the production of cell-associated polysaccharide was inhibited by antisera, while cell growth was actually increased. The adherence of S. mutans to a glass surface has also been shown to be inhibited by antiserum to whole cells (8). Experiments in our laboratory have shown that antisera to S. mutans will inhibit the glucosyltransferases present in S. mutans culture fluids.These enzymes synthesize polymeric dextrans from sucrose (9). Recently, evidence has been presented (10) showing that the extracellular or soluble glucosyltransferases of S. mutans become cell-associated as insoluble dextran is synthesized. These results suggest that there is a receptor on the bacterial cell surface which binds glucosyltransferase-dextran complexes. The finding that whole cell antisera inhibit

the adherence of S. mutans to wire and glass surfaces, inhibit the production of cell-associated polysaccharide synthesis while not inhibiting cell growth, and inhibit the
synthesis of polyglucan-containing polysaccharides from
sucrose by S. mutans glucosyltransferase enzymes suggests
that antibodies prevent S. mutans from colonizing dental
surfaces by interfering with the production of adherent
polysaccharide polymers. The studies to be reported here
show that the specificity of antibody-mediated inhibition
of S. mutans adherence, and inhibition of glucosyltransferase activity do not always follow the specificity of surface antigens which are used to classify strains of S. mutans (11). The evidence presented indicates that adherence does not depend upon an antigen common to all S. mutans and hence if caries immunization via inhibition of
adherence is to be successful, multivalent vaccines may be
required.

METHODS AND RESULTS

Anti-whole cell sera were prepared by intravenous injection of rabbits with washed S. mutans cells. S. mutans
cultures were kindly provided by Drs. R. Fitzgerald, P. Keyes,
and R. Gibbons. Rabbits were injected with 10^8 cells, six times
over a 2 week period, allowed to rest for varying periods of
time and then boosted with a single intravenous injection of
the same dose of cells and bled 1 week later. Groups of two
or three rabbits were immunized with S. mutans strains, 6715
(gr. "d"), FA-1 (gr. "b"), GS-5 (gr. "c"), and LM-7; the
latter reacts with Lancefield group E and is hereafter
termed gr. "e". The highest titered sera to each serotype
were selected on the basis of indirect immunofluorescent
titrations, and these bleedings were used throughout the
studies. Adherence of S. mutans to nichrome wires (12) and
to glass (8) was carried out in the continuous presence of
various dilutions of serum. Plaque formation on wires by S.
mutans 6715 was markedly inhibited when these wires were im-
mersed in media containing homologous antisera at dilutions
up to 1/320. At homologous antiserum dilutions of 1/10 cell
growth was 6.6 times that in the control tubes without added
serum. By contrast, cell-associated polysaccharide synthesis as measured by quantitative recovery of 0.5 N NaOH
extractible anthrone-positive material was markedly reduced.
Inhibition of S. mutans adherence to glass by homologous
antiserum as observed in a typical experiment, is shown in
Fig. 1.

This experiment was carried out in the presence of sucrose labeled with ^{14}C in the glucose moiety. After incubation, the cells were extracted with 0.5 N NaOH, and the 70% ethanol-insoluble radioactive polyglucan measured. This

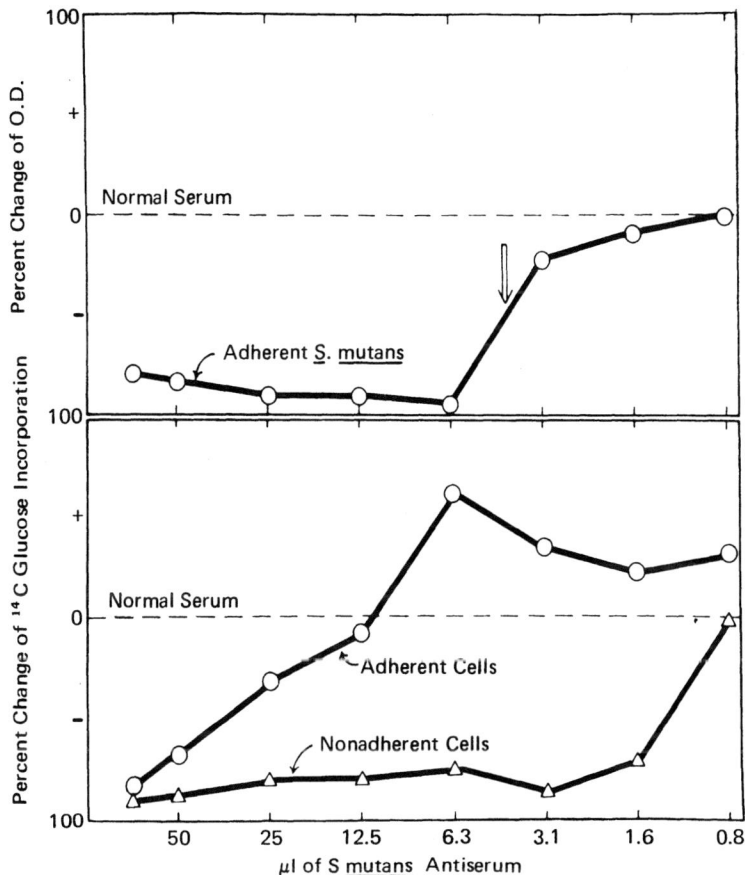

Fig. 1. The top portion represents the optical density of glass-adherent S. mutans st. 6715 cells grow in the presence of antiserum to st. 6715. The data are presented as % increase (+) or decrease (-) in cells compared to those grown in normal serum. The arrow represents the antiserum concentration at which 50% of the cells in the culture were adherent and 50% were free in the culture medium.

The bottom portion represents the change in cell-associated polysaccharide (CAP) synthesis of adherent and non-adherent st. 6715 cells grown in medium containing antiserum to st. 6715. CAP synthesis was assayed by measuring the amount of ^{14}C glucose released from the cells by 0.5 N NaOH. The culture medium contained sucrose labeled in the glucose moiety.

allowed measurement of cell-associated polysaccharide synthesis. There is a marked reduction in the number of adherent cells in the presence of antiserum as compared to non-immune rabbit serum. Non-adherent cells produced less cell-associated polysaccharide than adherent ones. Less antibody was required to reduce cell-associated polysaccharide synthesis (1.3 μl for 50% reduction) than was needed for a similar effect upon adherence (3.6 μl for 50% reduction). These results show that attachment of S. mutans to smooth surfaces can be markedly inhibited by homologous antibodies, and they suggest that inhibition of adherence is brought about by antibody-mediated interference with cell-associated dextran formation. In order to determine whether the antibodies could be functioning either by inhibiting glucosyltransferase activity or by preventing the attachment of glucosyltransferase-dextran complexes to a cell surface receptor, inhibition,by antiserum to st. 6715,of adherence to glass and cell-associated polysaccharide synthesis was measured. Organisms of the same (gr. "d") serotype, i.e. Kl-R, OMZ-176, and SL-1, as well as 6715 were used in the assay. It can be seen from data summarized in Table I that anti-6715 serum inhibited both adherence to glass and cell-associated polysaccharide formation by strains 6715, Kl-R and OMZ-176 but not by strain SL-1 cells. The simplest interpretation is that 6715, Kl-R and OMZ-176 contain common antigens responsible for adherence and that SL-1, even though it is in the same serogroup, lacks this antigen. Table I illustrates the failure of antisera to FA-1 (gr. "b"), GS-5 (gr. "c") and LM-7 (gr. "e") to inhibit adherence and cell-associated polysaccharide synthesis of st. 6715. These 3 antisera also failed to inhibit the adherence of st. 6715 to wires. As illustrated, antiserum to S. mutans st. E-49 (gr. "a"), inhibited the adherence of st. 6715 cells (gr. "d") to glass. This was a weak but significant reaction. This cross reaction did not extend to detectable inhibition of cell-associated polysaccharide synthesis.

The ability of these antisera to inhibit the activity of glucosyltransferases was investigated next since they appeared to inhibit polyglucan synthesis so effectively. Glucosyltransferase activity was assayed by measuring incorporation of the radiolabeled glucose moiety of sucrose into ethanol-insoluble polysaccharide as we have recently described (9). We have made numerous attempts to study the effects of anti-S. mutans sera on the activity of cell-associated glucosyltransferases which are released from the

Table I. Specificity of Inhibition of S. mutans Adherence
and Cell-associated-Polysaccharide Formation
by Rabbit Antisera.[a]

Strain of S. mutans	Inhibition					
	Anti-6715 (gr."d")[b]		Anti-FA-1(gr."b"), -GS-5(gr."c") -LM-7(gr."e")[c]		Anti-E-49 (gr."a")[d]	
	A[e]	P	A	P	A	P
6715(gr."d")	>10%[e]	>10%	<10%	<10%	>10%	<10%
K1-R(gr."d")	>10%	>10%	N.D.[e]		N.D	
OMZ-176 (gr."d")	>10%	>10%	N.D.		N.D.	
S1-1(gr."d)	<10%	<10%	N.D.		N.D.	

a   Adherence to glass was assayed by a modification of the procedures of Olson et al.(1971). Cell-associated polysaccharide production refers to the 0.5 N NaOH-extractible, cell-associated radioactive material produced when the bacteria are grown in sucrose radiolabeled in the glucose moiety. Most of this material is dextran or a dextran-levan polymer.

b   Gr. a,b,c,d, or e refers to the Bratthall serological group of the designated strain (11).

c   These antisera inhibited both adherence and cell-associated polysaccharide production of homologous organisms.

d   Since strain E-49 failed to adhere to glass, rabbit E-49 antiserum could not be tested on homologous bacteria.

e   "A" adherence, "P" cell-associated polysaccharide production, "N.D." not done; more than 10% inhibition was considered significant.

cell by sonication. However, we found enhancement, no effect and inhibition of activity depending on serum concentration and the individual antiserum used. Serum effects
on soluble glucosyltransferase were reproducible and showed
marked inhibition of enzyme activity. Rabbit antisera directed to S. mutans strains 6715 (gr. "d"), and GS-5 (gr.
"c") inhibit homologous soluble glucosyltransferases by 50%-
80%. Antisera to FA-1 (gr. "b") inhibits at a low but significant level (9). When soluble glucosyltransferase enzymes from st. 6715 are incubated with antisera directed to
whole cells of S. mutans strains LM-7 (gr. "e"), GS-5 (gr.
"c"), and FA-1 (gr. "b"), weak inhibition was observed (9).
From results in Table II, it can be seen that two anti-"d"
sera (anti-6715 and anti-OMZ-176) markedly inhibit enzymes
from 2 out of 3 group "d" strains of S. mutans. These antisera also showed substantial cross-reaction with enzymes
from S. mutans st. AHT and st. E-49, both of group "a".

It is of considerable interest that a similar pattern
of cross reactivity is seen when adherence inhibition, extracellular polysaccharide synthesis and glucosyltransferase
inhibition assays are carried out with antiserum to whole
cells. There are definite cross-reactions between group "a"
and "d" organisms with one notable exception. Antisera to
group "d" or group "a" strains do not inhibit adherence,
extracellular polysaccharide synthesis or glucosyltransferase activity of strain SL-1, a group "d" organism.

Boiling water extracts or boiling 0.1N HCl extracts of
S. mutans gr. "d" strains (6715, OMZ-176, SL-1) and gr. "a"
strains (AHT, E-49) were examined in gel-diffusion tests
with antisera to strains from gr. "a" and gr. "d". A cross-reacting
antigen was shared by strains 6715, OMZ-176, AHT and E-49.
Extracts of strain SL-1 have not shown this cross-reacting
antigen. The pattern of cross-reactions observed in the gel
diffusion assays and in the adherence assays suggests that
the antigenic determinant(s) shared by group "a" and "d" organisms are important in adherence.

The antibody nature of glucosyltransferase inhibition
by rabbit antisera is shown by the following: 1) preimmune
sera do not possess this activity; 2) homologous antisera
are markedly more inhibitory than heterologous ones, except
for the instances noted; 3) immunoglobulins, eluted at low
pH from S. mutans st. 6715 after incubation of these cells
in homologous rabbit antiserum, gave marked inhibition of st.

6715 glucosyltransferases; and 4) the inhibitory activity of immune serum could be removed by absorption of the serum with a glucosyltransferase-rich fraction of culture supernate (9).

Table II. Inhibition of S. mutans gr. "d" and "a" Glucosyltransferase Activity[a] by Rabbit Antiserum to gr. "d" cells

| Enzyme Source | Per Cent Inhibition[b] | | |
	Anti-6715	Anti-OMZ-176	NRS[c]
gr. "d"			
st. 6715	32	49	<10
st. OMZ-176	58	66	<10
st. SL-1	10	17	<10
gr. "a"			
st. AHT	52	4	<10
st. E-49	65	73	<10

[a] Whole culture fluids used as enzyme sources for these experiments.

[b] Calculated as the ratio of enzyme inhibition in test serum over that in normal serum, multiplied by 100.

The enzyme activity in normal rabbit serum was $\pm$ 10% of the activity in buffer without serum. Inhibition greater than 10% is thus considered significant. Counting error was less than 5% among replicates.

[c] Normal rabbit serum.

Vaccination studies with conventional and gnotobiotic rats have been done by Dr. M. Taubman. The effects on dental caries and plaque bacteria of various immunization procedures using S. mutans st. 6715 are reported elsewhere (13,15). Briefly, groups of conventional rats were immunized with formalized S. mutans st. 6715 cells in either the foot pads or in and around the salivary glands. Control groups were either sham immunized or left unimmunized. Immunization was repeated until salivary and serum antibody levels appeared to reach plateau levels in the experimental groups. At this time, they were infected with live S. mutans st. 6715. The mean caries scores of immunized rats were lower than the scores of sham-immunized rats. Also of considerable interest was the finding that the numbers of S. mutans st. 6715 were lower in the immune as compared to sham immunized animals (13,15). We have recently tested the serum and saliva of some of these animals for antibodies to glucosyltransferase. Serum and pilocarpine-

stimulated whole saliva from the non-immune control rats had
no effect on the activity of glucosyltransferases obtained
from S.mutans st. 6715 or st. GS-5. On the other hand, saliva and serum from rats immunized with st. 6715 cells markedly inhibited glucosyltransferase activity. Based upon the re-
producibility of the method, we consider greater inhibition
than 10% as significant. Using this criterion, serum from
each of six immunized rats inhibited glucosyltransferase
from st.6715. Only 2 out of these same 6 sera inhibited GS-
5 glucosyltransferase. Inhibition of 6715 glucosyltransferase was detected in 4 out of 6 salivas from immunized rats;
only 1 showed a cross-reaction with enzyme from st. GS-5.
These results confirm in a second animal species, the lack
of cross-reactivity of antibodies which inhibit glucosyltransferases from S. mutans groups "d" and"c" organisms.

After removal of immunoglobulins from saliva by incubation with excess antibody to IgA, inhibition of 6715 glucosyltransferase activity was considerably reduced. Rat saliva
samples were also absorbed with monospecific rabbit anti-rat
α-chain antisera and a similar reduction in inhibition of
glucosyltransferase activity was observed. These absorption
studies suggest that most if not all of the antibodies directed to glucosyltransferase in immunized conventional rat
saliva are of the IgA class.

SUMMARY

The experiments described here show that antisera directed to S. mutans cells can inhibit the adherence of these
cells to smooth surfaces. This new function of antibody is
not dependent upon killing of the bacteria. Inhibition of adherence correlates closely with inhibition of synthesis of
cell-associated polysaccharide and inhibition of glucosyltransferase activity. Studies of reactions among the various
S. mutans serotypes show extensive cross-reactivity between
strains of the Bratthall groups "a" and "d".

The evidence presented here and by others (14) shows
that strains of S. mutans "a" and "d" share an antigen,
termed the "a-d" antigenic determinant. Our findings that
adherence and glucosyltransferase activity of st. SL-1, a
group "d" organism is not inhibited with antisera to group
"a" or "d" organisms is of special importance since we and
others (14) found that this strain does not possess the

"a-d" antigenic determinant. Although direct evidence is lacking, it is likely that the "a-d" antigenic determinant is important in adherence of S. mutans strains of group "a" and "d".

The failure of our strains of group "c", "b", and "Lancefield E" to cross-react with group "d" organisms in adherence and glucosyltransferase assays may represent a true lack of cross reactivity. Further studies using antisera to other representatives of each serotype will be necessary to resolve this question.

The in vivo significance of antibodies to cell surface antigens of S. mutans is suggested by information from the rat experiments. We have shown that immunized rats have salivary antibodies of the IgA class which inhibit the activity of homologous glucosyltransferases. It is possible that these salivary IgA antibodies interfered with S. mutans colonization of the rat teeth by interfering with synthesis of adherent dextrans.

This work was supported in part by USPHS Grants DE-03888, 02814, 0617, and Contract No. NIH-NIDR-71-2333, and by a Public Health Service Research CareerDevelopment Award (to M.A.T.) KO 4 DE-70122.

REFERENCES

1. Jordan, H.V. and Keyes, P.H., Arch. Oral Biol. 11:793, 1966.
2. Gibbons, R.J. and Banghart, S.B., Arch. Oral Biol. 12: 11, 1967.
3. Guggenheim, B. and Newbrun, E., Helv. Odont. Acta 13: 84, 1969.
4. Scherp, H., Science, 173: 1199, 1971.
5. Makinen, K.K., Internat. Dental J. 22: 362, 1972.
6. de Stoppelaar, J.D., Konig, K.G., Plasschaert, J.M. and van der Hoeven, J.S., Arch. Oral Biol. 16: 971, 1971.
7. Genco, R.J. in Dayton, Small, Chanock, Kaufman and Tomasi, Secretory Immunologic System (Vero Beach Proc. 1969), p. 253 (U.S. Govt. Printing Office, Washington, 1971).
8. Olson, G.A., Bleiweis, A.S. and Small, Jr., P.A., Infect. Immunity 5: 419, 1972.
9. Evans, R.T. and Genco, R.J., Infect. Immunity, 7:237

    1973.
10. McCabe, M.M. and Smith, E.E., Infect. Immunity 7: 829, 1973.
11. Bratthall, D., J. Dental Res. 21: 143, 1970.
12. McCabe, R.M., Keyes, P.H., and Howell, A., Arch. Oral Biol. 12: 1653, 1967.
13. Taubman, M.A. in Comparative Immunology of the Oral Cavity, eds. H. Scherp and S. Mergenhagen, U.S. Govt. Printing Office, Washington, D.C., in press, 1973.
14. Mukasa, H. and Slade, H.D., Infect. Immunity, 8: 190, 1973.
15. Taubman, M.A. and Smith, D.J., Journ. Dental Res. Prog. and Abst. 52: 277, 1973.

We thank Mrs. J. Castine, C. Sadowski and J. Buckelew for excellent technical assistance.

SECRETORY ANTIBODIES IN MILK OF SWINE AGAINST TRANSMISSIBLE GASTROENTERITIS VIRUS[a]

Edward H. Bohl, Linda J. Saif,
R. K. Paul Gupta,[b] G. Thomas Frederick
Department of Veterinary Science
Ohio Agricultural Research & Development Center
Wooster, Ohio

Transmissible gastroenteritis (TGE) of swine is a highly contagious, enteric, viral disease characterized by severe diarrhea and high mortality in pigs under 2 weeks of age. TGE virus primarily infects the epithelial cells of the small intestine, resulting in an atrophy of the villi and a malabsorption syndrome (1). We have previously reported that TGE antibodies were primarily of the IgA class in milk from sows which had been exposed orally to virulent virus, but were primarily of the IgG class in those exposed parenterally to live attenuated virus (2,3,4). Also, passive immunity against intestinal infection was more closely associated with milk antibodies of the IgA than the IgG class. The present paper provides additional information, with emphasis on the contrasting features of the antibody response in animals which were orally versus intramammarily exposed to virulent TGE virus.

MATERIALS AND METHODS

Serum and milk were collected from swine which had

[a]Supported in part by an Agr. Res. Service Cooperative Agreement No. 12-14-100-11, 179(45) and a Public Health Service Research Grant AI 10735-01.
[b]Present address: Department of Veterinary Pathology, College of Veterinary Medicine, Haryana Agricultural University, Hissar, India.

been exposed, prior to parturition, with TGE viral preparations by different routes, as previously described (3).
The virulent virus used in these studies was a Miller strain
of gut origin, while the attenuated virus was a high cell-
culture passaged Purdue strain. Experimental oral exposure
was done by placing 5 ml of the virus in the mouth and 5 ml
on the feed of each animal approximately 30 to 45 days prepartum. For intramuscular injections, 5 ml of virus were
employed on each of two occasions, approximately 2 and 6
weeks prepartum. Intramammary injections were given into
three glands on the left side of the udder, using a total
of 5 ml of virus. Two injections were given, approximately
2 and 6 weeks prepartum. Data from injected glands given.

Neutralizing antibody titers were expressed as the
reciprocal of the specimen dilution resulting in an 80%
reduction in plaques (3). Gel filtration of milk was conducted using Sephadex G-200 columns, and fractions were
tested for TGE antibodies and for presence of IgM, IgA, and
IgG using monospecific antisera, as previously described (3).
To further delineate the immunoglobulin (Ig) class of TGE
antibodies, certain colostrum or milk samples were absorped
with monospecific rabbit anti-porcine IgG and IgA sera to
selectively remove the corresponding class of Ig and were
then tested for TGE antibody activity (4).

RESULTS

Oral Exposure with Virulent Virus

The serologic findings on two sows, which are representative of the results obtained on swine orally infected
with virulent virus, are given in Table 1. A characteristic feature was that antibody titers in milk persisted at
fairly high levels (>80) during the lactation period and
were invariably higher than in the corresponding serum
samples taken concurrently from the same animal.

Gel filtration studies on colostrum and milk samples
from animals in this group indicated that, throughout lactation, antibodies were always associated with IgA. In
contrast, antibodies were usually associated with IgG only
during the first few days of lactation. Figure 1 is representative of the gel filtration results obtained for animals of this group. In this sample, collected 5 days post

TABLE 1.--Antibody titers in serum and milk of swine exposed to virulent TGE virus by different routes

Exposure		Days post-	Antibody titers[a]	
Route	Sow no.	partum	Serum	Milk
Oral	107[b]	1.7	57	1100
		5	44	340
		13	35	98
	2[c]	4	45	105
I.Mm.	64-9[d]	0	560	2900
		5	570	90
		11	380	6
	55-5[e]	0	---	6600
		3.8	380	340
		11	360	20

[a]Reciprocal, plaque reduction 80%
[b]Virulent virus given 32 days prepartum
[c]Virulent virus given 39 days prepartum
[d]Intramammary, 43 and 16 days prepartum
[e]Intramammary, 42 and 17 days prepartum

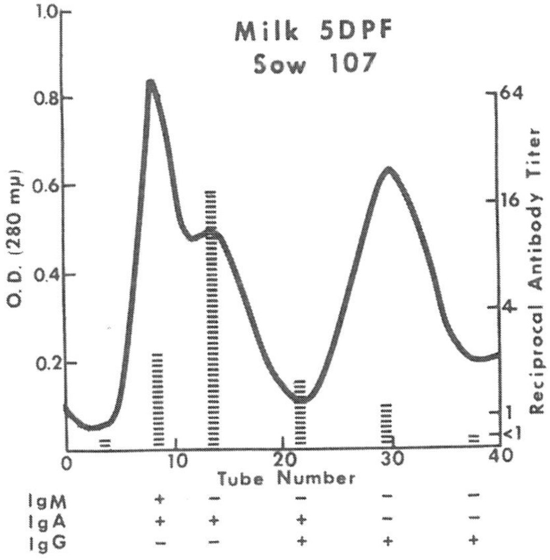

FIGURE 1.--Gel filtration on Sephadex G-200 of a 5-day post-farrowing (postpartum) milk sample from a sow which had been infected orally with virulent virus 32 days prepartum.

partum, antibody was associated almost entirely with the
IgA portion of the chromatogram. Such results were further
confirmed by evidence obtained from absorption studies.

Parenteral Exposure with Virus

Pregnant swine which had been injected either intramammarily with live virulent virus or intramuscularly with
live attenuated virus responded with relatively high antibody titers in serum and in colostrum. Thereafter, antibody levels in milk declined rapidly and markedly, so that
beginning 2 to 4 days postpartum, and thereafter, antibody
titers in milk were less than in serum. The serologic
findings on 2 sows which had been injected intramammarily
are presented in Table 1. They are representative of the
type of response observed in animals in this parenterally
injected group, with the exception that the antibody
response was usually greater in the intramammarily injected
animals.

Gel filtration studies on colostrum and milk samples
from animals in this group indicated that antibodies were
predominantly or entirely associated with the IgG portion
of the chromatograms, while being absent or in very low
titers in the IgA portion. Figure 2 is representative of

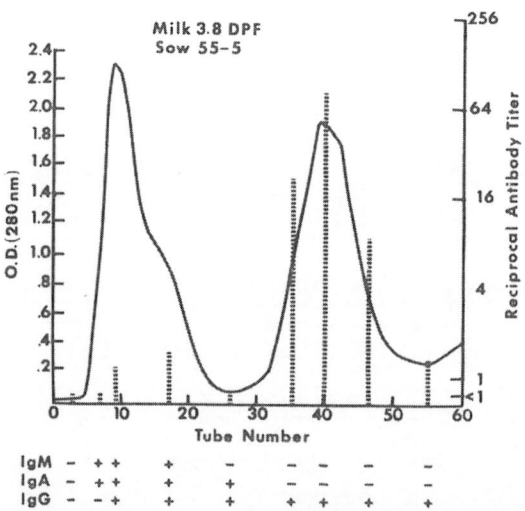

FIGURE 2.--Gel filtration on Sephadex G-200 of a 3.8 day
    postpartum milk sample from a sow which had been injec-
    ted intramammarily with virulent virus 17 and 42 days
    prepartum.

the gel filtration results conducted on these animals. This
sample was collected 3.8 days postpartum from a sow which
had been injected intramammarily with virulent virus. Antibodies were associated primarily, if not solely, with IgG.

To confirm this observation, colostrum from this sow
(no. 55-5) was absorbed with anti-porcine IgG, after which
a 52-fold reduction in the TGE antibody titer (to the limit
of the dilution factor) was observed. Following absorption
with anti-IgA, there was no significant reduction in antibody titer, further indicating most, if not all, of the
antibody activity was of the IgG class.

COMMENTS

TGE antibodies associated with IgG and IgA classes
have been detected in mammary secretions of swine (2,5). As
previously reported by us, a significant level of TGE antibodies of the IgA class has been consistently demonstrated
in colostrum and milk only after an infection of the gastrointestinal tract (2,3). One possible mechanism to account
for this observation is that antigenically sensitized
immunocytes from the lamina propria of the intestinal tract
may relocate and colonize the mammary gland, as we previously
suggested (2,3). A similar explanation was proposed by
Crabbe et al. (6) to account for the origin of IgA antibody-
producing cells found in extraintestinal sites following
oral immunization. Virulent TGE virus was injected intramammarily to determine if IgA antibodies could be locally
stimulated, as had been reported to occur in rabbits when
DNP-bovine gamma globulin was injected (7). However, antibody production appeared to be primarily, if not solely,
of the IgG class; as also occurred when live attenuated
virus was injected intramuscularly or intramammarily (4).

The maintenance of significant levels of TGE antibodies
in milk - at levels usually higher than in serum - during
the period of lactation probably indicates that such antibodies are predominantly of the IgA class. Whether this
characteristic is applicable with other infectious diseases
remains to be seen.

Highly effective passive immunity of the suckling pig
against enteric infection with TGE virus has been correlated
with the presence of antibodies of the IgA class in mammary

secretions (2,3,5). Such antibodies might be especially
suited for this function because of their enzymatic stability (8), their affinity for mucosal surfaces (9), their
predominance in milk throughout the lactation period (3)
and their role in inhibiting the adherence of pathogens to
mucosal surfaces (10).

These studies suggest that adequate passive immunity
against TGE - and possibly other intestinal infections -
will be provided to suckling pigs only when the sow has
been previously infected or vaccinated by the oral or
intestinal route.

REFERENCES

1. Haelterman, E. O. and Hooper, B. E., Gastroenterology,
   53:109, 1967.

2. Bohl, E. H., Gupta, R. K. P., McCloskey, L. W. and Saif,
   L. J., J. Am. Vet. Med. Ass., 160:543, 1972.

3. Bohl, E. H., Gupta, R. K. P., Olquin, M. V. F. and Saif,
   L. J., Infect. Immunity, 6:289, 1972.

4. Saif, L. J., Bohl, E. H. and Gupta, R. K. P., Infect.
   Immunity, 6:600, 1972.

5. Ristic, M. and Abou-Youssef, M., J. Am. Vet. Med. Ass.,
   160:549, 1972.

6. Crabbe, P. A., Nash, D. R., Bazin, H., Eyssen, H. and
   Heremans, J. F., J. Exp. Med., 130:723, 1969.

7. Genco, R. J. and Taubman, M. A., Nature, 221:679, 1969.

8. Cederblad, G., Johansson, B. G. and Rymo, L., Acta
   Chem. Scand., 20:2349, 1966.

9. Porter, P. and Allen, W. D., J. Am. Vet. Med. Ass.
   160:511, 1972.

10. Freter, R., Infect. Immunity, 5:556, 1970.

SECRETORY IgA AND DIRECT KILLING OF SHIGELLA BY SERUM COMPONENTS

William P. Reed, M.D.
Elizabeth L. Albright
Veterans Administration Hospital
Albuquerque, New Mexico

INTRODUCTION

Shigellosis is an enteric infection in which bacteria are restricted to the intestinal lumen and mucosa, and deeper systemic invasion is rare, even in nonimmune individuals. Spontaneous recovery is common, and subsequent resistance to reinfection may occur, but field trials with parenteral vaccines have shown systemic antibodies to be nonprotective. However, the effectiveness of oral vaccines suggests that local or intestinal immunity may exist. Since previous studies have shown large quantities of secretory IgA to be present in Shigella diarrhea stools (1), it seems possible that local immunity may be mediated by this immunoglobulin. The following studies investigate direct serum killing as one possible mechanism through which secretory IgA could exert an anti-Shigella effect.

METHODS

Shigella strains were obtained from 47 individuals with clinical shigellosis. Sera were from normal individuals as well as from patients recently recovered from Shigellosis. The serum bactericidal test was a modification of the phagocytic bactericidal test of Maaløe (2), but with the phagocytes omitted. Sufficient bacteria to make a final concentration of 2×10^6/ml were suspended in gel Hank's solution containing various dilutions of the serum being tested. A sample was removed by a 0.001 ml calibrated loop for colony counting, the mixture was incubated at 37°C, and additional samples were removed at 30, 60, and 120 minutes. Direct microscopy showed that decreases in colony counts could not be attributed to clumping of organisms.

Complement was inactivated by heat (56°C, 30 min), pre-incubation with cobra venom factor, and removal of C3 by Sepharose bound antiserum at 4°C in the presence of 0.01 M EDTA which was later dialyzed away. All techniques removed hemolytic complement activity, although it could be partially restored to the C3 depleted serum by the addition of C3 (Cordis). The early complement pathway was evaluated by using a naturally C2 deficient serum with no detectable hemolytic complement (supplied by Dr. Vincent Agnello, Rockefeller University). The alternate C3 activating path-way was inactivated by Sepharose bound anti-β_2 glycoprotein II (Behring) in the presence of 0.01 M EDTA. After removal of EDTA, the resulting serum had no detectable C3PA by immunoelectrophoresis, but still contained 30 CH_{50} units of hemolytic complement. Sera were also incubated with equal volumes of inulin at 37°C for 60 min which removed all detectable C3PA, but left hemolytic complement.

The role of immunoglobulins was evaluated by adding them to sera which had been depleted of Shigella antibody by overnight absorbtion at 0°C with heat killed organisms. The depleted sera had no detectable antibody to the strain of Shigella used for the absorbtions, but C3PA and hemolytic complement were present.

RESULTS

Many strains of Shigella were killed during two hours exposure to 10% fresh serum, with 42% of the strains susceptible (<5% survival), 30% intermediate (5-75% survival) and 28% resistant. All resistant strains were killed by all sera if leukocytes were added to the system. Results of the serum killing test were highly reproducible, and higher indirect hemagglutinating antibody titers did not increase the killing ability of a serum. All three complement inactivating techniques caused sera to lose their ability to kill even highly sensitive strains, thus indicating that complement including C3 was required. Addition of C3 partially restored the killing ability of C3 depleted serum.

The role of the early complement pathway was evaluated
by using the C2 deficient serum which had to be present in
eight times the concentration of a normal serum to kill at
the normal rate (Figure 1). Addition of purified C2 caused
it to kill at the normal rate. The role of the alternate
C3 activating pathway was evaluated by using the C3PA depleted serum which had approximately a four-fold reduction
in its bacteriolytic capacity (Figure 2). Similar results
were obtained with inulin treated serum. Serum from the C2
deficient patient failed to kill Shigella at all when the
alternate pathway was blocked.

The role of immunoglobulins was assessed by adding
immunoglobulin to Shigella absorbed serum which had lost
its ability to kill the absorbing strain, but retained the
ability to kill strains from other serotypes. The immunoglobulin preparations added included the 19S fraction from
a sucrose density gradient containing IgM, the 7S fraction
from the gradient containing IgG, the IgG containing fraction from a Sephadex G-200 column, and colostral 11S IgA
prepared in two different laboratories according to the
method of Tomasi (one prepared at the University of Minnesota by Dr. Folke Lindström). Results from these studies
indicate that as little as 0.02 mg/ml undiluted serum of the

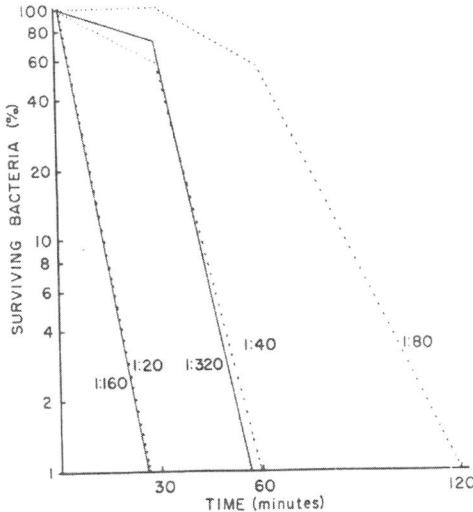

Figure 1: Bacterolytic capacity of C2 deficient serum
(dotted line) compared with normal serum (solid line).
Serum dilutions are given.

19S fraction restored full killing capacity, 12 mg IgG partially restored killing, but 4 mg 11S IgA failed to restore
any killing capacity (Figure 3).

DISCUSSION

The fact that all Shigella strains tested can be killed with any serum in combination with leukocytes may explain
why bacteremia is rare in Shigellosis, but these studies fail
to provide a mechanism for local intestinal immunity. Participation of both the early complement sequence and the
alternate pathway in bacterial killing was demonstrated, but
the in vivo contribution of each of the pathways is unknown.

The role of IgM in bacterial killing seems clear and
the fact that such small amounts are required may explain
why the killing power of various sera are independent of
the anti-Shigella titer. The role of IgG is less clear
since the presence of minute amounts of IgM in the preparation cannot be ruled out. Aggregated myeloma A protein is
known to activate the alternate complement pathway (3), so
even though secretory IgA fails to activate the classical

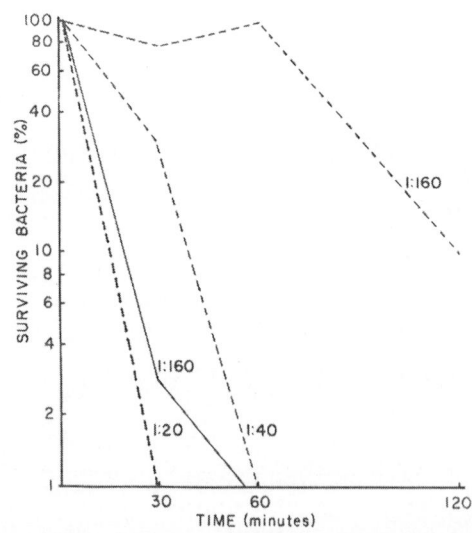

Figure 2: Bacteriolytic capacity of C3PA deficient serum
(dashed line) compared with normal serum (solid line).
Serum dilutions are given.

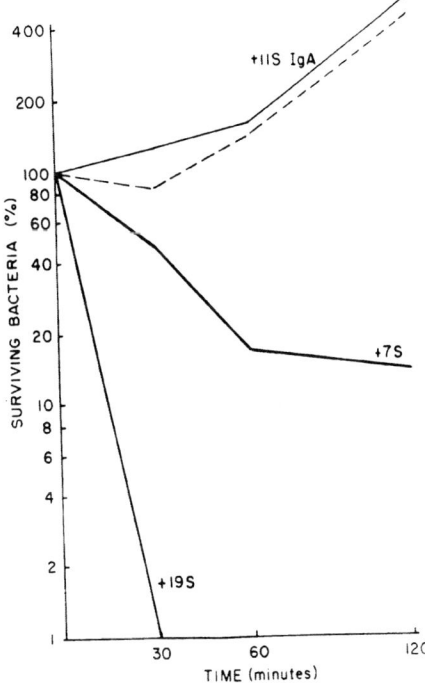

Figure 3: Effect of immunoglobulin in restoring bacteriolytic capacity of Shigella absorbed serum (dashed line).

early pathway, it has seemed possible that it might activate
the alternate pathway. However, two preparations of this
immunoglobulin failed to promote killing of Shigella. Hence,
it appears that under the conditions of these studies, secretory IgA has failed to activate the alternate pathway.

The fact that secretory IgA does not act in the serum
bactericidal reaction does not rule out its participation in
possible local immunity. It may act in another way such as
aiding mucosal elements in killing Shigella, or in preventing penetration of the organisms into mucosa.

REFERENCES

1. Reed, W. P., and Williams, R. C., Jr., Gastroenterology,
    61:35, 1971.

2. Maaløe, O., On the Relation Between Alexin and Opsonin,
    Munksgaard, Copenhagen, 1946.

3. Muller-Eberhard, H. J., in Progress in Immunology,
    Edited by B. Amos, Academic Press, Inc., 1971.

DISCUSSION

Dr. Rolf Freter (Initial Discussant) - Dr. Kraus, Ladies
and Gentlemen: I would like to briefly summarize some of
the data which you have heard in these two days, plus some
others which have not been mentioned, in order to see how
they can fit into a working hypothesis of the mechanisms
controlling bacterial growth on mucosal surfaces. I will
not say much about viruses. It is known that viruses in
tissue culture are "inactivated" by antibodies. Consequently,
there is no conceptual obstacle to assuming that this mechanism also operates on mucosal surfaces. Moreover, no extensive "normal" virus flora exists, i.e. viruses usually dis-
appear from the body at a time and under circumstances consistent with the assumption that effective local or systemic
immune mechanisms are at work. None of this can be said for
bacteria on mucosal surfaces. There is a serious conceptual
obstacle to accepting the idea of an effective local antibacterial immunity: The presence of a normal flora which
is constantly inhabiting the mucosal surfaces. A second
conceptual problem concerns the nature of local antibody
mediated antibacterial immune mechanisms. This difficulty
is the same whether we consider IgA or other local antibodies, because the accessory factors usually required for
antibody mediated immunity, e.g. complement or leukocytes,
are not usually present on mucosal surfaces. Progress has
recently been made with respect to the latter problem in
that two antibacterial mechanisms have been described which
are indeed able to function in the mucosal environment. You
have heard today about the first of these, namely, the inhibition of bacterial adhesion by antibodies. When we described
this phenomenon several years ago in experimental cholera,
I never dreamt that it would apply to so many different bacterial species, as has now been demonstrated by the work of
others. A second mechanism which operates on mucosal surfaces inhibits the growth of bacteria in the presence of
antibody. It is independent of complement and it requires
viable mucosal cells. It does not operate in mucosal scrapings or in the presence of metabolic inhibitors. It therefore appears to require an accessory factor which must be
continuously produced by the mucosa (J. Immunol. 111:395,
1973).

349

If you accept the idea that there are mechanisms based
on local antibody which can affect the implantation and survival of bacteria, then we have to examine next the factors
which control or modify the presence of antibodies on the
mucosa. These are (1) The inhibition of antigen absorption
by local antibodies, described by several speakers today.
This is a negative feedback mechanism which may limit the
degree of local immunity to microorganisms. (2) We know
that the secretion of local antibodies is intermittent. In
our very early work on human volunteers we found that antibodies in duodenal washings appeared only after a test meal.
(3) You have heard from Dr. Plaut the interesting finding
that a bacterial enzyme can specifically attack IgA. (4) We
know that mucosal antibodies are by no means exclusively of
the IgA type, but may also reside in serum-derived IgG and
IgM fractions. Dr. Fubara reported some time ago that the
stability of these IgG and IgM antibodies was controlled by
the presence of a normal flora (Infect. and Immun. 6:965,
1972). In its absence (i.e. in germfree mice) proteolytic
enzyme levels in the intestine were so high that IgM and IgG
were quickly inactivated, and only locally produced IgA antibody was present. In contrast, conventional animals had
lower intestinal enzyme levels, and serum-derived antibodies
of the IgG and IgM class contributed significantly to the
total intestinal antibody activity. Therefore, if the normal
bacterial flora is controlled by local antibodies, the reverse is also true: The appearance and stability of local
antibodies can be controlled by the normal flora. (5) You
have heard about another factor which may affect the stability of antibodies on mucosal surfaces: The antitrypsin
binding of IgA, the degree of which may conceivably be affected by variables in the mucosal environment. All these
are modifying factors which can determine whether the concentration of antibodies present on a mucosal surface under
a given set of circumstances will be sufficient to affect
bacterial colonization.

In spite of what I have said so far, there remains the
difficulty of reconciling the presence of a normal bacterial
flora on most mucosal surfaces with the idea that local antibodies can inhibit bacterial adhesion and growth. I brought
one slide that may have some bearing on this (Table). These
are experiments in which gnotobiotic mice were immunized
orally and then challenged by the same route with homologous
cholera vibrios. The cholera vibrio grows in these animals
like normal flora without causing pathology. Please note

EFFECT OF IMMUNITY AND BACTERIAL ANTAGONISM ON
THE GROWTH OF V. CHOLERAE IN THE CECUM OF GNOTOBIOTIC MICE

Expt. No.	Group	Route of immunization	Type of vaccine	Antagonistic flora present	No. of animals per group	Geometric Mean No. of vibrios per cecum***	Factor of difference (controls:immunized)
A12	A	oral	live	NONE	7	3.10×10^9	2.14
	B		NONE		7	6.59×10^9	
A13	A	i.p.	killed	NONE	12	4.35×10^9	1.55
	B		NONE		12	6.74×10^9	
A21	A	oral	killed	NONE	10	1.21×10^9	2.82
	B		NONE		10	3.42×10^9	
123	A	oral	live	NONE	8	4.62×10^9	1.79
	B		NONE		5	8.29×10^9	
125	A	oral	live	NONE	7	2.73×10^9	2.66
	B		NONE		4	7.25×10^9	
A11	A	oral	live	5 facult. aerobes*	5	7.11×10^6	4.79
	B		NONE		6	3.40×10^7	
A19	A	oral	killed	45 anaer-obes***	10	1.51×10^8	12.2
	B		NONE		10	1.83×10^9	
123	A	oral	live	5 facult. aerobes*	7	5.36×10^5	61.1
	B		NONE		8	3.28×10^7	
125	A	oral	live	5 facult. aerobes*	19	1.44×10^6	58.7
	B		NONE		8	8.45×10^7	

*Streptococcus fecalis, Aerobacter aerogenes, Proteus vulgaris and 2 strains of E. coli implanted
2 days before challenge.
**45 strains of gram negative strict anaerobes isolated from normal mouse cecum impoanted 1 week
before challenge.
***Counts were made 2 days after challenge
(A detailed account of these data will be published in J. Infect. Dis., March, 1974)

that the effect of immunization on the number of organisms
in the cecum of monoassociated animals (top 5 experiments)
was very small (1.55 to 2.82-fold decrease in vibrio population in immunized mice). In the presence of other bacteria
(bottom 4 experiments) the vibrio population in control AND
immunized groups was much smaller due to bacterial antagonism.
However, immunization caused in these animals a further reduction of the vibrio population, which was of considerably
greater magnitude (4.79 to 61.1-fold) than that observed in
the monoassociated mice. What can one say then about local
antibody and its effect on mucosal populations of bacteria?
It appears to be quite effective under circumstances where
other factors, such as the presence of an antagonistic
"normal" flora, already inhibit an invading microorganism
to a certain degree. In other words, local immunity may
have a major effect on bacterial colonization ONLY in the
presence of other antibacterial mechanisms which act synergistically with it. The predominant species of the normal
bacterial flora may be looked upon as growing in a situation
which is somewhat analogous to that of the vibrios in our
monoassociated mice: They are not subjected to inhibition
by other antagonistic bacterial species. If this assumption
is correct, one can easily see that local immunity may indeed
reduce the population size of the normal bacterial flora,
but that the degree of this reduction would be so minor that
it can escape detection. As Dr. Gibbons has pointed out,
successive antigenic mutants of intestinal bacteria may
overgrow the parent strain under the influence of local immunity (presumably by the successive deletion of antigenic
surface determinants). It seems to me, however, that this
process can continue only to a point where the bacterial
surface is not eroded to such a degree that the mutants can
no longer compete in the intestinal environment.

In summary then, it is consistent with the currently
available data to assume the following: (1) The predominant
species of the normal bacterial flora represent mutants which
have reduced their antigenic surface structures to the lowest
level compatible with survival. These bacteria exist in a
state of continuous but quantitatively very minor suppression
by local immune mechanisms. (2) Local antibacterial immunity
has a significant effect only when other antibacterial mechanisms (e.g. bacterial antagonism, mechanical removal) act
synergistically with it. (3) Local immunity is further modified by a variety of factors which affect the presence and
stability of local antibodies. Some of these factors are

in turn controlled by the bacterial flora. Control of bacterial flora on mucosal surfaces involves therefore a very
complex system in which IgA antibody is only one of many
factors and, under certain circumstances, may not even be
the controlling factor. It is easy to see, therefore, that
the control of bacterial populations on mucosal surfaces
cannot always correlate with the presence or absence of IgA
antibodies. Thank you for your attention.

Dr. Dalmasso - I would like to present additional information on the problem of the possibility of interaction of
secretory IgA with the complement system. In work that I
have done together with Dr. Manuel Kaplan (J. Immunol., 1972,
108:274), we have shown that S-IgA is capable of interacting
with the complement system, using a model which is somehow
similar to what Dr. Bienenstock has described but not identical. What we have used is the presence of anti-A or anti-
B blood group antibody activity in human colostrum. As a
target system we have employed human RBC treated with AET
(2-aminoethyliosthiouronium bromide) which behave similarly
to those of patients with paroxysmal nocturnal hemoglobinuria
in their extreme sensitivity to the hemolytic action of
complement. We have used highly purified colostrum S-IgA
from a type O mother who delivered an erythroblastotic type
B baby. She had high titer of anti-B in colostral S-IgA.
In the presence of fresh type B serum, the purified S-IgA
caused lysis of the PNH-like red cells and this was
complement-dependent. This required activation to the
complement system although we were unable to examine whether
this was due to the alternate or classical pathway. We were
also able to demonstrate complement activation by S-IgA in a
second system consisting of the complement-dependent opsonization of ABO-incompatible erythrocytes by S-IgA. With the
same purified S-IgA there was phagocytosis of B-type cells by
polymorphonuclear leukocytes and monocytes only in the
presence of complement. No phagocytosis could be mediated
by antibodies in the colostrum of 10 normal mothers. This
data may be pointing to a complex situation in which perhaps
one should look for qualitative differences in the type of
antibody. Perhaps immune S-IgA antibody may be more efficient
than naturally-occurring antibody in certain biological
properties, e.g. the ability to activate the complement system

Dr. Ørstavik - I have a question for Dr. Gibbons. I would
like to direct the attention to the possible importance of
non-immunological inhibitors of adherence to surfaces. We

have, in Dr. Kraus's laboratory, studied the adherence of
streptococci to the acquired pellicle on tooth surfaces. A
number of factors may act to inhibit the adherence of these
bacteria to this surface coating, which may be taken to be
an extension of the mucosal coating. One of the factors
that we have found to inhibit adherence is S-IgA purified
from whole saliva. However, by substituting the buffer that
was used to suspend the bacteria, with parotid fluid, we
get the same amount of inhibition and it seems that IgA is
not the factor in parotid fluid effecting this inhibition.
Since Dr. Gibbons has been working with salivary aggregating
factors other than IgA, I would like to ask his opinion on
the relative importance of these non-immunological mechanisms,
as opposed to the specific antibody activity of IgA, in the
phenomenon of adherence inhibition.

Dr. Gibbons - The mucinous glycoproteins in saliva appear
to bind to various bacteria. We have found that these
salivary mucins can also inhibit the attachment of certain
oral stroptococci to epithelial surfaces. These studies
have been carried out by Dr. Williams in our laboratories.
In our experience, strains of S. sanguis and S. mitis are
more commonly aggregated by salivary mucins than S. salivarius.
In addition, there appears to be considerable specificity
involved. One of the reasons we have focused upon S.
salivarius is that the strain used for the IgA inhibition
studies was not particularly prone to mucin-induced aggregation, and hence this organism seemed to be a good assay
for exploring IgA inhibition of adherence. Thus our data
concerning these mucins are in agreement with your findings.
I believe these non-immunological mechanisms will likely
prove of great significance in influencing the colonization
of bacteria on mucosal surfaces.

Dr. Ogra - Obviously, the data presented here are very
interesting and would suggest that probably the mechanism
of mammary gland IgA response is secondary to migration of
sensitized IgA cells to the mammary gland. These
data are somewhat contrary to our observations, and the
observations of Dr. Genco in rabbits where they immunized
intramammarily with DNCB and demonstrated local 11S antibody
response. In this context I would like to ask you four
questions. One, did you try to study the immune response in
the mammary gland which was not immunized and, second, did
you look at the response in the G.I. tract and quantitate the
gamma A response in the sera of these animals? The third

is, were all of these animals' sera negative for the TGE
antibody before the studies were started? The fourth is,
did you look at the distribution of the plasma cells of G,
A and M type in the mammary glands which were immunized by
different routes of immunization and in those not immunized?

Dr. Bohl - I'll try to answer some of these questions. One:
these animals were all serologically negative at the time
they were exposed to the TGE of viral preparations. We
examined milk from intramammarily-injected as well as non-
injected glands, and there did not seem to be very much
difference except the antibody titer in some cases was higher
in milk from the intramammarily injected glands. We have
not really made any exhaustive studies in reagrd to antibodies
in the gastrointestinal tract. Right now we are mainly
concerned with passive immunity. We have detected antibodies
in the stomach and intestinal contents of suckling pigs, but
this is obviously what remains from the milk that has been
ingested. We have not made examinations for presence of
IgA immunocytes in the mammary gland. Dr. Porter from
England has reported the presence of IgA immunocytes in
mammary glands of sows. Dr. Bourne from England reported
that 90% of the IgA in milk of sows originated from the
mammary gland.

Dr. Ogra - I have one more question for Dr. Gibbons. I
was wondering about the inhibitory mechanism of this antibody
interaction with streptococcal antigen. Is it somewhat
similar to a steric phenomena or like neutralization of
viruses? Have you tried any dissociation experiments where
you can still demonstrate infectivity of the streptococcus
after it is released from the antibody?

Dr. Gibbons - Our working hypothesis is that the antibody,
by coating surface antigens on the bacterial cells, probably
sterically hinders the attachment. I think this may well be
the same in the case of viral neutralization. I think that
it may simply be a steric hinderance. There is also another
possibility. The external fuzzy coat of these bacteria,
particularly the ones that have been studied in the mouth,
appears to consist, in part, of cell-bound enzymes, and it
is very likely, I feel, that these enzymes account, in part,
for the adsorption specificities which are quite remarkable
in these species. Dr. Genco and others have shown that
antibodies can inactivate these surface enzymes and in this
sense probably also sterically interfere with the affinity

of these enzymes to a substrate present on the mucosal surface.

Dr. Stone - Regarding TGE, there is a point that probably
should be made for general information; most of these
piglets are born virtually agammaglobulinemic. Within hours
of drinking or sucking colostrum, their sera reflect pretty
much what they drank or sucked. They will have the IgG and
IgA in their sera; neutralizing antibodies can also be
detected. However, if these piglets are removed from their
immune sows after challenge, they will die. They need the
continual ingestion of the immune colostrum to survive, in
spite of the fact that they may have immunoglobulins in their
sera. A second point: we are fractionating bovine sera now
and these sera are directed toward Brucella antigen. We are
able, in preliminary experiments, to show that the IgA fraction will fix complement.

Dr. McGhee - I'd like to ask Dr. Genco a question. In the
salivas you got from Dr. Taubman, how did he immunize his
rats? What were the antigens that he used?

Dr. Genco - The rats were immunized by foot pad immunization
or by salivary gland immunization. The results that I showed
were obtained with saliva from a salivary gland-immunized
animal.

Dr. McGhee - What was the antigen?

Dr. Genco - The antigen was formalin-killed whole cells of
Streptococcus mutans strain G715.

Dr. McGhee - Since you have purified the α antigen I was
wondering if you've looked at the IgA in saliva from these
immunized rats with this α antigen by any other immunological
methods?

Dr. Genco - Well what we showed was a gel diffusion with
extracts from boiled water or 0.1N HCl S. mutans. These
certainly are not pure antigens. However, the antisera were
absorbed with group A streptococci and Sephadex G-25 and
gave single bands.

Dr. Guggenheim - I have a question for Dr. Genco. Do you
think that your work implies that the glucosyl transferases
produced by the different Bratthall strains are immunologically
distinct?

Dr. Genco - Our work with rabbit antisera to S. mutans, and
more recently with monkey and rat sera to S. mutans, shows
that they markedly inhibit glucosyltransferase activity of
homologous strains, but give little or no inhibition of
enzyme from heterologous strains. The exceptions being, as
I described in my paper, the cross reactions between S.
mutans gr-"a" and gr-"d" organisms. All of these experiments
however have been carried out with whole supernate enzyme
preparations which have been shown to contain several
glucosyltransferase activities varying in isoelectric point
as well as in the type of dextran they produce. It is possible
that each strain of S. mutans produces varying proportions of
these glucosyltransferases and that antisera raised to one
set will not inhibit the activity of another set. Alternatively, and this is the interpretation I prefer, the antigenic
specificity of glucosyltransferases may be related to the
serologic group of the S. mutans strain from which they are
obtained.

Dr. Good - Two questions. One to Dr. Gibbons. As I remember
in the initial experiments of Rothbard and Watson, the
virulence of the group A streptococci was tested using a system
of parental immunization. Your evidence seemed to indicate
that the adherence of the group A streptococci which you
attribute to the M antigens and which you related to virulence
was to epithelial cells. Have you studied the capacity of
group A streptococci to adhere to cells other than epithelial
cells? Do you have anything that could explain these initial
observations of the association of the M protein with
virulence after intraperitoneal inoculation, for example?

Dr. Gibbons - Another characteristic of M protein which has
been studied widely is its ability to impede phagocytosis.
Many of the models that have been used to study group A
streptococcal infections have relied on intraperitoneal
inoculation. Under such systemic circumstances phagocytosis
is certainly an important characteristic. However, I would
also like to point out that Watson also carried out some very
nice experiments in monkeys. Watson immunized monkeys intranasally with virulent strains of Strep. pyogenes. The
organism colonized for several weeks, and then was eliminated.
These animals developed a type-specific immunity, because
when Watson tried to reinfect them with the same M type, the
challange organisms appeared to be rapidly cleared and they
could not be detected 24 hours after inocluation. However, if
these monkeys were infected with a different M type of S.

pyogenes the cycle of infection was repeated.

Dr. Good - Since phagocytosis involves adherence to phagocytic cells, it would be important to see whether or not an
adherence pehnomenon related to phagocytes would be explan-
atory.

Dr. Gibbons - Yes, that's right.

Dr. Good - Another question, I think this issue of IgA being
able to address the complement system is sufficiently important that we want to have the record very clear. Was
Dalmasso's IgA a highly purified 11 S IgA? I ask this
question because recent work Day has done in my laboratory with
Michael's group at Minnesota suggests that IgA can indeed
play an important role in the pathogenesis of disease
especially under circumstances where the complement system
can be activated via the alternate pathway.

Dr. Dalmasso - Yes, this was a highly purified S-IgA preparation, 11 S. Also, because of the possibility that perhaps
one might not be able to detect very minimal amounts of
IgG and IgM contaminants we employed colostral IgG and IgM
in concentrations slightly above the limit of the system
that we used to detect these possible contaminants. At
these concentrations colostral IgA and IgM did not mediate
opsonization of incompatible RBC. So the answer is that our
observations indicate that S-IgA is able to produce complement
activation.

Dr. Good - One final question, and that relates to the mammary
gland immunization. It was stated by Bohl that injections
into the mammary gland did not bring forward a response. Were
these diathelic immunizations involving IgA or were they
injections directly into the parenchyma of the gland?

Dr. Bohl - These were injected directly into the substance of
the gland. We did try to go into the cistern of the gland but
I am sure we got around some of the areas of the gland.
Whether this in itself might pose some difference in the type
of response I do not know but it's very difficult, in the case
of the non-lactating sow, to inject directly up into the teat
meatus.

Dr. Good - I ask this question because in the classical
experiments of Huddelson in 1917 in the cow, even injections

directly into the teat canal brought an antibody response to
that particular quarter in a matter of 4-6 hours. Only later,
24-48 hours, did an adjacent quarter produce antibody and
several days were required for the other two quarters to
get into gear. It would be very important to know if this
early response via teat canal were IgA antibody.

Dr. McNamara - I'd like to get Dr. Gibbon's comments on the
literature reports indicating that there was a low salivary
IgA level in the presence of high caries formation. The
reason I ask the question is that you would expect a fair
amount of antigen to be present during the formation of
caries. Would you not expect an S-IgA response to be
relatively high?

Dr. Gibbons - I have not been involved in experiments
concerning immunization against dental caries, but I would
like to make one point. One of the reasons why we have not
yet looked at the effects of antibody on events occurring
on the tooth surface is because the tooth surface does not
desquamate. As a result, I think it's likely that it will
be much more difficult to show effects of antibody against
bacteria colonizing a stable surface such as the tooth,
rather than on mucosal surfaces.

Dr. Lehner - In fact we published the paper about six years
ago that in patients with a high caries incidence, there is
a low salivary IgA and a high serum IgA and the reverse is
the case with a low caries incidence (Lehner, T., Cardwell,
J.E. and Clarry, E.D. 1967, Lancet 1, 1294). These studies
were confirmed by some and not others. I think a significant
finding was made by Zengo, A.N., Mandel, S.O., Goldman, R.
and Khurana, H.S. (1972, Archs. oral Biol., 16, 559) that the
whole salivary IgA level may well be related to the submandibular salivary secretion. Although we were able to show
this relationship with salivary IgA we were unable to confirm
this with antibodies to specific organisms such as Strep.
mutans.

Dr. Fudenberg - We have been talking about the secretory
immunologic system. I wonder if anyone has any data on
lactoferrin levels in saliva, mammary fluid and such, prefer-
ably before and after immunization by the oral, the nasal, or
the intramammary routes. Secondly, if so, does absence of
lactoferrin either by itself, or in the presence of secretory
IgA and/or lysozyme, exert an antimicrobial effect?

Dr. Freter - We had considered this in the intestinal system and this turned out not to be a factor; that is, addition of high amounts of iron had no effect on the bacteriocidal activity of local antibody.

Dr. Tomasi - I think the lactoferrin concentrations in new-born saliva and in adult saliva are nearly equal so that, if Dr. Fudenberg was implying any change by antigenic stimulation this data might help him.

Dr. Hanson - Dr. Gibbons mentioned the possibility that local antibodies could exert an influence on the microbial flora inducing mutations. We may have an additional example of this. We have seen secretory IgA antibodies in urine of patients with urinary tract infections which I will describe in some detail this afternoon. Now, following the type of bacteria in patients who have repeated infections or have an infection for a very long period, to our surprise we saw that these bacterial strains seemed to lose their surface antigens. They seem to lose what is supposed to be virulence antigens. Now the local antibodies, or at least what we think are locally produced antibodies, are directed against these surface antigens, especially the O antigens of E. coli. So could it be that these strains lose their surface antigens to try to evade the local immunity? What would you think about that Dr. Gibbons?

Dr. Gibbons - I believe that we develop immunity to indig-enous bacteria in a manner analogous to the way we develop immunity to pathogens. One reason for thinking this is this phenomenon of serotype conversion which appears to occur among indiginous bacteria. This has been very well documented for E. coli colonizing the intestinal canal, and as Dr. Freter also mentioned, it has been very well documented for vibrios colonizing gnotobiotic animals. Dr. Howell in our laboratory has been able to show changes in the antigenic composition of indigenous streptococci when they colonize gnotobiotic animals. I think indigenous bacteria colonize for periods of weeks or months, and then they are replaced by a different serotype which arise by mutation, or which may be introduced exogenously.

Dr. Newcomb - To come back to Dr. Fudenberg's question, we have reported attempts to measure levels of lactoferrin by Mancini's technique in which we found that the presence of either the sol or gel phase of sputum or of saliva interfered

with the measurement of lactoferrin by this technique. I
don't know how, but the exocrine fluids depressed the
apparent concentrations.

SESSION E

CLINICAL CONSIDERATIONS

CHAIRMAN: MAX D. COOPER

CURRENT KNOWLEDGE ON ALPHA CHAIN DISEASE

Maxime Seligmann and Edith Mihaesco

Laboratory of Immunochemistry, Research
Institute on Blood Diseases, Hopital
Saint-Louis, 75475 Paris Cedex 10, France

Since its first description in 1968 (1) alpha chain
disease (α CD) has been recognized in 59 patients to our
knowledge. Most of these cases have been detected or confirmed in our laboratory. Thus α CD is probably the most
frequent disorder among the group of heavy chain diseases
which, at present, includes diseases of the γ, α and μ types.

It is the purpose of this report to summarize the
clinico-pathological features of the disease and the immunochemical and structural studies carried out on a few α CD
proteins.

IMMUNOCHEMICAL AND STRUCTURAL STUDIES

We have previously emphasized that the laboratory diagnosis of α CD may be difficult (2,3). The serum electrophoretic pattern of these patients is not suggestive of a monoclonal type of Ig abnormality since the characteristic sharp
peak is always lacking. In only half of the 52 cases studied
in our laboratory, the electrophoregram showed an abnormal
broad band usually in the α2 and β region. In the other half
of the cases, the pathological protein was not noticeable on
the electrophoretic pattern. The various patterns obtained
at immunoelectrophoretic analysis have been previously described (2,3). In many instances, the protein abnormality
escapes routine immunoelectrophoresis with polyvalent antiserum to human normal serum. It should be emphasized that
the absence of precipitation of the anomalous IgA component

with antisera to light chains is not a sufficient criterion
for diagnosis since such a failure to precipitate has been
encountered with several IgA myeloma proteins. Selected
antisera specific for IgA and containing antibodies related
to the conformational specificity of the Fab region were
found to be very useful for the diagnosis of α CD by immunoelectrophoresis or Ouchterlony test (2). In doubtful cases,
the pathological protein should be purified in order to
demonstrate directly the lack of light chains. To add to
the difficulty of the diagnosis of α CD in a routine laboratory, the amount of pathological protein present in the urine
was found to be minimal when present. However, in most patients, the α CD protein has been found in the concentrated
urines. As expected in view of the involvement of the intestinal tract by the proliferative process, the α CD protein
was found in significant amounts in the jejunal fluid, and
it was associated with the secretory component (2).

Despite their electrophoretic heterogeneity, the pathological proteins are considered to be monoclonal because they
are all related to only one subclass of α chains. All 41
proteins which have been typed belonged to the α1 subclass.
The absence of a single case of α2 CD in this series is probably not accidental, but the meaning of this observation is
unknown.

When analysed in the ultracentrifuge, α CD proteins
appeared to consist either of dimers with a 3 to 4 S sedimentation constant or largely of multiple polymers of different sizes. The molecular weight of the basic polypeptide
subunit varied from patient to patient, the length of these
chains being greater than half and smaller than 3/4 of normal
α1 heavy chains (3). In these calculations, allowance was
made for carbohydrates since the carbohydrate content of α CD
proteins was usually high, showing individual variability (3).

Antigenic analysis (2) and preliminary chemical studies
including diagonal maps (3) indicated that the entire Fc
fragment was present in α CD proteins, that their carboxy-
terminus was identical to that of normal α1 chains and that
the heavy-light peptide was missing. The hinge region was
shown by chemical typing to be present in all 8 proteins so
far studied. All attempts to elicit individually specific
antibodies to α CD proteins have failed, indicating the
paucity of antigenic determinants of the variable portion of
the chain. In view of these results and of the molecular

weight data, the missing portion of the chain is located in
the Fd segment and involves both the V and C1 regions.

The N terminal residues of several α CD proteins were
shown to be heterogeneous (3). Even for those proteins
which seemed to be homogeneous at the N terminus, marked
heterogeneity became apparent after two steps. The N terminal residues were not similar to those found at the N
terminus of any of the subgroups of the variable regions of
heavy chains. The most likely explanation of this heterogeneity at the N terminus is that it is the consequence of
a post-synthetic proteolytic process. The fact that the N
terminal residues found in the seven proteins studied were
Val and/or Ileu in all instances suggests that the postulated degradation may stop at this level for some unknown
reason (enzyme specificity, steric hindrance, presence of a
carbohydrate moiety ?). The possibility of the synthesis of
normal α chains undergoing post-synthetic degradation seemed
unlikely, and we had postulated, in view of the demonstration
of a large internal deletion in a γ CD protein (4), that we
were dealing with a primary deletion followed and obscured
by a secondary limited aminoterminal proteolysis (3).

Recent structural studies on the α CD protein Def. (5)
have indicated that this hypothesis is correct. As for several other α CD proteins, attempts to obtain the NH2 terminal
sequence on an automated sequencer were unsuccessful. However the comparison between the amino acid sequence of the
hinge region of protein Def. and that of a normal IgA$_1$
showed that, after a short segment corresponding to the variable region, protein Def. displays a gap which comprises the
CH1 constant domain. Normal synthesis resumes at a Valine
residue in the hinge region just before a segment which contains a partially duplicated fragment and the inter-heavy
disulfide bonds. From there on, the molecule is apparently
normal with the exception of a substitution of Thr for Ser
in position 12. Protein Def. is therefore synthesized as an
internally deleted α1 heavy chain. It is of interest that
Val at position 9 of the hinge peptide, where the identity
with a normal α1 chain starts, could be the equivalent of
Glu at position 216 of γ chains, the site where normal synthesis resumes in several γ CD proteins with internal deletions (6).

If the primary defect is in fact a deletion affecting
in most instances and V and C1 regions of the heavy chains,

which are under independent genetic control, the mutant gene
could behave like polar mutants which affect the product of
two subsequent genes.

CELLULAR STUDIES

The results obtained in careful biosynthetic studies
are in accordance with the concept of a primary deletion followed and obscured by a very limited secondary intracellular
proteolysis since they have excluded the possibility of the
synthesis of a normal size α chain which would be sequentially degraded to a smaller fragment after its release from the
ribosomes (7). Studies of a non-sense mutant of alkaline
phosphatase of E. coli have shown that these incomplete
proteins are quite susceptible to cytoplasmic degradation
after ribosomal release (8).

Any genetic hypothesis about α CD proteins must take
into account the fact that the absence of light chains is
due to a lack of synthesis. Immunofluorescence studies and
radioimmunoelectrophoretic analyses of proteins synthesized
in vitro have failed to detect any light chain production in
the cells which secrete α CD proteins (2). The failure of
light chain synthesis has been confirmed by biosynthetic
studies of nascent Ig subunits in such patients (7). Since
light and heavy chains are under the control of non-linked
genes, the puzzling problem of a hypothetic factor controlling the function of both genes remains to be solved.

No membrane bound Ig chains were found at the surface
of the proliferating cells which synthesize α CD proteins (9).

CLINICO-PATHOLOGICAL PATTERN

The protein abnormality which defines α CD is associated
with a peculiar clinico-pathological pattern. Alpha CD
appears to be a condition affecting primarily the secretory
IgA system.

The clinical pattern of α CD has been strikingly similar
in the first reported patient (10) and in all but two subsequently recognized cases (all presently published cases are
reviewed elsewhere) (11). This pattern corresponds to the
intestinal form of α CD. The dominant clinical feature is
a severe malabsorption syndrome with considerable loss of
weight, chronic diarrhea, steatorrhea and hypocalcemia.

Abdominal pains are often a major presenting symptom, and
abdominal masses are palpable in several patients. Radio-
logical studies and multiple intestinal biopsies showed that
the whole length of the small intestine is usually involved.
When laparotomy was performed, diffuse mesenteric lymphaden-
opathies were usually found. At a late stage of the disease,
a tumoral symptomatology with possible intestinal obstruction
is frequent. These features are analogous to those reported
by Israeli authors who emphasized the frequency in their
country of abdominal lymphoma presenting as malabsorption
(12, 13). We believe that most cases of this so-called
"Mediterranean lymphoma" may well be α CD (14).

In contrast with these diffuse enteromesenteric lesions,
the involvement of other lymphoid organs (liver, spleen,
peripheral nodes) is usually absent in α CD or occurs at a
late stage. No osteolytic lesions at X ray examination have
yet been observed. A mild bone marrow invasion has been
found in two patients by immunofluorescence studies (2).

Two cases of α CD without detectable intestinal involvement have been reported. They probably represent the respiratory form of the disease (15, 16).

In all patients affected with the enteral form of α CD,
pathological examination of the intestine shows a diffuse
and massive infiltration of lymphoid cells in the lamina
propria. Mature plasma cells constitute the predominant
cell type. Medium size lymphocytes and reticulum cells are
also found. Secondary villous atrophy and crypt sparsity
is noted in all instances, whereas surface epithelial abnormalities are moderate. Sections of the mesenteric nodes may
show a similar plasmacytic proliferation.

In some patients, pathological features of "reticulum
cell sarcoma", "undifferentiated sarcoma" or an histologic
picture somewhat similar to that of Hodgkin's disease are
found in the small bowel and mainly in mesenteric nodes.
The relationship between the lymphoplasmacytic proliferation
and the relatively frequent occurrence of reticulum cell
sarcoma is still open to question. Although the possibility
of a biclonal proliferation is not ruled out, the hypothesis
of a direct filiation between the two proliferative processes
seems more likely. The plasmacytic proliferation and the
reticulum cell sarcoma picture can be intimately intricated
both in the nodes and in the gut (14). Some ultrastructural

features of plasma cells may be found in the so-called reticulum sarcoma cells.

The neoplastic nature of the plasmacytic proliferation
of α CD has been convincingly demonstrated in a few cases
(14). Moreover the hypothesis of a non-malignant process
seems unlikely in those patients with high and rising levels
of serum monoclonal Ig. However, the malignant nature of
the plasma cell infiltration in the so-called "Mediterranean
lymphoma" appeared questionable (17), and the early intestinal and node biopsies of a patient affected with α CD who
died later with disseminated reticulum cell sarcoma were considered as non-malignant (14). Thus the non-malignant nature
of the condition at its relatively early stage constitutes a
real possibility, and α CD may well represent a model of a
lymphoma characterized by a continuous chain of events ranging from an apparently benign and reversible proliferation
to a truly malignant process. In this respect the occurrence of a long lasting and apparently complete clinical and
histological remission of the disease with disappearance of
the Ig abnormality in two patients who had been treated only
with antibiotics is of great interest (18, 19), especially
in view of some etiological considerations.

ETIOLOGICAL CONSIDERATIONS

The age distribution of α CD is in sharp contrast to
that of multiple myeloma since it occurs mainly in the second
and third decade of life. The sex distribution shows a moderate predominance of males.

The geographic origin of patients affected with α CD
(Table 1) shows a very striking predilection for some populations. The common denominator to these patients is that most
originated from and had been living in areas with a high rate
of infestation by intestinal microorganisms. It should be
emphasized that the two patients from Netherlands and United
States were those without detectable intestinal involvement.
This geographic distribution strongly suggests that environmental factors which provide a sustained local antigenic
stimulus do play a role in the etiology and pathogenesis of
α CD. This hypothesis does not exclude a possible interference with predisposing genetic factors. Limited parasitolog-
ic, virologic and bacteriologic studies in patients with α CD
have been unrewarding. In view of the structural data, there
is little chance to demonstrate any antibody activity in the

Table 1. Geographic origin of 59 patients

North Africa		South America	
Algeria	13	Colombia	1
Tunisia	10	North Argentina	1
Morocco	1	**Europe**	
Libya	1	South Italy	4
Middle East		Spain	4
Israel	8	Yugoslavia	1
Syria	1	Greece	2
Iran	4	Finland	1
Lebanon	1	Netherlands	1
Iraq	1		
Far East		**North America**	
Pakistan	2	U.S.A.	1
Cambodia	1		

α CD proteins. The specific or nonspecific nature of the postulated antigenic stimulus is open to question.

It is remarkable that this enteral stimulus appears to lead always to α CD and never to IgA myeloma. Whether this is related to the nature of the triggered cells or to that of the triggering agent is presently a matter of speculation. The possible reversibility of the hyperplastic process after withdrawal of a postulated triggering agent is obviously of great theoretical and practical interest.

Acknowledgment: These studies were supported in part by Grants from Institut National de la Sante et de la Recherche Medicale (INSERM) and Centre National de la Recherche Scientifique (CNRS).

REFERENCES

1. Seligmann, M., Danon, F., Hurez, D., Mihaesco, E. and Preud'Homme, J.L., Science 162:1396, 1968.
2. Seligmann, M., Mihaesco, E., Hurez, D., Mihaesco, C., Preud'Homme, J.L. and Rambaud, J.C., J. Clin. Invest. 48:2374, 1969.
3. Seligmann, M., Mihaesco, E. and Frangione, B., Ann. N.Y. Acad. Sci. 190:487, 1971.
4. Frangione, B. and Milstein, C., Nature 224:597, 1969.

5. Wolfenstein-Todel, C., Mihaesco, E. and Frangione, B., Proc. Nat. Acad. Sci. USA (in press).

6. Frangione, B. and Franklin, E.C., Seminars Hematol. 10: 53, 1973.

7. Buxbaum, J.N. and Preud'Homme, J.L., J. Immunol. 109: 1131, 1972.

8. Natori, S. and Garen, A., J. Mol. Biol. 49:577, 1970.

9. Preud'Homme, J.L. and Seligmann, M., Blood 40:777, 1972.

10. Rambaud, J.C., Bognel, C., Prost, A., Bernier, J.J., Le Quintrec, Y., Lambling, A., Danon, F., Hurez, D. and Seligmann, M., Digestion 1:321, 1968.

11. Seligmann, M., in International Myeloma Symposium, Arch. Int. Med. (in press).

12. Ramot, B., Shanin, N. and Bubis, J.J., Israel J. Med. Sci. 1:221, 1965.

13. Eidelman, S., Parkins, R.A. and Rubin, C., Medicine 45: 111, 1966.

14. Bognel, J.C., Rambaud, J.C., Modigliani, R., Matuchansky, C., Bognel, C., Bernier, J.J., Scotto, J., Hautefeuille, P., Mihaesco, E., Hurez, D., Preud'Homme, J.L. and Seligmann, M., Rev. Europ. Et. Clin. Biol. 17: 362, 1972.

15. Stoop, J.W., Ballieux, R.E., Hijmans, W. and Zegers, B.J.M., Clin. Exp. Immunol. 9:625, 1971.

16. Faux, J.A., Crain, J.D., Rosen, F.S. and Merler, E., Clin. Immunol. Immunopath. 1:282, 1973.

17. Rappaport, H., Ramot, B., Hulu, N. and Park, J.K., Cancer 29:1502, 1972.

18. Roge, J., Druet, P. and Marche, C., Path. et Biol. 18: 851, 1970.

19. Monges, H., Aubert, L., Chamlian, A., Remacle, J.P., Bernard, D., Mathieu, B. and Cougard, A., Arch. Franc. Mal. App. Dig. (in press).

THE CELLULAR BASIS OF IgA DEFICIENCY IN HUMANS

Alexander R. Lawton, L. Y. Frank Wu, and
Max D. Cooper
Spain Research Laboratories, Depts. of
Pediatrics and Microbiology, University of
Alabama in Birmingham, Birmingham, Alabama

Isolated deficiency of IgA is by far the most commonly identified defect of the immune system in humans. It occurs in individuals who are otherwise entirely healthy, but has also been frequently associated with such diverse disease states as congenital viral or parasitic infection, chromosomal abnormalities, and autoimmune diseases. Family studies have suggested that this condition may be inherited either as an autosomal dominant or recessive trait.

In 1969 Oppenheim, Rogentine, and Terry made the very interesting observation that monkey antiserum to human IgA stimulated blast transformation of lymphocytes from 3 IgA deficient subjects to the same extent as lymphocytes from normal donors (1). They suggested that these IgA deficient individuals had lymphocytes in peripheral blood which expressed IgA determinants. Subsequently Grey et al., using direct immunofluorescence, demonstrated IgA-bearing B-lymphocytes in 3 IgA deficient patients (2). We initiated a study of IgA deficient patients in anticipation of being able to subdivide this group into those who had and those who lacked IgA-bearing B-lymphocytes. Although our patients included individuals whose IgA deficiency was familial, sporadic, or associated with congenital rubella syndrome, all were found to have normal proportions of IgA B-lymphocytes (3). At this time B-lymphocyte studies on more than 40 IgA deficient patients have been reported; none have lacked lymphocytes expressing IgA determinants (reviewed in 4).

These results imply that most instances of isolated

IgA deficiency reflect an abnormality of cell differentiation rather than a deletion or major structural anomaly of
the gene for the constant region of the α chain. This paper
will review our studies on the differentiation capabilities
of lymphocytes from IgA-deficient patients (5, 6) and present some perspectives - but no final answers - on the
pathogenesis of this defect.

MATERIALS AND METHODS

Eleven children with isolated deficiency of IgA have
been studied. One had congenital toxoplasmosis and one
congenital rubella. Circumstantial evidence for a heritable
defect was obtained in six patients. One of these had
ataxia-telangiectasia, and the others had a family member
with deficiency of IgA or other immunoglobulin classes. One
patient had chronic active hepatitis. For the remaining
three, no environmental or genetic factors were implicated.
Excepting the child with ataxia-telangiectasia, none of
these patients had a demonstrable gap in humoral or cell
mediated immunity other than IgA deficiency. Clinical data,
immunologic profiles, and results of B-lymphocyte assays on
most of these patients have been reported previously (3).
The differentiation capacity of B-lymphocytes was
assayed by their in vitro response to pokeweed mitogen
(PWM). The precise methods used in processing peripheral
blood lymphocytes, establishing cultures, and analyzing the
results are presented in detail elsewhere (6). In brief,
10^5 lymphocytes purified by Ficoll-Hypaque gradient centrifugation were cultured in microplate wells in 0.2 ml of
tissue culture medium supplemented with 20% agammaglobulinemic human plasma. An optimal dose of PWM was added to half
the cultures. ^{14}C thymidine was added after 6¼ days incubation at 37^0 in a 5% CO_2 atmosphere; cultures were harvested
at 7 days. DNA synthesis was measured by determining the
radioactivity of TCA precipitates of cultured cells. Repli-
cate cultures were layered onto slides using a cytocentrifuge, fixed, and stained with fluorochrome-labeled anti-
immunoglobulins for determination of cells containing cytoplasmic immunoglobulins. In some experiments, in vitro
biosynthesis of immunoglobulins was measured by the classical technique of immunoelectrophoresis-radioautography.
Newly synthesized immunoglobulins were labeled by incorporation of ^{14}C lysine and isoleucine added to cultures 18
hours prior to termination. Culture supernatants, or cell

lysates and supernatants, were dialyzed and concentrated by lyophilization. The 10-fold concentrates were electrophoresed with normal serum as a carrier and developed with antisera specific for IgM, IgG, and IgA. Radioautographs were prepared by exposing the washed stained plates to high speed film.

RESULTS

PWM-stimulated cultures of peripheral blood lymphocytes from normal donors contain substantial numbers of cells exhibiting bright cytoplasmic fluorescence when stained with anti-immunoglobulins. The median frequencies of these cells in cultures from 27 normal donors were 2.3% for IgM, 1.6% for IgG, and 1.7% for IgA. Unstimulated cultures had fewer than 0.1% fluorescent cells. A similar low frequency of cells containing detectable cytoplasmic immunoglobulin was found in fixed preparations of lymphocytes prior to culture. The stained cells had the morphologic appearance of lymphoblasts (Fig. 1). Mitotic figures were occasionally observed.

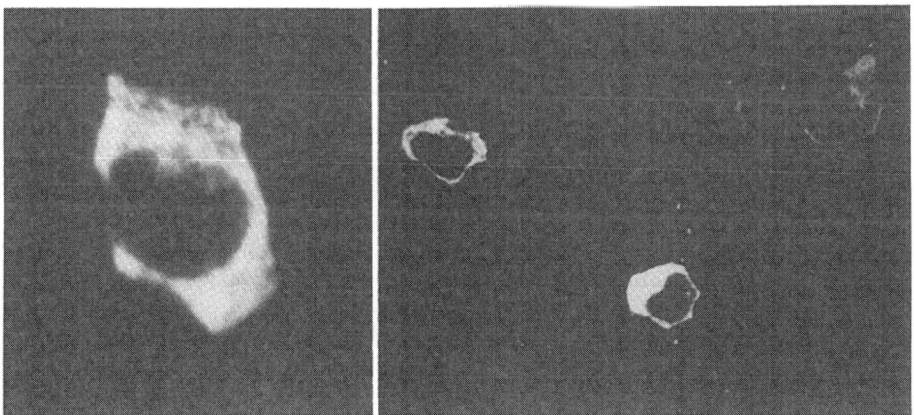

Fig. 1. Cells from pokeweed mitogen stimulated lymphocyte cultures stained with fluorescine-labeled anti α. Left: Normal donor culture, final magnification x 5000. Right: Culture from a boy with IgA deficiency and ataxia-telangiectasia, x 1920.

Simultaneous cultures from individuals were assayed for immunoglobulin biosynthesis by incorporation of ^{14}C amino acids. PWM-stimulated cultures produced much more intense labeling of immunoglobulins than did unstimulated cultures. Comparison of the extent of labeling in culture supernatants with that in the cell sap indicated that most of the newly synthesized immunoglobulin had been secreted.

No immunoglobulin-containing cells were found when lymphocytes from 3 boys with X-linked agammaglobulinemia (who had few or no B-lymphocytes) were cultured with PWM. DNA synthesis by these cultures was similar to that observed in cultures from normal individuals.

At the time of study 9 of the 11 IgA-deficient patients had no serum IgA detectable by radial immunodiffusion (lower limit < .03 mg/ml) or by a more sensitive Ouchterlony technique; the other 2 had levels of 0.07 and 0.11 mg/ml. The percentage of lymphocytes bearing membrane-bound IgA ranged from 1.5 to 13, well within the normal range. None of these children had detectable serum antibodies to IgA, but several had antibodies to goat proteins.

The response of peripheral lymphocytes from these patients to PWM was strikingly similar to that of normal cells. Without exception, PWM-treated cultures contained cells with easily detectable cytoplasmic IgA, as well as cells which stained for IgM or IgG. The range of IgA positive cells was from 0.4 to 7.9% of total recovered cells. These data are graphically summarized in Figure 2.

In 7 patients biosynthesis of IgA was also assessed by immunoelectrophoresis and radioautography of culture fluids. Fluids from PWM-stimulated cultures showed distinct labeling of the IgA arc; the remaining culture was one in which few (0.6%) IgA-containing cells were found by immunofluorescence.

The possibility that in vivo failure of terminal differentiation was caused by a serum inhibitor tested in one of our IgA deficient patients. Development of IgA-containing cells was similar in cultures supplemented with either autologous or pooled agammaglobulinemic serum.

Culture supernatants and cell pellets (disrupted by repeated freezing and thawing) were individually analyzed for IgA biosynthesis. As was the case in normals, the supernatant fluids contained more labeled IgA than did the cells. As the ^{14}C amino acids had been added only 18 hours prior to termination of cultures, we conclude that PWM-stimulated cells are capable of both synthesis and active secretion of IgA.

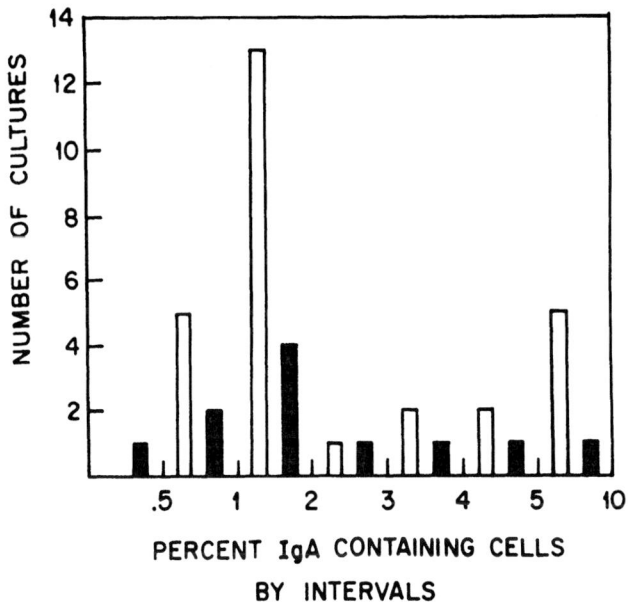

Fig. 2. Frequency of IgA containing cells in PWM stimulated
cultures from normals (open bars) and IgA deficient patients
(closed bars). The modal frequency and distribution for the
two groups is similar.

DISCUSSION

Differentiation implies a correlated change in morpho-
logy and function. By these criteria, pokeweed mitogen
stimulation may be said to induce terminal differentiation
of B-lymphocytes in vitro. Ultrastructural changes resulting from PWM stimulation include formation of an extensive
network of rough endoplasmic reticulum connecting to the
Golgi apparatus which is characteristic of differentiated
plasma cells. B-lymphocytes, for the most part, lack these
structures; although they synthesize immunoglobulin, incorporate it into their membrane, and shed it at a slow rate,
they do not contain a sufficient cytoplasmic pool to be detected by immunofluorescence after fixation. The immunofluorescence assay used in these studies thus offers a
clear-cut advantage in assessing differentiation. It can
distinguish a small increase in the rate of immunoglobulin

synthesis and shedding by a large population of B-lymphocytes from true differentiation of lymphocytes to plasma
cells synthesizing and secreting immunoglobulins at a high
rate.

These experiments have shown that a population of B-
lymphocytes from IgA deficient patients can be triggered by
PWM to differentiate to cells synthesizing large quantities
of IgA. A major part of the newly synthesized IgA is secreted into the culture medium. This response is qualitatively and quantitatively indistinguishable from that of
cells from normal donors. We assume, but have not proven,
that the precursors of these secretory cells are IgA-bearing
B-lymphocytes, which are present in normal numbers in the
circulation of our patients. It is difficult to avoid the
interpretation that the in vivo defect in IgA synthesis is
not related to an intrinsic abnormality of the B-lymphocyte.

These observations perhaps become more meaningful when
compared to results of similar studies on patients with
other types of immune deficiency (6). We have observed
patients with normal proportions of B-lymphocytes but marked
deficiency of the corresponding serum immunoglobulin classes
in whom PWM did not stimulate B-lymphocyte differentiation.
One patient was agammaglobulinemic; PWM induced DNA snythesis
in her cultured lymphocytes, but no immunoglobulin-containing cells were found. Another had normal serum IgM but very
low IgG (0.2 mg/ml) and undetectable IgA. Normal numbers of
IgM-containing cells, but almost none staining for IgG or
IgA were found in PWM-stimulated cultures. We have also
found that fetal lymphocyte preparations containing normal
proportions of B-lymphocytes of the three major classes are
triggered to synthesize IgM normally, but very few IgG
or IgA-containing cells are found. In this case the in
vitro response to PWM mimics the ontogeny of immunoglobulin
synthesis in vivo.

Serial observations on some of our IgA deficient
patients have indicated that their in vivo defect in IgA
synthesis may be reversed under certain circumstances. Congenital toxoplasmosis was diagnosed in one boy after his
cord blood IgM was found to be elevated. He had normal
levels of serum IgA for this age up until 6 months, but has
had none detectable on serial observations during four subsequent years. A six year old girl had normal serum IgA
(1.25 mg/ml), together with a marked elevation of IgG (> 30
mg/ml) during the early stages of chronic active hepatitis.
Her hypergammaglobulinemia resolved on steroid therapy, but
IgA disappeared completely from her circulation.

It has become popular among immunologists, when faced with an observation for which there is no ready explanation, to blame it on the T-lymphocyte. We are no exception. There is abundant evidence in the literature suggesting a special relationship between IgA synthesis and thymic function (reviewed in 6). Perhaps the most striking example occurs in the congenitally athymic nude mouse, in which IgA synthesis is markedly deficient despite the presence of IgA bearing B-lymphocytes (7, 8). The sum of these observations would seem to be that T-lymphocyte "helper function" is required to a greater extent in triggering IgA than IgG responses, which are in turn more thymic dependent than IgM responses. It is conceivable that defective T cell regulatory function might explain the frequent association of IgA deficiency and autoimmune disease (9).

SUMMARY

Despite the heterogenicity of clinical circumstances in which it occurs, isolated IgA deficiency seems to have a fairly uniform cellular basis. B lymphocytes bearing surface IgA are present in normal numbers, and can be triggered in vitro to differentiate to IgA secreting cells. This information suggests that the failure of IgA production in vivo involves a potentially reversible block in terminal differentiation of precursor B-lymphocytes which may be related to abnormal function of another cell line.

This work was supported by USPHS Grants Al CA 11502, RR 3213, HD 00102, and CA 13148.

REFERENCES

1. Oppenheim, J.J., Rogentine, G.N., and Terry, W.D., Immunology 16:123-138, 1969.
2. Grey, H.M., Rabellino, E., and Pirofsky, B., J. Clin. Invest. 50:2368-2375, 1971.
3. Lawton, A.R., Royal, S.A., Self, K.S., and Cooper, M.D., J. Lab. Clin. Med. 80:26-33, 1972.
4. Cooper, M.D., Keightley, R.G., Wu, Frank Liang-Yeh, and Lawton, A.R., Transplant. Rev. In press.
5. Wu, L.Y.F., Lawton, A.R., Greaves, M.F., and Cooper, M.D., in Proceedings of the Seventh Leucocyte Culture Conference, ed. Daguillard, F., Academic Press, N. Y., p. 485-495, 1973.

6. Wu, L.Y.F., Lawton, A.R., and Cooper, M.D., J. Clin.
     Invest. In press.
7. Bankhurst, A.D. and Warner, N.L., Aust. J. Exp. Biol.
     Med. Sci. 50:661, 1972.
8. Crewther, P. and Warner, N.L., Aust. J. Exp. Biol. Med.
     Sci. 50:625-635, 1972.
9. Ammann, A.J. and Hong, R., Medicine 50:223, 1971.

ALPHA CHAIN DETERMINANTS ON THE MEMBRANE OF IMMUNOGLOBULIN SYNTHESIZING CELLS

W. Hijmans, Henrica R.E. Schuit, J. Radl and
J.M.J.J. Vossen

Institute for Experimental Gerontology T.N.O.,
Rijswijk (Z.H.) and Department of Pediatrics,
University of Leiden, The Netherlands

INTRODUCTION

In a study of surface immunoglobulins (Ig) on lymphocytes from patients with paraproteinemia (1), we observed that a variable number of plasma cells not only contained intracellular Ig, but also had Ig on their surface, as shown in the vital technique of immunofluorescence. Moreover, in the bone marrow specimens from persons without paraproteinemia, the Ig class on the membrane was not always indentical with the Ig class within the cell.

Here we report on a systematic study in which two questions were asked. First, to what extent do human Ig-secreting cells, i.e. differentiated lymphocytes and plasma cells, carry surface Ig; and, second, whether there is a correspondence between the class of Ig within the cell and on its surface.

MATERIALS AND METHODS

The preparation of cell suspensions from bone marrow and tissues as well as the preparation and the specificity testing of the conjugates has been described (2).

The staining for membrane bound immunoglobulins was done by the vital technique at room temperature for 30 min. Only TRITC labeled conjugates were used. After washing the cells, cytocentrifuge or sedimentation chamber slides were

prepared. The standard acetic acid-ethanol fixation was not
applied because dissociation of the antigen-antibody complex
on the cell surface could occur at low pH. Therefore, the
slides were fixed in acetone at $-20^{\circ}C$ for 15 min, washed,
and subsequently stained with FITC labeled conjugates. The
essential information on the conjugates which is necessary
for the evaluation of the results is presented in Table I.
Details on the markers used to detect dimeric IgA are given
elsewhere (4). Information concerning a conjugate against
human serum albumin (HSA) used as a control reagent has also
been published (5). Two anti-α conjugates were also used
after ultracentrifugation at 100,000 x G for 30 min to exclude the possibility that positive reactions were due to
the uptake of aggregates.

Bone marrow specimens from 8 normal individuals and 2
myeloma patients, as well as 2 spleens and 5 tonsils from
immunologically normal persons were tested. Only differentiated, large lymphocytes and plasma cells with clear cytoplasmic fluorescence were studied in each slide.

The slides were examined under epi-illumination and the
two wavelength method was applied (6). In this way, one can
distinguish the fluorescein and the rhodamine dye with a
high degree of efficiency. An HBO 100 lamp served as the
light source. In order to facilitate the presentation and
the discussion of the results, the following coding will be
used: cells with cytoplasmic staining will be designated by
the capitals A, M, G, D and the corresponding small Greek
letters will be used to indicate surface staining for that
particular Ig class.

RESULTS

In the first series of experiments, the percentage of
cells with cytoplasmic staining for any of the Ig classes
from bone marrow, spleen, and tonsil which also showed surface fluorescence with the anti-α conjugate was calculated.
The results (Table II) show the presence of the α-determinants
on an appreciable number of cells, regardless of the class of
Ig within the cytoplasm. These cells were large lymphocytes
or plasma cells. The surface fluorescence was distinctly
granular, and usually covered the entire or almost the entire
surface (Fig.1). The number of A + α cells was always higher
than the number of A cells with surface determinants of the
other Ig classes.

TABLE I

Specification of conjugates

no.	specifi-city	material used for immunization	antiserum raised in	pre-paration	fluor	reference for method or source
1	α	secretory IgA from human milk	sheep	antibody	FITC TRITC	(3)
2	α	heterogenous serum IgA	goat	IgG fraction	FITC RB 200	Nordic 2-171
3	α	IgA paraprotein	rabbit	globulin fraction	TRITC	(2)
4	α	mixture of 3 IgA paraproteins	rabbits	antibody	TRITC	(3)
5	γ	IgG paraprotein	sheep	antibody	FITC TRITC	(3)
6	γ	heterogenous serum IgG	goat	IgG fraction	FITC	Nordic 2-372
7	γ	heterogenous serum IgG	rabbit	IgG fraction	FITC	Nordic 871
8	μ	heterogenous serum IgM	rabbit	antibody	FITC TRITC	(3)
9	μ	no data available	horse	globulin fraction	FITC	Roboz, adsorbed
10	δ	IgD paraprotein	rabbit	antibody	TRITC	(3)
11	δ	IgD paraprotein + heterogenous IgD	swine	globulin fraction	FITC	Nordic 1-668
12	κ	pool of 3 κ Bence Jones	rabbit	globulin fraction	TRITC	(2)
13	λ	pool of 2 λ Bence Jones	rabbit	globulin fraction	TRITC	(2)

Cell suspensions from the same sources were also tested for the other combinations (Table II). It is clear that the combinations with α on the surface were always more prevalant than the other combinations with the exception of D + δ.

A clear capping phenomenon was never seen in any of the synthesizing cells in contrast to the presence of this phenomenon in nonsynthesizing precursor cells in the same slides.

The presence of surface bound light chains was determined in 4 bone marrow samples. Three were from IgA myeloma patients and one from a four-year old child. Only in one myeloma case could surface bound light chains be detected, but they were on such a small number of cells that these could easily be due to the presence of residual normal cells. In this group, the percentage of cells with surface α determinants ranged from 10 to 98%.

The molecular form of the IgA on the membrane was tested with the three specific markers for the dimeric (polymeric) form (4). More than 300 cells which were positive for the α determinants were analyzed but the presence of determinants of the dimeric form could not be detected.

One sample of cells from tonsillar tissue was investigated with 2 anti α-conjugates. Tests were made on A, M, G, and D cells, both before and after ultracentrifugation of these conjugates. No influence of ultracentrifugation was observed.

One bone marrow and one spleen sample was tested with an antibody preparation of an anti α-conjugate in serial dilution. The data give an indication of a prozone effect which is followed by a decrease in titer to zero at a dilution of approximately 1:1,000.

Finally a bone marrow specimen of a 2 year old boy with an IgA deficiency was tested. Cells containing IgA in the cytoplasm were absent, and neither could α determinants be detected on the surface of the cells synthesizing other immunoglobulins.

TABLE II

Combined presence of cytoplasmic and surface immunoglobulins

Combined staining for:		Percentage of Ig containing cells[b] with surface staining in:		
cytoplasmic Ig^a	surface Ig^a	Bone marrow	Spleen	Tonsil
A +	α	67(60-82)	68(50-72)	68(60-82)
A +	μ	2(1-4)	10	16(2-42)
A +	γ	2(0-4)	7	25(0-44)
A +	δ	n.t.	n.t.	0
M +	α	38(25-42)	23(22-27)	16(2-42)
M +	μ	12(0-14)	15	8(0-17)
M +	γ	1(0-7)	0	2(2-5)
M +	δ	25	n.t.	n.t.
G +	α	22(16-24)	8(6-10)	43(33-52)
G +	μ	1(0-2)	0	2(2-3)
G +	γ	2(0-2)	0	2(2-3)
G +	δ	2	n.t.	n.t.
D +	α	30	n.t.	50(48-52)
D +	μ	10	n.t.	25
D +	γ	10	n.t.	10
D +	δ	93(90-96)	n.t.	72

a) Cells were first processed for surface and then for cytoplasmic staining. Capitals are used to indicate cytoplasmic staining and Greek letters for surface fluorescence.

b) The numbers between brackets indicate the range. When no range is given, only a single test was performed.

n.t. = not tested.

DISCUSSION

The most prominent finding in this study was the detection of Ig determinants on the surface of a large number
of cells which contained Ig within their cytoplasm. Furthermore, there was an excess in the number of these cells with
α determinants on their surface in comparison with the other
heavy chains, regardless of the class of Ig within the cells.
The results indicate that these surface bound α molecules
lack the dimer specific determinants. Capping was never
observed. Light chains were not detected in a limited series.
Because of the preponderance of the α determinants, we shall
focus on this Ig in the discussion.

Extensive control experiments were performed to exclude
artifacts. The conjugates had been tested for specificity on
monoclonal bone marrow cells and had been proved to be specific in a large number of different tests. They could be used
in high dilution. Moreover, 2 of our conjugates were isolated
antibody preparations of which the background and nonspecific
staining were minimal. They did not show activity against
the secretory component or the J chain. No influence of
ultracentrifugation was seen. Ultracentrifugation was performed in order to remove any aggregates, if present, as the
possible cause of surface fluorescence.

Comparable results were obtained with 4 conjugates which
had been prepared from different sources. Negative controls
included an IgA deficient patient, and cells from 25 patients
with chronic lymphatic leukemia which did not react with the
anti α-conjugates on vital staining. Also the percentage of
surface α positive cells in peripheral blood lymphocytes
from normal persons was less than one (7) which is in the
same range as the low estimates reported by other workers.
Suspensions treated with a conjugated antiserum against
human serum albumin prepared in the same way as the antibody conjugates were consistently negative. Fluorescence was
also absent with an anti α dimer conjugate and a conjugate
against the secretory component prepared from the same crude
antiserum as one of the anti α conjugates (3,4).

These considerations lead us to conclude that we are
not dealing here with an artifact but with α chains most
probably of a monomer or part thereof not likely in association with light chains.

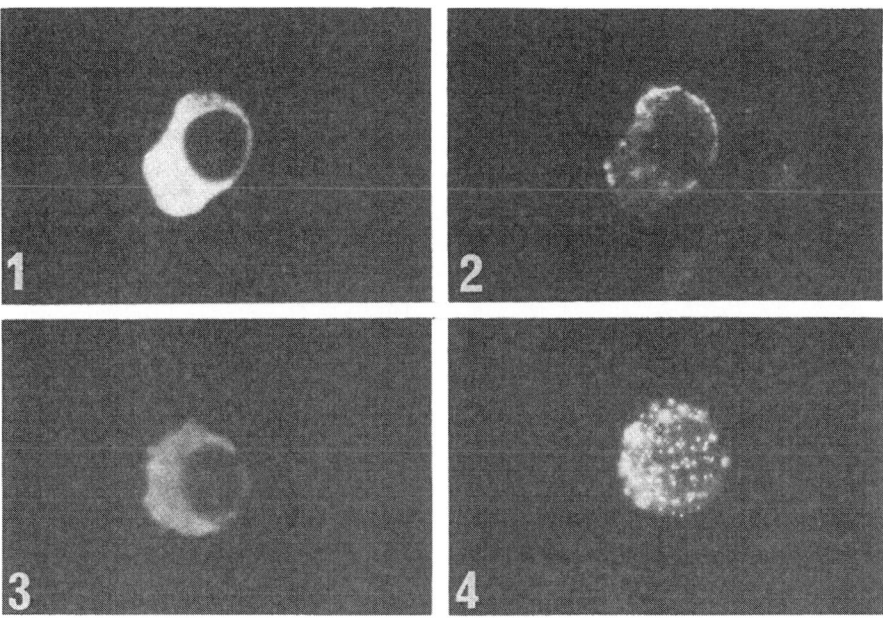

Fig. 1. Cells from tonsil (1,2) and bone marrow (3,4). Cytoplasmic staining with anti α FITC (1), and the same cell with surface staining with anti α TRITC (2). Cytoplasmic staining with anti δ FITC (3), and the same cell with surface staining with anti α TRITC (4). Details of photography: Ilford HP4 film, excitation of FITC at 500 mm, of TRITC at 546 nm Final magnification: x 1,000.

The absence of capping also indicates that these surface structures on the Ig containing cells are different from the IgA on the receptor bearing lymphocyte without cytoplasmic Ig. The possibility that this surface fluorescence represents Ig or immune complexes bound *in vivo* by the Fc receptors cannot be excluded. This explanation is not very plausible, however, because light chains were not detected, nor would one then expect an excess of α determinants over those of other classes of Ig. This phenomenon could represent a certain stage of differentiation into mature plasma cells or perhaps a switch in the synthesis of Ig. Whether the α molecules exert a special and so far unknown function in the process of differentiation or activity of the Ig secreting cells remains to be determined.

SUMMARY

A high percentage of immunoglobulin (Ig) containing cells from human bone marrow, tonsils, and spleen carry Ig on their surface which mainly belong to the α class. Further immunofluorescence studies showed that these α molecules do not contain the determinants specific for the polymeric form. Negative results in the tests for Ig light chains and the absence of capping point to the possibility that these surface components are different from the surface IgA seen on lymphocytes without cytoplasmic Ig.

Acknowledgements. The authors are indebted to Miss P. van den Berg for her assistance in the preparation of the conjugates and to Mrs. P.C. Moree-van der Linde for her help in immunofluorescence.

REFERENCES

1. Knapp, W., Schuit, H.R.E., Bolhuis, R.L.H. and Hijmans,W., in preparation.
2. Hijmans, W., Schuit, H.R.E. and Klein, F., Clin.exp.Immunol. 4:457, 1969.
3. Rádl, J., v.d.Berg, P., Voormolen, M., Hendriks, W.D.H. and Schaefer U.W., Clin.exp.Immunol., in press.
4. Rádl, J., Schuit, H.R.E., Mestecky, J. and Hijmans, W., this volume.
5. Hijmans, W., Schuit, H.R.E., Yamashita, T. and Schechter, I., Eur.J.Immunol. 2:1, 1972.
6. Hijmans, W., Schuit, H.R.E. and Hulsing-Hesselink, E., Ann.N.Y.Acad.Sci. 177:290, 1971.
7. Knapp, W., Bolhuis, R.L.H., Rádl, J. and Hijmans, W., J.Immunol., in press.

SECRETORY AND SERUM IgA IN CHILDREN WITH PROTEIN-CALORIE MALNUTRITION

Stitaya Sirisinha, Robert Suskind,
Robert Edelman, Chairat Asvapaka, and
Robert E. Olson

Department of Microbiology, Faculty of Science,
Mahidol University, and SEATO Medical Research
Laboratory, Bangkok; Anemia and Malnutrition
Research Center, Chiang Mai, Thailand

INTRODUCTION

The incidence and the severity of infection is often increased in children with protein-calorie malnutrition (P.C.M.) (1-3). Several groups of investigators have demonstrated an impairment of the cell-mediated immune function, of the inflammatory response, and of the complement and C3-activating systems in these children (4-9). However, there is no unanimous agreement on the effect of P.C.M. on the humoral immune mechanism. In general, the serum immunoglobulin levels are not reduced (10-13).

Because of the clinical impression that malnourished children are prone to infections that occur at the body surfaces (1-3, 14), it seems reasonable that local host defenses may be defective in children who have severe P.C.M. The present study was designed to evaluate the effect of P.C.M. on the immunoglobulins of secretions that contribute to the adequacy of the local surface defenses (15). Emphasis was placed on immunoglobulins of the IgA class because these are predominant among the immunoglobulins in secretions (15). The level of secretory IgA (S-IgA) was determined in the nasal washings of children with P.C.M. on admission and during dietary treatment. In addition, S-IgA and serum IgA were compared in the same patients to evaluate the entire IgA system.

MATERIALS AND METHODS

Malnourished Patients

The patients, aged 1 to 5 years, were admitted to the research ward of the Anemia and Malnutrition Research Center where they remained throughout the 84-day study period. All of the 24 children admitted had primary malnutrition and weighed between 3 and 12 kg. On admission, the patients were classified (16) as having marasmus (M), marasmus-kwashiorkor (MK), or kwashiorkor (K). Ten patients also suffered from clinical vitamin A deficiency manifested by xerophthalmia and follicular hyperkeratosis. Patients were treated for fluid and electrolyte imbalance during the first hospital days and received supplemental vitamins and minerals.

The patients' 84-day hospital course was divided into 4 main periods. During the stabilization period (days 1-7) patients were given a caloric intake which gradually increased from 25 cal. and 1 g protein/kg body-weight/day, at day 1, to 100 cal. and 1 g protein/kg/day, at day 7. The stabilization period was followed by a 3-week dietary study period (days 8-29) when patients were randomly assigned to 1 of 4 dietary treatment schemes (Table 1). All patients again

TABLE I
Dietary treatment and clinical status of P.C.M. children.

Dietary Group	Dietary Intake (days 8-29)		No. Children			
	Cal./kg/d.	G.protein/kg/d.	K	M	MK	Total
1	100	1	1	3	1	5
2	100	4	2	1	4	7
3	175	1	1	1	1	3
4	175	4	4	2	3	9
All groups			8	7	9	24

received the same diet (175 cal. and 4 g protein/kg/day) during the third period (days 30-70). During the last period (days 71-84) the patients were given an ad lib solid food diet having the same quantity of calorie and protein content as the third-period diet. All patients had recovered

clinically 8 weeks after admission. A follow-up study was
performed on the nasal washings 15 to 22 months after discharge.

Normal Children

The "normal" controls in this study were healthy
children and mildly anemic children who attended the Anemia
and Malnutrition Clinic but were otherwise clinically well-
nourished; all were from the same geographical area as the
patients suffering P.C.M.

Collection and Processing of Specimens

Nasal washings were collected on day 1 or 2 of admission
and at intervals during hospitalization. Blood was routinely
collected within 1 or 2 days of the nasal washing. At least
5 pairs of nasal wash and serum specimens were collected
during the 84-day period from 20 of the 24 children. Only
1 nasal wash was obtained from each of the control children.

To obtain nasal washings, the child was positioned on
one side with the neck extended and the head tilted downward.
Five ml of 0.85% NaCl was slowly instilled deep into the
upper nostril with an ear syringe. After a few seconds, the
saline was aspirated from the nasopharynx through a No.8
French plastic catheter inserted through the lower nostril.
The same procedure was repeated with the patient lying on the
other side.   The nasal washings were centrifuged at 1000 G
for 30 minutes at 4°C, and the supernatant was stored at
-20°C until analyzed. Specimens that were bloody were dis-
carded.

Immunoglobulin Determinations

The concentrations of IgG and S-IgA in the nasal washings
were determined by electroimmunodiffusion (17). The lower
limit of sensitivity of this technique in our laboratory was
approximately 1 mg per 100 ml for both proteins. S-IgA used
as a standard was purified as described (18). To aid comparison of values between individuals and groups, the absolute values were converted to per cent of the total protein
concentration. The concentration of serum IgA was determined
by radial immunodiffusion (19). Antiserum to purified salivary IgA was made specific for S-IgA by absorption with normal

serum until further addition of serum no longer precipitated
the antiserum. The absorbed antiserum (anti-SC) reacted only
with S-IgA in immunodiffusion and immunoelectrophoresis, and
its precipitating activity was removed only with purified
S-IgA.

Other Techniques

Albumin in the nasal wash specimens was determined by
radial immunodiffusion (19). The limit of sensitivity was
1.7 mg%. Human serum albumin (Miles Laboratories, Inc.,
Kankakee, Ill., U.S.A.) was used for the calibration of a
standard curve. Total protein was determined by the biuret
method (20) using albumin as standard. Immunodiffusion (21)
and immunoelectrophoresis (22) were used for the qualitative
analyses of nasal wash proteins.

RESULTS

Immunoglobulins in the Nasal Washings of Malnourished Children

The nasal washings of malnourished children were indistinguishable from those of the normal children by immunoelectrophoresis, using polyvalent antiserum to normal serum.
At least 3 or 4 bands of precipitation were consistently
detected in unconcentrated nasal washings from both groups.
Some of the bands of the malnourished children seemed,
however, less pronounced. Further analysis with monospecific
antisera revealed the presence of IgA, IgG, albumin and
transferrin in most nasal washings. The nasal washings of
P.C.M. children also contained a component that reacted with
anti-SC and that gave a reaction of complete identity with
purified S-IgA. In addition, when the nasal washings were
tested with anti-SC and anti-α chain antisera by immunodiffusion, a single line of complete identity resulted; the
reactivity disappeared when anti-α chain, but not anti-γ
chain, was added to the specimens before immunodiffusion
(Fig. 1). These observations indicated that both antisera
reacted with the same molecule and suggested both that the
IgA component of the nasal washing was associated with secretory component (SC) and a detectable amount of unbound SC was
not present in the nasal washings of either the malnourished
or the normal children. IgG and albumin in the nasal washings
from both groups were indistinguishable from the corresponding
serum components. No nasal washings reacted with antiserum to
IgM.

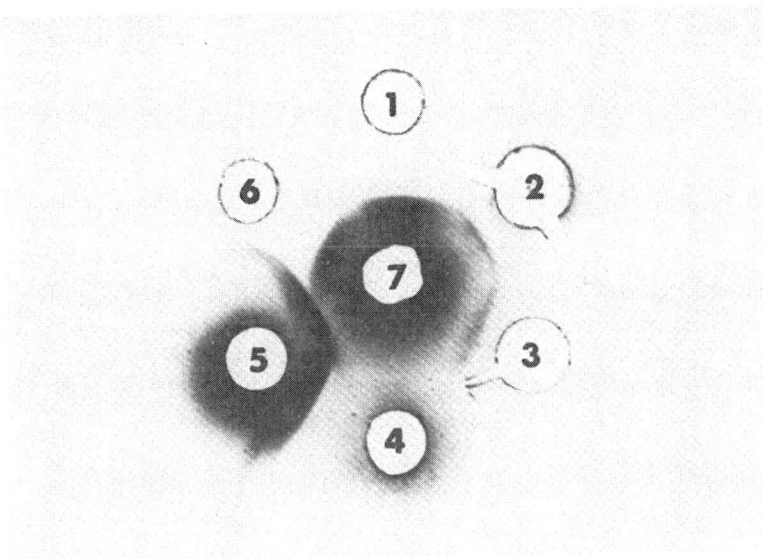

Figure 1. Immunodiffusion analysis showing that the reactivity of nasal washing from P.C.M. children (3) with anti-SC
(7) could be specifically inhibited by previous exposure of
the specimen with anti-α chain (4) but not with anti-γ chain
(5) antisera. The heavy bands that formed between wells 5
and 7 and between well 5 and 4 were due to the reaction of
anti-γ chain in well 5 with excess IgG used for the absorption
of anti-SC and anti-α chain. Well 2 contained pooled nasal
washing from normal children.

S-IgA was the prominent protein in the nasal washings
from both groups of children. More than 90% of the 140 nasal
washings collected from 24 malnourished children during the
84-day hospitalization period contained detectable S-IgA and
albumin. IgG was detected in only two-thirds of the samples.
Less than 10% of the nasal washings tested were positive for
α-amylase by immunodiffusion, suggesting that salivary contamination was insignificant and that S-IgA found in the
nasal wash samples was not of salivary origin.

Quantitative Comparison of the Nasal Washings of Malnourished
                  and of Normal Children

The relative concentrations of S-IgA in all nasal washings
from the 24 P.C.M. children were significantly lower than that
of specimens from the "normal" children (16.1% vs 24.3%,
p<0.01 by "t" test) (Fig. 2). The values of S-IgA in serial
nasal washings from any one subject varied considerably during

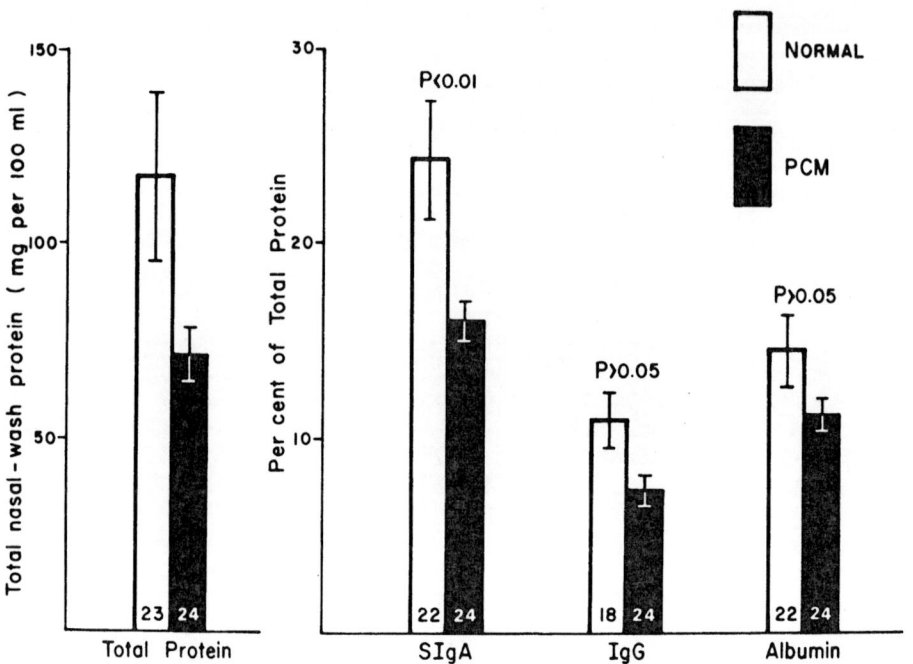

Figure 2.   Diagramatic representations of total protein, S-IgA,
IgG and albumin in the nasal washings of P.C.M. and normal
children.   Bars and lines represent mean ± S.E.M.; the number
at the base of each bar represents the number of children.
Individual values used for calculating the group means were
the average concentrations determined from serial samples
collected during the 84-day hospitalization period.

the hospitalization period.   When the data were pooled according
to hospital day, the relative concentrations of days 1-2, 1-8,
29, 50-70 and 71-84 samples were not strikingly different from
the total value, although slight improvement was observed by
day 29.   However, when the late follow-up samples from some
of these children were analyzed, a noticeable increase in the
S-IgA level was observed; the mean concentration of 20.6% was
not significantly different from the normal value of 24.3% at
the 5% level.   The relative concentrations of S-IgA in nasal
washings determined at intervals during dietary treatment did
not differ significantly between the 4 dietary treatment schemes

In contrast to S-IgA, the relative concentrations of IgG
and albumin in the 2 groups of children were similar.   The level
of IgG and albumin were correlated (correlation coefficient,
r, = 0.55, p<0.01), but the levels of S-IgA and albumin were
not (r = 0.06, p>0.05).

S-IgA, IgG, and Albumin in the Nasal Washings of Malnourished Children with Different Clinical Status

The S-IgA levels in nasal washings of the various clinical groups among the malnourished children were not significantly different. In samples collected during the first 48 hr, the relative concentrations of S-IgA from P.C.M. children with no clinical manifestations of vitamin A deficiency were slightly higher than those from children who also had vitamin A deficiency (19.2% vs 13.7%); the difference was not, however, statistically significant at the 5% level. The S-IgA level did not seem related to the presence or absence of acute upper respiratory disease or generalized infections in the children.

Serum IgA in P.C.M. Children

The mean admission level of serum IgA in the malnourished children was significantly higher than the value in normal children of the same age (Fig. 3). The high admission level gradually returned to the "normal" level during dietary treatment. Electroimmunodiffusion analysis failed to disclose the presence of secretory component (SC) in these serum samples. There was no correlation between the serum IgA and the S-IgA in the nasal washings.

DISCUSSION

The present results demonstrate a deficiency of S-IgA in the nasal washings of children with P.C.M. Some improvement was observed after prolonged treatment with 175 cal. and 4 g protein/kg/day. Because concentrations of IgG and albumin in the nasal washings were normal, the low level of S-IgA was selective and not due to either a general reduction of all proteins in the nasal secretions of the P.C.M. children or to unusual degradation of proteins by enzymes in the nasal fluids. The possibility of enhanced clearance of normally synthesized S-IgA in these children cannot yet be excluded, however. It seems unlikely that S-IgA was returning to the circulation because no component reactive with anti-SC was detected in the serum of these children as was detected in other conditions (23, 24).

The low S-IgA concentration in children with severe P.C.M. could relate to the clinical observations that malnourish children seem prone to develop mucosal infections (1-3, 14).

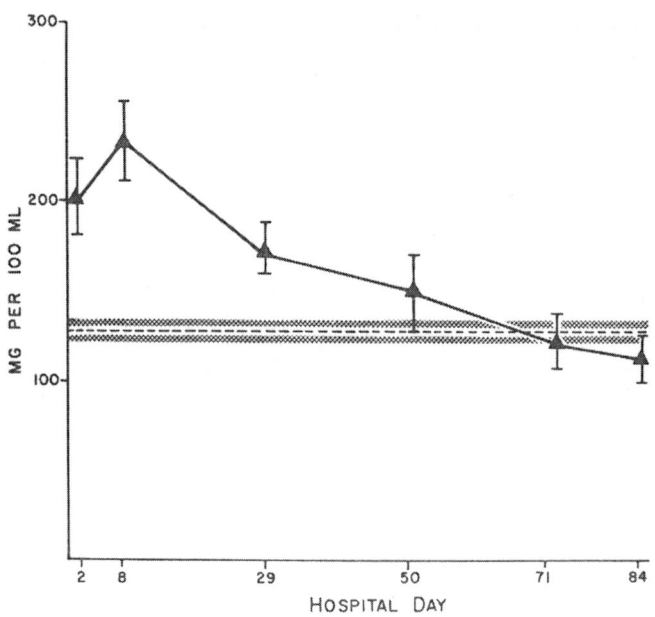

Figure 3.   Serum IgA concentrations (mean ± 1 S.E.M.) in
P.C.M. children.   Horizontal line and shaded area represent
mean ± 1 S.E.M. from normal children of the same age group
and from the same geographical area.   Differences from the
mean of the normal children at admission and on day 8 and 29
were statistically significant (p<0.05).

It has been suggested that S-IgA in the gastrointestinal tract
may be responsible for the localization of the enteric organisms
to the intestinal lumen (25) and thereby reducing the incidence
of gram-negative septicemia, a condition that is fairly common
in children with P.C.M. (2, 14).   These suggestions are also
consistent with the observations that well-nourished children
who had selective IgA defect from some other causes appeared to
have suffered more respiratory infection than normal (26) and
that resistance to respiratory virus infection correlated with
the presence of antibody of S-IgA class in respiratory tract
secretion (15).

SUMMARY

The local immune system of children suffering P.C.M. was
investigated by analyzing the level of immunoglobulins in the
nasal washing of these children on admission, and repeatedly
during the 84-day hospitalization period.   The mean concentration of IgA in nasal washings of P.C.M. children was significantly lower (p<0.01) than that of normal children from the

same geographical area. The defect in S-IgA was selective
because (i) the IgG and albumin concentrations of nasal
washing in the P.C.M. children were not different from those
of normal children and (ii) serum IgA was markedly elevated
at the time of admission and decreased to normal during
dietary treatment; S-IgA was not detected in any of the serum
samples. The low levels of S-IgA were only partially corrected
during prolonged treatment with 175 cal. and 4 g protein/kg/day
but appeared to return to normal within 1 to 2 years after
discharge. These findings could relate to the clinical
observations that malnourished children seem prone to develop
mucosal infections.

REFERENCES

1. Scrimshaw, N.S., Taylor, C.E. and Gordon, J.E., Am. J. Med
    Sci., 237:367, 1959.
2. Phillips, I. and Wharton, B., Brit. Med. J., 1:407, 1968.
3. Scrimshaw, N.S., Taylor, C.E. and Gordon, J.E., Monograph
    Ser. W.H.O. 57, 1968.
4. Edelman, R., Suskind, R., Olson, R.E. and Sirisinha, S.,
    Lancet 1:506, 1973.
5. Smythe, P.M., Schonland, M., Brereton-Stiles, G.G.,
    Coovadia, H.M., Grace, H.J., Loening, W.E.K., Mayfoyane,
    A., Parent, M.A. and Vos, G.H., Lancet 2:939, 1971.
6. Sirisinha, S., Suskind, R., Edelman, R., Charupatana, C.
    and Olson, R.E., Lancet, 1:1016, 1973.
7. Chandra, R.K., J. Pediat., 81:1194, 1972.
8. Suskind, R., Edelman, R., Sirisinha, S., Pariyanonda, A.
    and Olson, R.E. (manuscript in preparation).
9. Geefhuysen, J., Rosen, E.U., Katz, J., Ipp, I. and Metz,
    J., Brit. Med. J., 4:527, 1971.
10. Suskind, R., Sirisinha, S., Edelman, R. and Olson, R.E.
    (manuscript in preparation).
11. Alvarado, J. and Luthringer, D.G., Clin. Pediat. 10:174,
    1971.
12. Keet, M.P. and Thom, H., Archs. Dis. Childh., 44:600,1969.
13. Pretorius, P.J. and De Villias, L.S., Am. J. Clin. Nut.,
    10:279, 1971.
14. Hutt, M.R.S., J. Trop. Pediat., 15:153, 1969.
15. Bienenstock, J. and Perey, D.Y.E., Med. Clin. N. Am., 56:
    391, 1972.
16. Gomez, F., Galvan, R.R., Cravioto, J. and Frenk, S., Adv.
    Pediat., 7:131, 1955.
17. Lopez, M., Tsu, T. and Hyslop, N.E., Immunochemistry, 6:
    513, 1969.

18. Sirisinha, S. and Charupatana, C., Infec. Immun., 2:29, 1970.
19. Fahey, J.L. and McKelvey, E.M., J. Immunol., 94:84, 1965.
20. Kabat, E.A. and Mayer, M.M., Experimental Immunochemistry. 2nd Edi., Charles C. Thomas, Springfield, Ill., 1967.
21. Ouchterlony, O., Acta Path. Microbiol. Scand,, 25:186, 194
22. Grabar, P. and Burtin, P., L'analyse immunoelectrophoretiq Masson et Cie., Paris, 1960.
23. Thompson, R.A., Asquith, P. and Cooke, W.T., Lancet, 2: 517, 1969.
24. Waldman, R.H., Mach, J.P., Stella, M.M. and Rowe, D.S., J. Immunol., 105:43, 1970.
25. Stites, D.P., Levin, A.S., Lauer, B.A., Costom, B.H. and Fudenberg, H.H., Am. J. Med., 54:260, 1973.
26. Collins-Williams, C., Lamenza, C. and Kokubu, H., Can. Med Ass. J., 275:1145, 1966.

STUDIES OF SECRETORY ANTIBODIES TO E. COLI IN HUMAN URINE COMPARED TO THE SERUM ANTIBODY CONTENT

L.Å. Hanson, S. Ahlstedt, B. Carlsson, U. Jodal,
U. Lindberg and A. Sohl
Department of Immunology, Institute of Medical
Microbiology and Department of Pediatrics,
University of Göteborg, Sweden

INTRODUCTION

Antibodies in urine can either originate from serum or from local production in the urinary tract. In rabbits with experimental pyelonephritis a local response of IgG and occasionally of IgA antibodies has been detected (1). In experimental bladder infections in dogs a local antibody production has been seen (2).

In humans, antibodies in urine have mainly belonged to the IgG class (3-6), also when appearing as antibodies against E. coli bacteria causing urinary tract infection, UTI (5,6). In healthy individuals antibodies to E. coli of the secretory IgA type have been observed as well (7). Since increased levels of secretory IgA are found in the urine of patients with UTI (8-10), a search for secretory IgA antibodies against the infecting agent in such patients might provide information of diagnostic value. Furthermore, it might aid in the understanding of the pathogenesis of UTI (11).

Previous studies have usually employed techniques that require concentration of the urine samples to be analyzed. Such procedures confer a great risk of protein loss and denaturation (12,13). In the present work a sensitive enzyme-linked immunosorbent assay (14) has been employed which permits determination of antibodies of different immunoglobulin classes in unconcentrated urine samples. This technique has been useful in recent studies of the occurrence and synthesis of colostral antibodies to E. coli (15).

MATERIALS AND METHODS

The patient material consists of 35 infants and children with significant bacteriuria ($>10^5$ bacteria/ml). Of these 27, 7-16 years old, had "asymptomatic" infections without signs of renal involvement such as lowered renal concentrating capacity or increased levels of agglutinating serum antibodies against the infecting agent (16). Among the 8 remaining patients were five girls, 4/12, 4, 6 and 9 years of age, with acute attacks of symptomatic pyelonephritis (16). They had lowered concentrating capacity and increased serum antibody levels to the infecting E. coli strain. Three boys, 1, 2 and 5 months of age, with acute pyelonephritis were included as well. In agreement with earlier findings the youngest infants did not show the striking serum antibody response seen in older children with attacks of acute pyelonephritis (17). All the patients had normal BUN, no proteinuria (Albustix) and no signs of urinary tract abnormalities on intravenous pyelography or micturating cystourethrography. Morning urine specimens were collected from all the patients and from 16 control children, 2-16 years old, without bacteriuria or history of urinary tract disease. Serum samples were obtained from all the patients, the 16 controls, and from 10 healthy blood donors. All samples were immediately frozen at $-20^{\circ}C$ without addition of preservative. Before analysis the urine portions were centrifuged at 2000 x g for 10 minutes.

Antibodies were recorded by the enzyme-linked immunosorbent assay (ELISA) as described by Engvall and Perlmann (14). Antisera specific for IgG, IgM, IgA and secretory component, SC, (Dacopats AS, Copenhagen, Denmark) tested as described elsewhere (17) were conjugated with alkaline phosphatase (Sigma Chemical Co., St. Louis, USA) with a specific activity of 320-380 IU/mg. This was made according to Engvall and Perlmann (14) except that immunosorbent-purified anti-antibodies were not used. A serum with a high content of IgG, IgM and IgA antibodies against a pool of eight O antigens representing common E. coli serotypes (18) was included in each run, and titres of tested samples were expressed in relation to this. As standard for the determinations with the anti-SC serum, a pool of human milk containing secretory IgA antibodies to E. coli was employed (15).

The highest enzyme activity of any dilution of the samples
was expressed in percent of the enzyme activity of the same
dilution of the standard serum. All determinations were
made in duplicate. The accuracy of the titre determinations
was within ± 10% ($p < 0.05$) according to previous results (17).

Somatic 0 antigens were prepared from the E. coli
strains isolated from the patient's urine (16). For the
standard serum and the sera and urines from the healthy
controls a pool of the eight most common 0 antigens was
used (18). Twelve of the patients with asymptomatic bacteriuria were also investigated for antibodies against the cap-
sular E. coli antigen K1 which is common among strains causing UTI (19).

Human colostrum was fractionated on Agarose Biogel A-5m
(Bio-Rad. Lab., Richmond, USA) as previously described (20)
for purification of secretory IgA antibodies. The secretory
IgA-fraction was used to examine the relationship between
the results obtained with the anti-IgA- and the anti-SC-
enzyme conjugates. For selective immunoadsorption anti-IgA
was attached to cyano-activated Sepharose (AB Pharmacia,
Uppsala, Sweden).

RESULTS

The Application of ELISA for Analysis of Secretory IgA
Antibodies

The sensitivity of ELISA was illustrated by detection
of antibodies against E. coli 0 antigen in sera from healthy
blood donors diluted $1/10^5$ using the anti-IgA-enzyme conjugate. The same antiserum showed IgA antibodies in the
standard milk pool diluted $1/10^4$. In unconcentrated urines
of some UTI patients IgA antibodies could be found in dilutions 1/1 - 1/10. No measurable anti-0 activity was obtained in serum with the anti-SC-enzyme conjugate. Only in
undiluted urines from some UTI patients did this anti-SC
detect E. coli antibodies.

Control experiments were performed to investigate how
the two different antiserum conjugates, detecting SC and IgA
respectively, recorded secretory IgA antibodies. This was
made by parallel analyses of colostral secretory IgA antibodies against E. coli purified by gel filtration through
Agarose A-5m. Analyzing this secretory IgA fraction the

enzyme activity with the anti-SC conjugate was 20 percent of
that obtained with the anti-IgA conjugate. The lower values
obtained for the same antibody sample with the weaker anti-SC
conjugate were further accentuated when related to the standard since the serum standard gave a value which was only
73 percent of what the anti-IgA gave with the milk standard.

The anti-SC and anti-IgA conjugates were compared after
the secretory IgA fraction had been treated with an anti-IgA
immunosorbent. A good correlation was obtained since the
reading with the anti-IgA conjugate decreased by a mean of
66 percent and with anti-SC by 68 percent after the absorption.

Antibody Determinations in Serum and Urine of Normals and
                    Patients with UTI

Unconcentrated urines from normals did not contain any
antibodies of the IgA class detectable with the ELISA, but
6/16 had trace amounts of IgG antibodies (Fig. 1). In serum
from healthy individuals IgG as well as IgM and IgA antibodies
were found in agreement with previous results obtained by the
indirect hemagglutination technique (18).

In the five older patients with pyelonephritis, increased
levels of serum IgM, IgG and IgA antibodies were found. In
their urines antibodies were detected with anti-IgG, IgA
and SC (Fig. 1 and patient I in Fig. 2A). The youngest infants, 1 and 2 months of age, showed no increase of serum
antibodies and only insignificant amounts of IgG antibodies
in urine (Fig. 1 and patient II in Fig. 2A).

Among the patients with asymptomatic bacteriuria, two
major groups could be discerned. One group had IgG but no
IgA antibodies in serum. Of these 17 patients 14 had IgA
antibodies in urine (Fig. 1 and patient II in Fig. 2B). In
the other group of 10 children rather low levels of serum antibodies to E. coli were found of the IgG and IgA types. All of
these had IgG antibodies in urine, and 7 of them also had IgA
antibodies against E. coli O antigen (patient I in Fig. 2B).

The weaker anti-SC conjugate gave lower values than the
anti-IgA, but a good correlation was seen between the results
of the two antibody conjugates with the urines using the
Spearman rank correlation test ($r = 0.61$; $p < 0.01$) as illustrated (Fig. 3A). In contrast no relationship was seen
between the levels of serum and urine IgA antibodies against

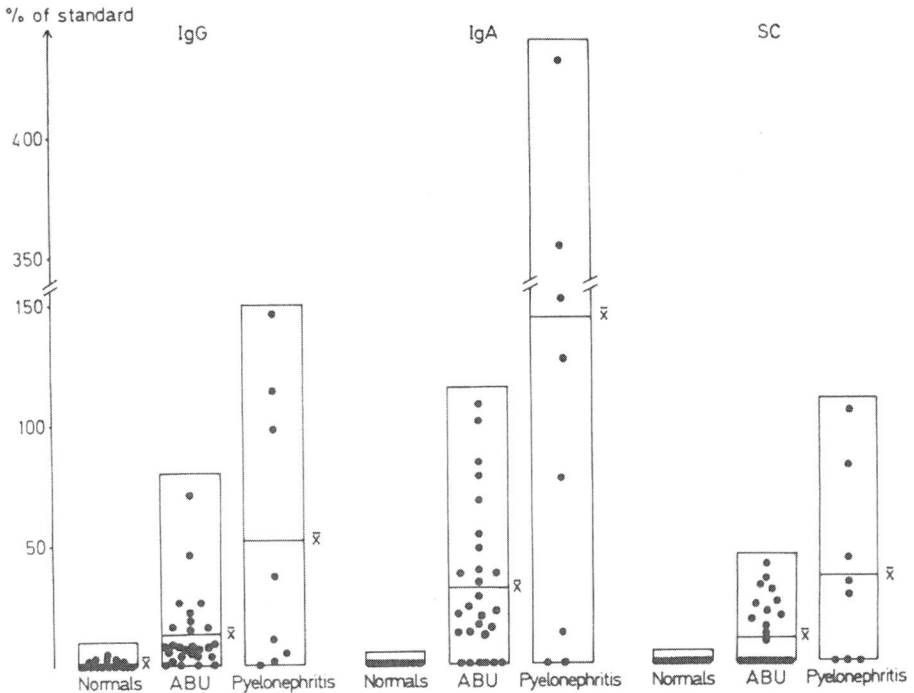

Fig. 1. Levels of antibodies to E. coli 0 antigen in urine samples from healthy individuals and from patients with asymptomatic bacteriuria (ABU) or acute pyelonephritis as determined with ELISA. The levels obtained with the anti-IgG and anti-IgA conjugates are related to a serum standard, those obtained with the anti-SC conjugate to a milk standard.

E. coli 0 antigen (r = -0.05; not significant) as shown in Fig. 3B.

IgM antibodies were not found in urine from any normal or UTI patient. The anti-SC conjugate indicated the presence of E. coli antibodies in 12 of the 21 patients with asymptomatic bacteriuria who had IgA antibodies in urine (Fig. 1).

Serum and urine from 11 patients were also analyzed for the presence of antibodies to the E. coli Kl antigen. The results correlated well with those obtained with the 0 antigens using the anti-IgG as well as the anti-IgA and anti-SC conjugates when tested by the Spearman rank correlation test (r = 0.91 - 1.00; p< 0.001) for the 0 and K antibodies of

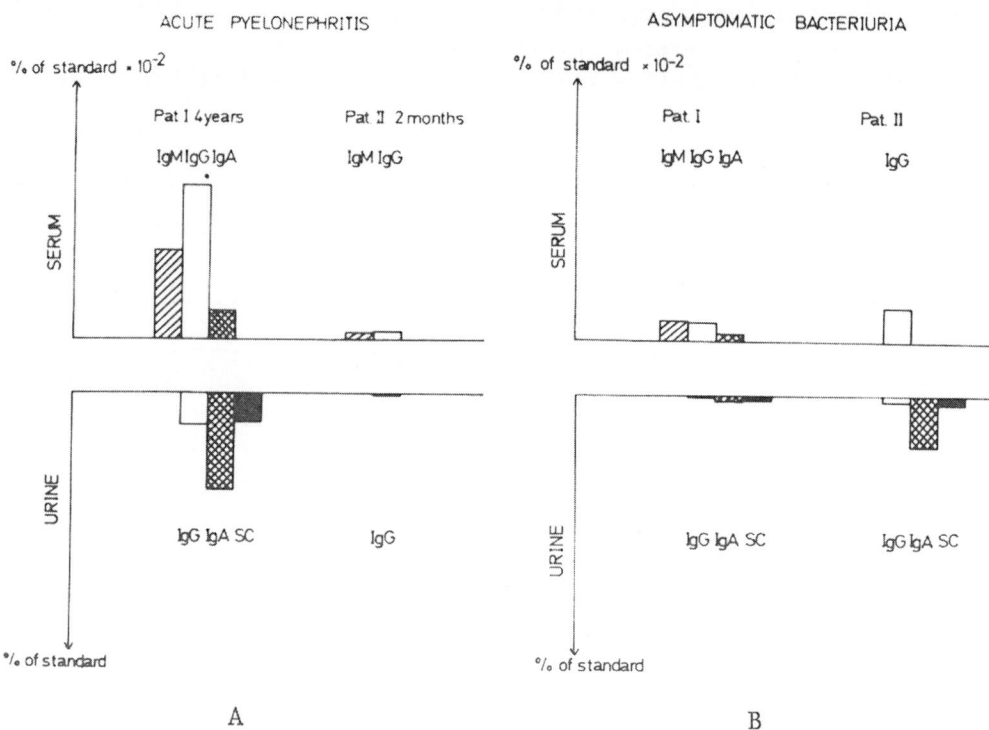

Fig. 2.   (A) Serum and urine antibodies to the 0 antigen of
the infecting E. coli strain in two patients with acute pyelonephritis as determined with ELISA.   (B) Similar represen-
tation as in (A) of two children with ABU.   Patient II has
urine IgA antibodies but no detectable serum IgA antibodies.

DISCUSSION

The enzyme-linked immunosorbent assay (ELISA) was
employed in the present work on antibodies against E. coli
in urine and serum, since it permits determination of antibodies of different immunoglobulin classes in samples of
various origins such as serum, urine and milk (15).   Its
sensitivity made it possible to detect IgA antibodies to
E. coli in unconcentrated urine from infants and children
with UTI but not in normals.   Procedures to concentrate the
urine have previously been found often to denature and cause
protein loss (12,13) which thus can be avoided.   Antibody
detection in urine might also provide a possibility for
immunological diagnosis of UTI without blood sampling.

Previous studies of UTI have shown a serum antibody
response in patients with pyelonephritis, but not with

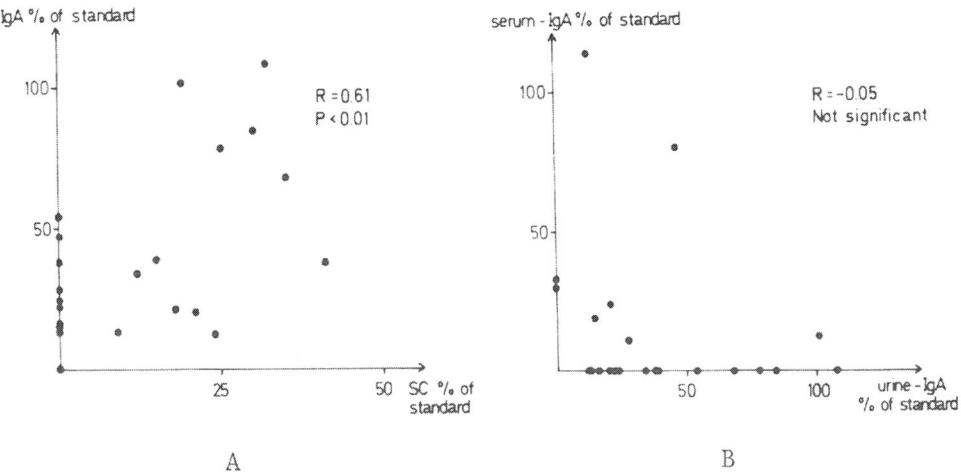

Fig. 3. (A) The scattergram shows the correlation between the urine antibodies to E. coli O antigen determined with the anti-IgA conjugate and the anti-SC conjugate (r = 0.61; p<0.01). (B) The scattergram shows the lack of correlation (r = -0.05; not significant) between the levels of IgA antibodies to E. coli O antigen in serum and urine of patients with asymptomatic bacteriuria.

cystitis (16,18). The present work shows that patients with acute pyelonephritis and with asymptomatic bacteriuria without signs of renal involvement have antibodies in the urine against the infecting agent. Further studies may show if their detection can be of diagnostic use in UTI and if their presence can influence the appearance and course of the infections (11). Such an effect might be expected from the recent observations of a protective capacity in experimental infections of serum antibodies to E. coli O and K antigens (21,22). Secretory IgA antibodies from colostrum against E. coli were also found protective in an experimental model (15).

The fact that urinary IgA antibodies against the infecting E. coli bacteria could be found in the absence of serum IgA antibodies supports the assumption that these antibodies are synthesized in the urinary tract. This is further supported by the finding that many of the patients with urinary IgA antibodies had such antibodies detectable with anti-SC as well. According to control experiments, the anti-IgA and anti-SC conjugates employed reacted in a similar fashion with secretory IgA antibodies although the anti-SC was much weaker and gave lower values. This may explain why some of the samples with urinary IgA antibodies did not react with anti-SC. Another possibility is that these urines contained more 7S IgA, since this has occasionally been observed in an earlier study of urines from UTI patients (6).

An alternative explanation for the occurrence of IgA-antibodies in the urine in the lack of detectable serum IgA antibodies could be a selective renal filtration of serum IgA antibodies. In such a case they should not be expected to carry SC determinants since neonates who after exchange transfusion have serum IgA in urine do not combine it with their free urinary SC to a complete secretory IgA molecule (23). Furthermore, there was no relationship between the serum and urine IgA antibody values of the UTI patients, but between the urine antibody values obtained with the anti-IgA and anti-SC conjugates.

Continued studies are needed to evaluate the implications of this suggested local secretory IgA antibody response in humans with urinary tract infections.

SUMMARY

A sensitive and discriminative enzyme-linked immunosorbent assay (ELISA) was employed to analyze antibodies of different immunoglobulin classes to E. coli O and K antigens in serum and unconcentrated urine of normals and of infants and children with urinary tract infections.

No IgA antibodies and only occasionally very low levels of IgG antibodies were found in urine of normals. In patients with pyelonephritis high levels of serum and urine antibodies were seen. In patients with asymptomatic bacteriuria without signs of renal involvement SC-containing IgA antibodies to E. coli were often found in the urine in the absence of detectable serum IgA antibodies suggesting a local antibody response of secretory IgA antibodies.

Acknowledgments: The skillful technical assistance of Mrs. B. Andersson was appreciated. The work was supported by grants from the Medical Faculty, University of Göteborg and the Swedish Medical Research Council (Grant No. 19X-215).

REFERENCES

1. Lehmann, J.D., Smith, J.W., Miller, T.E., Barnett, J.A. and Sanford, J.P., J. Clin. Invest. 47:2541, 1968.
2. Uehling, D.T., Barnhart, D.D. and Seastone, C.V., Invest. Urol. 6:211, 1968.
3. Hanson, L.Å. and Tan, E.M., J. Clin. Invest. 44:703, 1965.
4. Turner, M.W. and Rowe, D.S., Immunology 12:689, 1967.
5. Vosti, K.L. and Remington, J.S., J. Lab. Clin. Med. 72:71, 1968.
6. Hanson, L.Å., Holmgren, J., Jodal, U., Kaijser, B., Lönnroth, I and Wadsworth, C., in The Secretory Immunologic System, Edited by D.H. Dayton, Jr., P.A. Small, Jr., R.M. Chanock, H.E. Kaufman and T.B. Tomasi, Jr., U.S. Government Printing Office, Washington, D.C., 1971, p. 367.
7. Tourville, D., Bienenstock, J. and Tomasi, T.B., Jr., Proc. Soc. Exp. Biol. Med. 128:722, 1968.
8. Burdon, D.W., Clin. exp. Immunol. 6:189, 1970.
9. Kaufman, D.B., Katz, R. and McIntosh, R.M., Brit. Med. J. 4:463, 1970.
10. Uehling, D.T. and Stiehm, R.E., Pediatrics 47:40, 1971.
11. Hanson, L.Å., J. Infect. Dis. 127:726, 1973.
12. Migasato, F. and Pollak, V.E., J. Clin. Lab. Med. 67: 1036, 1966.
13. Peterson, P.A., Ervin, P.-E. and Berggård, I., J. Clin. Invest. 48:1189, 1969.
14. Engvall, E. and Perlmann, P., J. Immunol. 109:129, 1972.
15. Hanson, L.Å., Carlsson, B., Ahlstedt, S., Svanborg, C. and Kaijser, B., in Milk and Lactation, Second International Congress of the International Organisation for the Study of Human Development, 1973 (in press).
16. Winberg, J., Andersen, H.J., Hanson L.Å. and Lincoln, K. Brit. Med. J. II:524, 1963.
17. Ahlstedt, S., Holmgren, J. and Hanson, L.Å., Immunology (in press).
18. Hanson, L.Å., Winberg, J., Andersen, H.J., Holmgren, J., Jodal, U. and Kaijser, B., in Renal Infection and Renal Scarring, Edited by P. Kincaid-Smith and K.F. Fairley, Mercedes Publ. Co., Melbourne, 1971, p. 117.
19. Kaijser, B., Jodal, U. and Hanson, L.Å., Int. Arch. Allergy 44:260, 1973.
20. Holmgren, J., Svennerholm, A.-M. and Ouchterlong, Ö, Acta Path. Microbiol. Scand. Sect. B 80:489, 1972.

21. Kaijser, B., Holmgren, J. and Hanson, L.Å., Scand. J.
     Immunol. 1:27, 1972.
22. Kaijser, B. and Olling, S., J. Infect. Dis. 128:41,
     1973.
23. Hanson, L.Å., Motas, C., Barrett, J., Wadsworth, C.
     and Jodal, U., in Proceedings of the Second International
     Symposium on Immunology of Reproduction, Bulgarian
     Academy of Science Press, Sofia, 1973, p. 687.

SECRETORY IgA: AN ADOLESCENT COMING OF AGE

Richard Hong

Department of Pediatrics and Medical
Microbiology, University of Wisconsin,
Center for Health Sciences, Madison,
Wisconsin 53706

INTRODUCTION

The various immunoglobulin classes of man differ not
only in their primary structure but quite radically in their
biological roles. As a group, all immunoglobulins possess
the capability of responding to specific antigens in one of
several ways. There may be a physical combination with the
antigen or the synthesis of the immunoglobulin may be stimulated or even suppressed by these same antigens. Individual
Ig classes, however, react quite differently after the antigenic combination. Some are especially efficient in activating the complement system, some are potent opsonizers, others
initiate histamine release, some block cytophilic antibodies,
some enhance tumor growth and some initiate cytotoxic reactions. Exactly how each Ig class fits into the human protective scheme evolved by Nature is still not fully understood. IgA has been known as an immunoglobulin for nearly
15 years (1) and thus is in its stormy adolescence. This
may explain why dealing with IgA in the clinical setting is
so capricious.

There can be little question that IgA is a major system
of immunoglobulin defense having its primary area of activity
along the lining of the secretory surfaces (2). Although
there is good response to direct stimulation and better correlation of susceptibility to infection with secretory IgA
antibody levels than with serum titres, the true importance
of this mechanism pales in the light of known cases of

selective IgA deficiency who enjoy normal health (3). If
other defense mechanisms, immune or otherwise, can easily
compensate for the IgA system, what has been the selective
evolutionary pressure for its persistence? On the other
hand, the asymptomatic cases of selective IgA deficiency
should not a priori lead us to a generalization of the
clinical insignificance of that state. Recently Spitler
et al. (4) described a woman with at least 14 years of
hypogammaglobulinemia and no evidence of normal cell-mediated
immunity. Yet, she had no diarrhea nor any unusual susceptibility to infections. Surely we cannot discard the role
of the immune system in the hundreds of patients described
in the past 19 years with symptomatic B and T cell deficiencies on the basis of this kind of negative corroboration.
Nevertheless, the biological role of IgA needs much clarification. At this juncture, a number of questions seem most
provocative to me: 1) What is the clinical consequence of
loss of IgA protection? 2) What is the significance of selective elevation of IgA? 3) What is the significance of the
"scavenger" role of IgA? 4) Is IgA deficiency a sign of a
subtle thymic defect?

CLINICAL CONSEQUENCES OF LOSS OF IgA

Although IgA is an antibody and antibody deficiency is
usually manifested by excess numbers of infections, it seems
quite clear that absence of IgA does not uniformly result
in excessive respiratory or gastrointestinal infections.
The usual explanation is that appropriate compensation prevents undue infection. Certainly, the interstitial tissues
seem to be appropriately replaced by IgM, and in some cases,
IgG containing cells under the conditions of gamma A deficiency (5,6). In view of the proposed switch mechanism and
recent experiments showing a prior state of IgM dominance
in ontogeny (7,8), one might ask whether the accumulation
of IgM containing cells represents a failure of the switch-
over rather than compensation. We might further ask whether
the IgM is as competent in the local area as is IgA. The
evidence that some of the IgM found in the secretions under
these conditions is 7S IgM (9) might lead one to postulate
that the antibody produced might be qualitatively different
from the usual 19S protein.

It seems quite clear now that materials other than
infectious agents are controlled in their access to the systemic immune system by virtue of the local antibody system.

This has been well documented in man by the work of Rothberg (10) and in animals by Walker et al. (11). We have suggested that the consequence of uncontrolled access leads to auto-immunity (12).

The association of the gluten sensitive sprue syndrome with selective IgA deficiency may or may not be one of chance. Further insight into this matter can be gained from ascertainment for the presence of HL-A8 which exhibits such a marked preponderance in gluten sensitivity occurring in IgA normal individuals (80% cf 20%). In two cases that have been studied by Dr. Warren Strober, one was found to have HL-A8 while the other did not. Thus, we must await further data to see what sort of pattern emerges. Finally, the possibility that IgA deficiency may predispose to malignancy in those areas protected by the secretory Ig system must be entertained. Five cases have so far been reported (13).

ELEVATION OF IgA

Although elevations of immunoglobulin are usually asso-ciated with chronic inflammatory reactions, some of the most impressive elevations of IgA are seen in an immunodeficiency disorder, Wiskott-Aldrich syndrome. Although the defect in this disorder has been thought to be an antigen processing defect (14), the gradual loss of T and B cell function is poorly explained. As the disease reaches its full intensity, a characteristic pattern of low IgM and extremely high IgA develops. Extensive study of the functional capability of this elevated fraction has not been carried out, although it appears not to be monoclonal. In another immunodeficiency state, ataxia-telangiectasia, deficiency of IgA is usually the case but extreme elevations have been reported. Appro-priate investigation of these states may give us some in-sight into the normal responsivity of the IgA system or even perhaps into the mechanism of immunoglobulin synthesis and secretions in general. Elevation of IgA may herald a silent cirrhosis (15). In anaphylactoid purpura elevated levels have been recorded, and in some instances immunofluorescent studies reveal prominence of IgA in the kidney (16,17). What specifically "turns on" IgA?

SCAVENGER ACTIVITY

A "scavenger" role of IgA was first described by Heremans and was noted for albumin and haptoglobin (18).

Subsequent to that time, however, many interactions with various other proteins have been described. The interactions can be covalent in nature involving disulfide interchange (19), but this is not a firm requirement for the union to occur. Generally speaking, this phenomenon does not result in interference with normal biologic activity, although in one case a coagulation abnormality was reported after union of an IgA myeloma with antihemophiliac globulin (20). Recently, in collaboration with Dr. Theodore Goodfriend, we have found binding of angiotensin to IgA in approximately 5% of hospital patients. We are at present investigating the possibility that IgA may bind angiotensin receptors. A recent demonstration that complement was activated in the cold by an IgA-containing fraction in a patient with focal glomerulonephritis is also extremely provocative (21). We wonder whether the IgA in that situation may have been complexed with some substance which was able to activate the complement system resulting in persistent disease and attack upon the kidney. What could be the biologic advantage of such phenomena?

THYMUS DEFICIENCY

Although major development of the immunoglobulin system can occur with minimal thymic influence, recent studies suggest that the IgA system may be more thymic dependent confirming experimental data obtained previously. Thymectomized mice, rats and rabbits and the congenitally athymic ("nude") mice are selectively deficient for IgA (22,23,24,25,26). In humans diminished T cell function shown by deficient lymphocyte response to phytohemagglutinin (27) and decreased sheep red blood cell rosette formation (28) have been observed in IgA deficiency. We have observed two patients with selective IgA deficiency with extremely high IgE elevation. In view of Okumura and Tada's (29) observation of T cell suppression of IgE production, uncontrolled IgE production may further suggest a thymic defect. We have also observed occasional patients with absent IgA who have virtually uncontrolled asthma. Is it possible that excessive IgE production secondary to a thymic fault in association with selective IgA deficiency could be expressed clinically as unusually severe allergy?

The above observations bring forth but a few of the fascinating questions which are still unexplained. Antibody roles in body processes ought to be straightforward, but

they are not. There has been a great leap forward in
elucidation of immunoglobulin structure. Hopefully, the
next few years will be followed by equal advancement of our
knowledge in the mechanistic aspects of immunoglobulin
activities and their functional roles in human biology.
Like an adolescent, IgA at this moment seems impossible to
understand but fascinating to study.

(Some of the work cited was supported by grants from
USPHS, AM-15086 and HD-07778).

REFERENCES

1. Heremans, J.F., Heremans, M.T. and Schultze, H.E.,
    Protides Biol. Fluids 6:166, 1958.
2. Tomasi, T.B., Jr. and Bienenstock, J., Adv. Immunol.
    9:1, 1968.
3. Rockey, J.H., Hanson, L.A., Heremans, J.F. and Kunkel,
    H.G., J. Lab. Clin. Med. 63:205, 1964.
4. Spitler, L.E., Levin, A.S. and Fudenberg, H.H., Amer.
    J. Med. 54:371, 1973.
5. Crabbe, P.A. and Heremans, J.F., Gut 7:119, 1966.
6. Brandtzaeg, P., Fjellanger, I. and Gjeruldsen, S.T.,
    Science 160:789, 1968.
7. Kincade, P.W. and Cooper, M.D., Science 179:398, 1973.
8. Allen, W.D. and Porter, P., Immunology 24:493, 1973.
9. Stobo, J.D. and Tomasi, T.B., Jr., J. Clin. Invest.
    46:1329, 1967.
10. Rothberg, R.M., J. Pediat. 75:391, 1969.
11. Walker, W.A., Isselbacher, K.J. and Bloch, K.J., Science
    177:608, 1972.
12. Ammann, A.J. and Hong, R., Clin. Exp. Immun. 7:833,
    1970.
13. Ammann, A.J. and Hong, R., in Immunologic Disorders in
    Infants and Children, Edited by E.R. Stiehm and V.
    Fulginiti, W.B. Saunders Co., 1973.
14. Cooper, M.D., Chase, H.P., Lowman, J.T., Krivit, W.
    and Good, R.A., Amer. J. Med. 44:499, 1968.
15. Tomasi, T.B., Jr. and Tisdale, W.A., Nature (London)
    201:834, 1964.
16. Trygstad, C.W. and Stiehm, E.R., Pediatrics 47:1023,
    1971.
17. Berger, J., Transplant. Proc. 1:939, 1969.
18. Heremans, J.F., Les globulines seriques du systeme
    gamma. Leur nature et leur pathologie, Arscia, Brussels,
    and Masson, Paris, 1960.

19. Mannik, M., J. Immun. $\underline{99}$:899, 1967.
20. Glueck, H.I. and Hong, R., J. Clin. Invest. $\underline{44}$:1866, 1965.
21. Day, N.K., Geiger, H., McLean, R., Resnick, J., Michael, A. and Good, R.A., J. Clin. Invest. $\underline{52}$:1698, 1973.
22. Arnason, B.G., St. Cyr Cole, V. and Relyveld, R.H., Int. Arch. Allergy $\underline{25}$:206, 1964.
23. Grundmann, E. and Hobik, H.P., in Germinal Centers in Immune Responses, Edited by H. Cottier, N. Odartchenko, R. Schindler and C.C. Congdon, Springer-Verlag, 1967.
24. Perey, D.Y.E., Frommel, D., Hong, R. and Good, R.A., Lab. Invest. $\underline{22}$:212, 1970.
25. Clough, J.D., Mims, L.H. and Strober, W., J. Immun. $\underline{106}$:1624, 1971.
26. Good, R.A. and Wortis, H.H., in Progress in Immunology, Edited by B. Amos, Academic Press, Inc., 1971.
27. Lawton, A.R., Royal, S.A., Self, S. and Cooper, M.D., J. Lab. Clin. Med. $\underline{80}$:26, 1972.
28. Horowitz, S. and Hong, R., Proceedings of the Second International Workshop on Primary Immunodeficiency Diseases in Man, St. Petersburg, Florida, February, 1973.
29. Okumura, K. and Tada, T., J. Immun. $\underline{107}$:1682, 1971.

DISCUSSION

Dr. Cooper - We will start with a general discussion of the first papers that have been given this afternoon. The first person I would like to call on is Dr. Tom Waldmann, who has some remarks relevant to IgA deficiency.

Dr. Thomas Waldmann - My comments are related to Dr. Lawton's presentation. We also have been very interested in defining the nature of defects leading to IgA deficiency in man and in the study of mechanisms of promoting synthesis and secretion of IgA by lymphoid cells from such patients. I would like to emphasize first that using techniques similar to those discussed by Dr. Lawton, we have also found that most patients with isolated IgA deficiency have normal numbers of IgA bearing cells. We support his view that these patients have a basic defect in the terminal differentiation of these cells. However, in the few moments that I have, I would like to focus first on results derived from a different technique for quantitating lymphocyte IgA biosynthesis, and second to discuss rare patients who have deficiency patterns other than those which have already been discussed, and that provide interesting insights in addition to those that have been presented.

We have cultured peripheral blood lymphocytes from patients and controls in media free of human serum proteins, and have quantitated immunoglobulin synthesized and released into the media using double antibody radioimmunoassay procedures. In these studies we have washed sedimented human leukocytes 12 times and cultured them for a period of 7 days at 2×10^6 lymphocytes per culture vial, in the presence of fetal calf serum or human serum deficient in IgA, and in the presence or absence of pokeweed mitogen. The synthesis and release of each class of the immunoglobulin was then quantitated by determining amounts of IgA, IgG, and IgM in the supernatant fluids of these cultures with a double antibody radioimmunoassay procedure sensitive to high picogram quantities of these proteins. This technique has the disadvantage that the cells must be cultured in fetal calf serum or media free of human IgA but has significant advantages. First, it is a quantitative technique. Second, it does not have the

major problem plaguing the Hochwald radioimmunoelectrophoresis technique, i.e. it does not have false positive values
due to nonspecific co-precipitation of radioactivity. Cells
from normal individuals synthesize 300 nanograms of IgA/2 x
10^6 lymphocytes in the 7-day culture period in the absence
of pokeweed mitogen and about 2300 nanograms of IgA when
pokeweed mitogen is added.

The patients with IgA deficiency show a number of patterns when all techniques are utilized. The first pattern
is exemplified by one patient with no serum IgA and an
exceedingly high titer of anti-IgA antibodies. This patient
had no demonstrable circulating IgA bearing cells; he made
no IgA in the cytoplasm in response to pokeweed mitogen as
assessed by cytoplasmic immunofluorescence and released no
IgA into the media as assessed by radioimmunoassay. Normal
cells cultured in his serum and fetal calf serum in the
presence of pokeweed mitogen also did not demonstrate cytoplasmic IgA nor did they secrete IgA into the media. This
patient is the only one that we have studied who lacks IgA
bearing cells. We feel that he has a circulating factor
inhibiting maturation of IgA bearing B cells into cells
synthesizing and releasing IgA. This factor may or may not
be related to his anti-IgA antibodies.

The second pattern is exemplified by a child with
extreme thymic deficiency and marked reduction in serum IgA
levels. The cells of this patient made very low quantities
of IgA, i.e. 40 nanograms/2 x 10^6 lymphocytes, when stimulated with pokeweed mitogen alone. However, in the presence
of T cells from a patient with the Sezary syndrome or derived
from normal individuals by the use of T cell rosette technique, the patient's lymphocytes synthesized 10,000 nanograms
of IgA per 2 x 10^6 cells, an approximately 500-fold increase.
This isolated observation supports the concept that Dr.
Lawton and others have proposed, that T cells cooperate with
B cells to promote their maturation to a state where they
produce and release large quantities of IgA. I would like
to conclude with a discussion of the third pattern of results, that observed in the majority of patients with isolated IgA deficiency or with ataxia telangiectasia and IgA
deficiency. We would agree with Dr. Lawton and co-workers
that these patients have normal numbers of IgA bearing B cells
and that they have normal numbers of cells that stain for IgA
in their cytoplasm following 7-day cultures in the presence
of pokeweed mitogen. However, using the radioimmunoassay
procedure of the culture supernatants, we found that their
cells either did not produce and secrete any IgA into the

media in the presence of pokeweed mitogen, or had a very
reduced response. Thus we feel that at least in the culture
conditions we utilized, none of the groups of patients we
studied with isolated IgA deficiency could be stimulated by
pokeweed mitogen to undergo complete maturation of IgA
bearing B cells into cells that synthesize and secrete
significant quantities of IgA.

Dr. Cooper - We have spent quite a bit of time discussing
these differences with Dr. Waldmann, and feel that we have
to do more experiments and sharing of materials in order to
find out just what is the basis for the discrepancy. We
could not come to any logical conclusion as to exactly what
it might be, but perhaps you can see the data and decide for
yourself or make suggestions as to how the conflict might be
resolved.

Dr. Fudenberg - I have questions directed to each of the
speakers, and I will take each one in turn. First, Dr.
Seligmann, you said you had 59 patients with alpha chain
disease; your slide showed data on 57 who had the abdominal
form. I assume, then, that the two others had pulmonary
alpha chain disease.

Dr. Seligmann - I said, the two with respiratory forms were
included in the table; hence 57 is an error of my secretary.
It should read 59.

Dr. Fudenberg - Second question, Maxime. Do you know whether
the ratio of all alpha 1 is the same in these pulmonary alpha
chain proteins as it is in normal population?

Dr. Seligmann - Proteins from all patients were of the alpha
1 subclass. I have never seen a single case of alpha 2 chain
disease.

Dr. Fudenberg - What I really wanted to make sure of in my own
mind was whether pulmonary alpha chain proteins were also
alpha 1.

Dr. Seligmann - One of the pulmonary cases I have looked at
was Dr. Ballieux's and it was alpha 1. The other is from
Fred Rosen - I did not study it, but he told me it was also
alpha 1.

Dr. Fudenberg - Thirdly, with regard to your geographic
medicine slide listing the various places where these people
came from, I would be more interested in their ethnic origin
rather than where they reside. I know, for example, that
one patient was from Colombia - was it a part of Colombia
which was settled by Spanish Jews in about 1600? I wonder
if you have ethnic data as well as geographic? Was the
Boston patient of Jewish descent?

Dr. Seligmann - I have been interested also in this, especially because of the cases that were described originally
by the Israeli authors. They did not include immunoglobulin
studies but we guess many were alpha chain disease cases.
They stated very strongly that this disease occurred only in
Arabs and in Sephardic Jews, but not in Ashkenazic Jews
inside Israel. For this reason, at the beginning of our
studies, we looked for a possible genetic factor and for the
ethnic origin of these patients. But now it appears, from
reports from many countries as well as from our data, that
the ethnic origin of the patients is extremely diverse, and
we are unable to define anything precise in terms of ethnic
origin.

Dr. Good - Several questions and a couple of comments. First
of all, with respect to Dr. Seligmann's presentation, one has
to be deeply impressed with the gastrointestinal manifestations of this disease in which it appears that light chains
are not produced. On a recent visit to Switzerland Barandun
and his associates presented some very interesting data to
me on an extraordinary gastrointestinal syndrome associated
with inability to form one or the other light chain class.
These patients had normal amounts of immunoglobulin, but were
lacking in ability to produce the lambda chain or the kappa
chain. Here again, selective clinical disease associated
with the gastrointestinal tract and essentially intractable
diarrhea occurred. These patients differed, of course, very
sharply from the patients with alpha chain disease in that
the circulating lymphocytes, the B lymphocytes, had normal
distribution of kappa and lambda chain. It was just the
plasma cells of the marrow and gut that were lacking either
kappa or lambda chains. This is, I think, a striking Experiment of Nature that may have something to do either with
the selectivity in the process of terminal differentiation
or with a separate origin of the secretory cells from the
circulating B lymphocytes.

The nutritional work presented here this morning is, I think, extremely important. It is, however, very, very difficult to interpret what is happening with nutritional deprivation in the field. Under field conditions we have observed in patients with severe protein calorie malnutrition, complex vitamin deficiencies and complex influences of extraordinary infections, everything ranging from agammaglobulinemia to extreme hypergammaglobulinemia. We have also seen selective depression of cellular immunity and even selective increase of cellular immunity. The immunological state of the malnourished child also depends on the age at which the onset of the nutritional deprivation occurs. Thus we felt that it is not only difficult but perhaps just impossible to sort out the variables from field study. In sorting things out in the laboratory, a fairly clean picture seems to emerge, i.e. where nutritional deprivation is acute, where there is a stressful situation, very marked deficits of T cells and T cell immunity function can be demonstrated. When one encounters chronic protein deprivation of a low grade nature where there is no evidence of acute stress, in laboratory studies one may find evidence of inability to form antibodies. This need not be associated with depression of the immunoglobulin levels. Balancing factors in immunoglobulin catabolism may be playing a role here. Under these same conditions cellular immunity may remain quite intact. With extreme chronic deprivations of protein or even specific amino acids, both antibody and cell-mediated immunity may be deficient. I think that the infections and the variety of intoxications one encounters in the field can have influences that make field observations of nutritional influence very difficult to interpret. I think it is fair to point out that in the material where a deficit of secretory IgA was demonstrated, this was a relatively moderate or mild quantitative deficiency that had reached a level of statistical significance. A deficiency of albumin and total protein was also observed in those secretions. I would, from long experience with this kind of investigation, want to see studies that have included analysis of response to antigeneic stimulation and see some experimental studies designed to address this clinical contention. As another example, we have made sharply different observations in the laboratory on the complement system than appears from these field studies. In the field studies, however, undefinable circumstances of infection and intoxication that go along with the nutritional deprivation may be responsible for the differences observed.

Dr. Plaut - I would like to make one comment about Dr. Seligmann's paper and then ask him a question. It is surprising how many gastrointestinal illnesses are treatable by antibiotics, and now Dr. Seligmann tells us that alpha chain disease also seems to clear up with antibiotics. It is known that tropical sprue and Whipple's disease are gastrointestinal ailments which seem to clear up on antibiotic therapy. I would just like to raise the possibility, as a speculation, that antibiotics may not be eliminating a microorganism which is causing the disease but rather is eliminating a microorganism that is interfering with the proper function of the immune system. Once this interfering microbe is eliminated, the immune apparatus can cope with the etiologic agent.

The question I had for Dr. Seligmann is this: Since there is a proteolytic cleavage in the alpha chain, do you have any information as to exactly where cleavage is occurring? Is this intracellular, at the cell membrane, or does it occur after the secretion of the alpha chain protein from the cell? What can you tell us about that?

Dr. Seligmann - All I can say is that there is no evidence for an extracellular cleavage, since we found no proteolytic activity in serum from these patients and since by radio-immunoelectrophoretic analysis and biosynthesis experiments, we found that the alpha chain disease protein was secreted as such. Presumably this is an intracellular limited proteolysis, but it has not been directly proven. It could be something similar to what has been described some years ago in the Journal of Molecular Biology for a mutant of E. coli phosphatase. These studies showed that such incomplete proteins are very susceptible to intracellular proteolysis.

Dr. Seligmann - May I address a question to Willy Hijmans? If I understood well the very interesting data presented by Dr. Hijmans, they were from the study of normal individuals' marrows. I would like to ask him if his findings also apply to monoclonal proliferations. We should expect from these data that in 30 percent of patients with macroglobulinemia, we should find alpha chain on the surface of the cells, and in 22 percent of patients with IgG myeloma we should expect to find alpha chains on the cells. However, I would like to state that in our studies with macroglobulinemia and myeloma, this appears not to be the case. In 40 cases of macroglobulinemia, we never found alpha chain determinants on the cells. In IgG myeloma we never found alpha chains on the

surface of the cells containing IgG myeloma proteins. What
we found in a few cases of myeloma was the presence of mu
chain determinants at the surface of myeloma cells containing
either IgG or IgA, or solely Bence-Jones proteins which would
fit well with some switch hypothesis and which recalls some
of the findings of Pernis in rabbits. We have found, in more
than 100 patients with CLL, a single case with alpha chain
determinants on the surface of the cells.

Dr. Hijmans - There are a number of discrepancies between our
findings. First of all, the chronic lymphocytic leukemia.
We did not find any alpha determinants on the cells in chronic
lymphocytic leukemia. I would like to stress again what we
reported - this concerns cells which do contain immunoglobulins, i.e. differentiated plasma cells and lymphocytes, and
not the early forms such as are found in chronic lymphocytic
leukemia. However, we do find cells from a number of chronic
lymphocytic leukemia patients without any surface staining,
but that is another story. Second, the figures we presented
give the percentages of positive cells per individual, and
not the percentage of positive cases.
     Now you asked about our findings in myeloma. In four
patients with IgA myeloma we did find this alpha determinant
on from 10 to 98 percent of the cells. In one patient we
investigated twice, before and after treatment, and there
was a drop from 95 to 10 percent. In six patients with IgG
myeloma, cells with gamma chain on the surface varied from 0
to 60 percent.

Dr. Seligmann - Did you find alpha chain on IgG myeloma cells?

Dr. Hijmans - No alpha chain there, no. In the two cases we
investigated we found only one percent and six percent,
respectively, of myeloma cells with alpha chain determinants
on the surface.

Dr. Strober - We have been focusing attention on IgA deficiency, but Dr. Hong has pointed out that there are certain
instances of elevated IgA levels in serum. One large group
that he did not mention but which I think deserves some
consideration is patients with gastrointestinal disease of
various kinds. For instance, in gluten-sensitive enteropathy
or celiac disease there is very regularly an elevation of IgA
and this is usually associated with IgM deficiency. Whether
or not there is some sort of reciprocity between IgA and IgM
levels that is brought about by these diseases is not known.

Also interesting is another situation in which one finds an isolated IgA elevation in a disease, and that is in hereditary sensory neuropathy. This condition is a rare familial disease of wide geographic distribution in which the only demonstrable immunoglobulin abnormality that could be found is an elevation of IgA. This disease is characterized by a very severe sensory neuropathy leading to complete loss of sensation over the extremities and a leprosy-like picture with loss of limbs and digits. Dr. John Whitaker and I studied patients from a number of kindreds and have found that the affected members of the family have IgA elevations, whereas unaffected members of the family have normal IgA. We have carried these studies further and have shown that the GI tract has increased production of IgA, using a radio-isotope incorporation technique. Apparently the elevated IgA in the serum is the result of increased production of IgA at a local GI site. We have looked at the molecular species of IgA in the serum, and in fact it proves to be a 7S IgA just as it is in other inflammatory diseases of the bowel. Hereditary sensory neuropathy, although primarily a neurological disease, turns out to have a gastrointestinal component.

Dr. Parkhouse - In the past it has been suggested that the light chain may function in immunoglobulin biosynthesis by effecting either the release of heavy chain from polyribosomes or by functioning as a label for secretion. Now, as Dr. Seligmann has told us, these alpha chain disease cells do not make light chain. This fact would argue against such a mandatory role for light chain in heavy chain biosynthesis and secretion. While I am here I would like to make a point in relation to Dr. Hijman's presentation. I think it would be a good idea in the light of increasing evidence from various systems in which immunoglobulin is cytophilic for cells to extend these observations by first of all stripping the surface immunoglobulin from these cell types with an enzyme and then looking for resynthesis of immunoglobulin molecules.

Dr. McGhee - I have a question for Dr. Sirisinha. I was wondering, in relation to what Dr. Good has said, whether the production of SC or the amount of SC that is in the epithelial cell could be a limiting factor on the amount of secretion of S-IgA in these malnourished patients?

Dr. Sirisinha - There is this possibility, because it has
been reported that in epithelial cells, during or even after
malnutrition, there are biochemical malfunctions. In many
of these cases even after they nutritionally recover, the
malfunction still persists for a long time in the epithelial
cells.

Dr. Lehner - I should like to ask a question of Dr. Seligmann.
Familial Mediterranean Fever is found in Sephardic but not
Ashkenazic Jews. Now some of these have amyloid in the
gastrointestinal tract and may present as a malabsorption
syndrome. I should like to ask whether he has looked for
amyloid in alpha chain disease, although amyloid to a large
extent may well be a light chain disease.

Dr. Seligmann - In all those cases where amyloid was looked
for, no amyloid was found. However, I must say for the
patients in Paris that we have some problems, since a very
old law forbids us to perform any post mortem studies on
Moslem patients.

Dr. Lehner - Can I also ask, while I am here, a question of
Dr. Hanson? His data suggested an independent association
of serum and urinary antibodies to E. coli. Would he care
to speculate on the possible feedback inhibition of these
antibodies?

Dr. Hanson - We have some information from the very nice
experimental work by Dr. Jim Smith who is present. In experimental pyelonephritis a local antibody response occurs
first in the kidneys. Dr. Smith showed that this response
was followed by seeding of cells, for example, to the spleen
where a similar response then followed. Now in humans, of
course, we would not know this yet; we know that in pyelonephritis there is a very evident serum response, and as I
showed, there is probably as well a local response. In
cystitis there is no indication of a serum response, but we
do see, as I indicated, a local response. In this case there
would be a dissociation.

Dr. Ballieux - I have additional information in relation to
Dr. Good's remark on the fascinating patients of Dr. Barandun.
We reported recently at the Meeting of the European Society
for Clinical Investigation (abstract Europ. J. Clin. Invest.
7 (1972) 294) data on a patient with cystic fibrosis who was
lacking completely kappa chains but had normal levels of

immunoglobulins. We isolated the light chains of the
immunoglobulins, and Don Capra analysed the sequence of the
N-terminal first 20 amino acids. There was no indication of
restricted heterogeneity as far as we can see. What is very
interesting is that the patient's sister also had the same
disease or abnormality. Intracellular kappa chains in plasma
cells were absent, but kappa chains were found on the surface
of lymphocytes. What we must do now is stimulate her cells
with pokeweed mitogen.

Could I ask one short question of Dr. Good? Recently
we have been studying the kappa:lambda ratio of the surface
immunoglobulins on peripheral lymphocytes. We have found in
a few patients with immunoglobulin deficiency that there was
a marked shift of the kappa:lambda ratio on the surface of
the peripheral lymphocytes toward the lambda type. I wonder
if similar data has been obtained by other people working
in this field.

Dr. Good - I would just ask you whether or not your patient
had severe gastrointestinal disease as the Barandun cases
had?

Dr. Ballieux - He had cystic fibrosis. He had steatorrhea,
but it may have been related to pancreatic insufficiency.

Dr. Good - The striking finding in those cases was an extraordinary watery diarrhea.

Dr. Ballieux - Well, you know there is a third case which
was published by George Bernier et al (Blood 40 (1972) 795).
This was also a kappa chain deficiency. I do not recall if
this patient did have gastrointestinal disease (note added
after the meeting: the patient did have diarrhea that at
various times "could be partially relieved by fat restriction,
gluten restriction and lacrose restriction").

Dr. Seligmann - Just a reply to Dr. Ballieux about his kappa:
lambda ratio in immune deficiency patients. I would like to
recall that in 1967, if I remember well, both Dr. Hong and
ourselves independently showed that there might be such
abnormality in the kappa:lambda ratio in serum Ig with a
prevalence of lambda chain bearing molecules in immunodeficiency patients, and I suppose he has seen the same
phenomenon at the lymphocyte level.

Dr. Ballieux - Well, that is the reason I asked this, Maxime, and I saw that Dick Hong was smiling when I asked the question. I would like to know if there is a reflection on the lymphocyte surface of this phenomenon which you and Dick Hong observed years ago in the serum.

Dr. Cooper - Apparently no one can answer the question at this time.

Dr. Good - This question constantly plagues me. All the evidence is accumulating indicating that the T cells are essential for the development of cells that can synthesize and secrete IgA and perhaps some of the other immunological responses of humans, as is the case with certain experimental animals. The question that keeps returning is that raised by patients with the most extreme deficiencies of T cells, namely the patients with the DiGeorge syndrome. When we study those patients, we are hard put to find any circulating T cells. Yet they may have quite normal IgA levels, and they surely have very well developed IgA producing and secreting lymphocyte and plasma cell populations in the circulation, bone marrow and lamina propria. I am perfectly willing to accept that there is some association between T cells and levels of IgA and IgA secreting plasma cells. These patients, however, make me raise the question: "What is substituting for T cell in the DiGeorge patient?"

The other issue is the relationship of hyperimmunity states. Wherever we find an apparent hyperimmunity state, for example, an IgA elevation, if we look hard enough we find an immunodeficiency that is leading to excessive stimulation of one or another of the remaining systems. To this point, the recent studies of Bo DuPont and Versild in multiple sclerosis are, I think, so pertinent. They have shown that multiple sclerosis is linked to a particular allele controlled at what we call the MLRS locus, i.e. a locus outside the HLA system which controls lymphocyte-determined histocompatibility response. Further, patients with multiple sclerosis failed to respond with cellular immunity to the paramyxo viruses, e.g. measles, mumps, while responding well with cellular immunity to other viruses. Their other immune responses, however, are perfectly all right and yet they fail to respond with cellular immunity to these antigens. They have a segmental immunodeficiency. Associated with that deficiency, you see evidence of excessive antibody response to antigens of these very same organisms. This is the real criticism I have of interpretation of rheumatic fever data,

rheumatoid arthritis data, and all the rest where diseases
are thought to be due to immunological excess. I think in
most of these circumstances we will find that the critical
issue will, in most instances, be immunologic deficiency,
be that deficiency segmental or more generic.

Dr. Rowe - As a brief question, I did not hear anyone say
whether the IgA positive lymphocytes which are present in
the IgA deficient individuals have light chain determinants
on their surface or not. Is that known?

Dr. Lawton - We have not done any double staining, but the
proportions add up; I mean they have cells that stain with
light chains, and if one adds the M, G, and A, it is in
reasonable agreement with kappa plus lambda.

Dr. Good - We have done double staining experiments, and
they have light chains on their surface.

Dr. Seligmann - We have done double staining experiments,
and we found light chains.

Dr. Hong - Concerning Dr. Good's objections, I would like
to comment as follows. I think until we know, first of all,
that the IgA immunoglobulin that is produced in DiGeorge
patients is in fact functional gamma globulin, we cannot say
that the IgA system is normal in its extent. The other
point which would relate to this situation is that in the
DiGeorge patients we are never sure how much thymic function
there is or was. In one example, there was a spontaneous
remission of the entire disease, and there have also been
cases described in which there was no immunologic abnormality
at all. So I think the DiGeorge is probably a very bad
clinical situation to cite as an isolated T cell deficiency.
In the most unambiguous situation that I know of, where a
chromosomal defect leads to thymic deficiency, that is, the
nude mice, it seems that IgA deficiency is rather constant.

Dr. Brandtzaeg - I have a question for Dr. Seligmann related
to alpha chain disease. I am a little bit worried about your
statement that you have an association between secretory
component and the alpha chain. Have you looked for J chain
in these preparations? Since these proteins are produced by
cells which are gland associated, it might be expected that
they would produce dimers. Could you comment on the physico-
chemical properties of these alpha chain proteins?

<u>Dr. Seligmann</u> - First, about the association to secretory
component, we have shown it in our very early papers, but
we have not performed any study in order to know if secretory component found on the alpha chain disease proteins
was or was not covalently linked to it. Second, as far as
J chain is concerned, we have indeed found J chain in all
preparations of alpha chain disease purified proteins we
have studied.

TYPES OF SIZE HETEROGENEITY OF IgA MOLECULES ISOLATED FROM MYELOMA AND NORMAL HUMAN SERUM

J. M. Fine, P. Lambin and D. Frommel

Centre National de Transfusion
75015 Paris, France

INTRODUCTION

In normal human serum IgA is present in a series of polymeric forms; the largely predominant monomeric 7S form coexists with components of increasing sedimentation coefficients (1,2). This size heterogeneity was also observed in serum of IgA myeloma (3,4). In 1964, studying 32 isolated IgA myeloma proteins, we reported that starch gel electrophoresis revealed 3 different types of polymerization - type I, II and III (5). More than 95% of 165 IgA M-components analyzed in this laboratory could be ascribed to one of these types. In our experience the type of polymerization remains stable for any given IgA myeloma. Taking advantage of a procedure for IgA purification which avoids the sieving effects or gel filtration (6), we confirmed and extended our previous findings (7). In this communication we present data concerning the types of size heterogeneity observed in monoclonal and polyclonal IgA preparations.

MATERIALS AND METHODS

IgA was isolated as described (6) from 14 myeloma sera and from the sera of 12 individual blood donors. Molecular heterogeneity remained unchanged from the starting serum to the final step of purification. IgA proteins obtained from myeloma sera were free of contaminants whereas those obtained from normal sera contained some IgM. These 26 preparations were compared by means of analytical ultra-

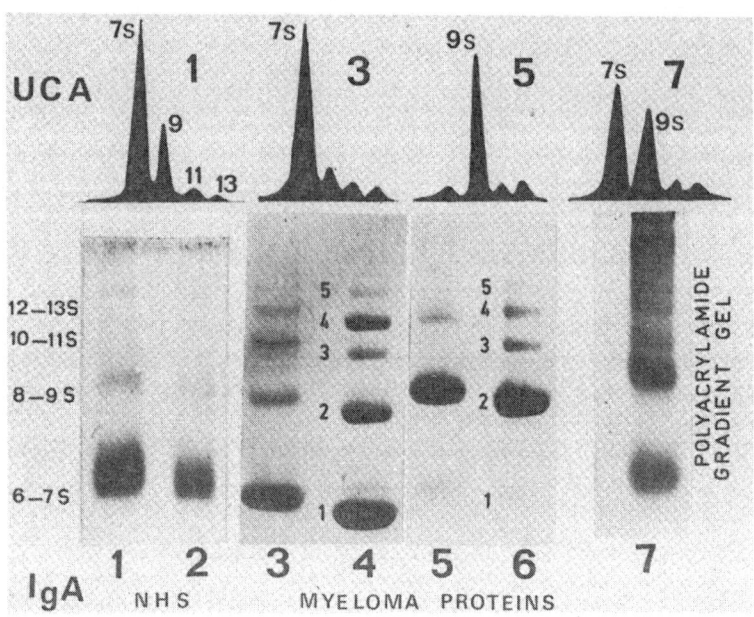

Figure 1. Types of size heterogeneity of IgA preparations.
Top: diagrams of analytical ultracentrifugation (UCA).
Bottom: electrophoretic patterns in polyacrylamide gels.
Samples 1 and 2: IgA from 2 different blood donors; 3 to 7:
monoclonal IgA. Major 7S component in 3 and 4; predominant
9S component in 5 and 6; marked increase of both 7S and 9S
components (type III) in 7.

centrifugation, electrophoreses in starch gel and in polyacrylamide gradient gel, and immunochemical analyses (7).

RESULTS

Three different types of polymerization of IgA molecules
were observed both in ultracentrifugation and in polyacrylamide gel. The type with a predominant 7S component (type II
in ref. 5) is encountered with an incidence of about 55%;
the one defined by a major 9S component (type I in ref. 5)
occurs in 35%; and the third type, characterized by 7S and
9S components at approximately equal ratio, makes up with few
exceptions the remainder. Minor 7S or 9S components, and
polymers of higher order, usually in a quantitative ratio decreasing in proportion to molecular size, are present at
low concentrations in all 3 types. J chain was detected in

all polymers. In IgA from normal serum, the 7S component
is predominant; as a consequence of the polyclonal nature of
normal IgA, the different components give broader bands in
acrylamide gel. Immunochemical analyses of individual IgA
preparations by two-dimensional electrophoresis (first separation in starch gel, electro-immunodiffusion in the second
dimension) using antisera specific for alpha chain, or in
the case of myeloma protein for idiotypic determinants,
showed that all components separated by virtue of their difference in size, shared isotypic and idiotypic determinants.
Thus the monoclonal nature of the polydispersed IgA myeloma
proteins does not appear to be questionable.

DISCUSSION

Contrasting with the regular size distribution of IgA
in normal serum, the many types of size heterogeneity observed in IgA myeloma proteins raise many questions. As J
chain was found to be a component of all IgA polymers, a
shift towards polymer formation as seen in myeloma, probably
reflects an increase of the J chain pool, this change being
related to the malignant process. In analogy to the polymerization of haptoglobins, types 2-1 and 2-2, which result
from different mechanisms of molecular association, mechanisms additional to J chain or related to its presence, might
also play a role in the distribution of IgA proteins into
polymers.

REFERENCES

1. Heremans, J.F., Les globulines sériques du système gamma,
    Arscia, Bruxelles, 1960.
2. Vaerman, J.P., Fudenberg, H.H., Vaerman, C. and Mandy,
    W.J., Immunochemistry 2:263, 1965.
3. Fine, J.M. and Creyssel, R., Rev. Franc. Et. Clin. et
    Biol. 6:766, 1961.
4. Laurell, A.H.F., Acta Med. Scand. Suppl. 367:69, 1961.
5. Fine, J.M., Boffa, G.A. and Creyssel, R., Clin. Chim.
    Acta 9:526, 1964.
6. Fine, J.M. and Steinbuch, M., Rev. Europ. Et. Clin. et
    Biol. 15:1115, 1970.
7. Fine, J.M., Lambin, P. and Frommel, D., Biomedicine 18:
    145, 1973.

DISTRIBUTION OF IgA SUBCLASSES IN SERA AND BONE MARROW PLASMA CELLS OF 21 NORMAL INDIVIDUALS

F. Skvaril and A. Morell

Institute for Clinical and Experimental Cancer Research, University of Berne, 3004 Berne, Switzerland

I would like to report some experiments which Dr. Morell and I have recently performed in Berne, Switzerland. We compared the distribution of the two IgA subclasses in the sera and in the IgA containing cells in the bone marrow of normal individuals. We are indebted to Dr. Hijmans for his help in the immunofluorescence studies of the bone marrow.

The IgA subclass specific antisera were prepared in rabbits by immunization with isolated myeloma proteins. After extensive absorption the antisera were specific for the heavy chains of either IgA_1 or IgA_2. The serum concentrations of the two subclasses were determined by a solid phase radioimmunoassay as previously described for quantitative analyses of IgG subclasses (1). As a control, total IgA in the sera was measured by radial immunodiffusion tests on Partigen plates (Behringwerke).

For conjugation, the subclass antisera were absorbed with antigens insolubilized by glutaraldehyde (2) until they were found to be specific by immunodiffusion tests. Then the globulin fraction was isolated by ammonium sulfate precipitation and conjugated with TRITC according to the method of Hijmans et al (3). The specificity of the conjugates was tested with bone marrow of myeloma patients who had monoclonal IgA protein of a known subclass in the serum.

Sera and bone marrow of 21 normal individuals were collected. The sera were kept frozen at - 20° C until the immunoglobulins were determined. Preparations of bone marrow cells were made according to Hijmans' procedure (3). The washed cells were placed on glass slides by use of a cytocentrifuge. Each preparation contained about 50,000 nucleated cells. These slides were stored at - 70° C. When used, they were fixed by ethanol:acetic acid (100:5, v/v) mixture and stained with the conjugated reagents. They were evaluated with a Leitz Orthoplan Microscope equipped with a Pleom-epiilluminator for fluorescence microscopy.

The results are summarized in Table I. The numbers presented are the arithmetical means. The sum of IgA$_1$ and IgA$_2$ concentrations in sera (in mg/ml) as determined in radioimmunoassays corresponds to the total IgA concentration measured in radial immunodiffusion. The means of both these values agree quite well. In individual sera, however, some differences could be seen but, in general, in sera with low IgA levels the sym of IgA$_1$ + IgA$_2$ was proportionally low and in sera with high IgA content the IgA$_1$ + IgA$_2$ value was high. In the Table it can be seen that the total IgA consists of approximately 82 percent IgA$_1$ and 18 percent IgA$_2$. When the percentage distribution of IgA$_1$ and IgA$_2$ in the serum was compared with the percentage of IgA$_1$ and IgA$_2$ positive cells in bone marrow, only small differences could be detected. The ratio of IgA$_1$:IgA$_2$ positive cells (88:12) was similar to the concentration ratio of these subclasses in the serum (82:18).

In a previous paper the metabolic properties of IgA$_1$ and IgA$_2$ were reported (4). The synthetic rate for IgA$_1$ was 24 mg/kg/day or about 85 percent of the total serum IgA synthesis. For IgA$_2$, the synthetic rate was 4.3 mg/kg/day or 15 percent of serum IgA. Thus we see that the percentage distribution of the two subclasses as found in the serum, their synthetic rates and numbers of plasma cells in bone marrow for each are similar. This fits into the concept that the bone marrow can be considered as the major source of circulating IgA immunoglobulin.

Table I.   Distribution of IgA subclasses in sera and bone
           marrow plasma cells of 21 normal individuals

	IgA_1	IgA_2	$IgA_1 + IgA_2$	IgA
Serum concentrations in mg/ml	2.1±0.9	0.5±0.3	2.6±1.2	2.6±0.7
(range)	(0.7–3.8)	(0.1–1.4)	(1.2–5.3)	(1.3–3.9)
Serum concentrations in percent	82±6	18±6	100	--
(range)	(72–91)	(9–28)		
Positive cells in bone marrow in percent	88±4	12±4	100	
(range)	(76–94)	(6–24)		

REFERENCES

1. Morell, A. and Skvaril, F., Protides of the Biological
    Fluids, 19th Colloquium Brugges, pp.533-540, Pergamon
    Press, Oxford, New York, 1972.

2. Avrameas, S. and Ternynck, Th., Immunochemistry 6:53,
    1969.

3. Hijmans, W., Schuit, H.R.E. and Klein, F., Clin.exp.
    Immunol. 4:457, 1969.

4. Morell, A., Skvaril, F., Noseda, G. and Barandun, S.,
    Clin.exp. Immunol. 13:521, 1973.

SELECTIVE IgA DEFICIENCY AND CHRONIC OBSTRUCTIVE PULMONARY DISEASE--A FAMILY STUDY

D. Robert Webb

The Mason Clinic

1118 Ninth Avenue, Seattle WN 98101

A 43 year old housewife with far advanced chronic obstructive pulmonary disease (COPD) was referred for evaluation of alpha$_1$ antitrypsin (AAT) type because of the early onset of her disease and her family history. Gradually progressive dyspnea on exertion and productive cough had been present for six years. There had been frequent upper respiratory infections and a mastoidectomy in the past. She had been a 2 pack per day cigaret smoker for years. On physical exam she was a cachectic woman in moderate respiratory distress. Breath sounds were almost absent at the lung bases and scattered wheezes and rhonchi were present. The chest film showed hyperexpansion and a suggestion of cyst formation at the bases. Pulmonary function testing showed severe obstruction which did not respond to bronchodilators. AAT quantitation and phenotyping by starch gel electrophoresis and subsequent crossed electrophoresis were normal. Quantitative immunoglobulin determinations revealed less than 4 mg./100 cc. of IgA in serum (adult normals 50-250) and slightly elevated IgG and IgM. IgE level was 44 ng./cc. (Normal--less than 500) Concentrated parotid secretions also showed no IgA.

The patient's large family (see family tree) was subsequently studied. Four of her eight children had no detectable IgA in serum. These children were sired by three different men; two were studied and both had normal IgA levels. Of the patient's six siblings, one died of per-

tussis pneumonia at two years of age. Three and perhaps
four of the five surviving siblings had borderline low
levels of IgA. Two nieces had definite low values (28 and
44 mg./100 cc.). Both of the proband's parents had normal
IgA levels. Consanguinity was present in this family; the
proband's mother had married her paternal uncle (her father's
brother). IgG, IgM, and IgE levels were normal in all family members.

The proband's mother and two older brothers had obvious COPD by history, physical examination, and physiologic
evaluations. The sister had elevated airway resistance but
no abnormality of flow rates. These four all were cigaret
smokers. The 38 year old brother was a non-smoker and had
slightly increased residual volume but no other abnormality.

Family with ↓ IgA and COPD

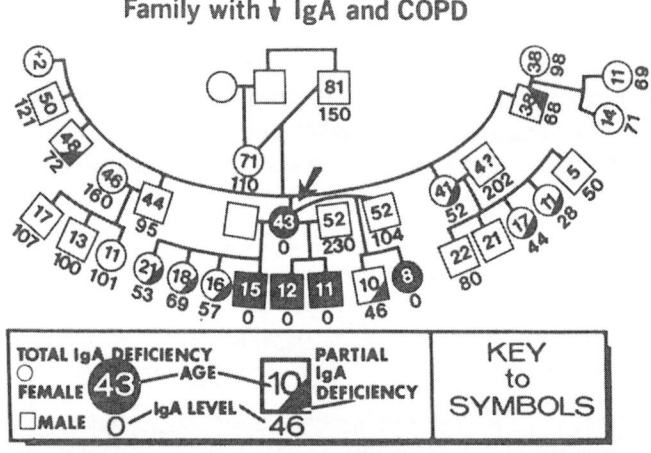

The genetic transmission of IgA deficiency in this family and the possible interaction between the IgA deficiency
and familial obstructive lung disease warrant discussion.
Initial evaluation of this family suggested a sporadic appearance of IgA deficiency in the proband, which was passed
in dominant fashion to 4 of 8 children. However, intermediate inheritance is suggested by 1) consanguinity, which
allows an unusual trait (IgA deficiency here) to occur in
both parents of the proband and thus become apparent, and 2)
borderline low IgA levels, which may represent partial deficiency. At least 3 of 4 siblings, 2 nieces, and the remaining 4 children had IgA levels in serum which were near or
below the lower limits of normal for their age. If intermed-

iate transmission is accepted, the parents of the proband
are obligate heterozygotes, but they have normal IgA values.
Similarly all fathers of completely deficient children must
carry the partial deficiency; this is statistically very unlikely. The two fathers studied had normal IgA levels but
IgA could have been falsely elevated by alcoholic liver disease. Although intermediate inheritance is suggested, it can
not be proven in this family.

COPD has not previously been associated with IgA deficiency. Early onset COPD is well documented in this family
as is selective IgA deficiency. Causal linkage between the
two entities is attractive. Predisposition to COPD in
patients with IgA deficiency would fit nicely into the proteolytic hypothesis of emphysema. Proteolytic enzymes in the
lung are hypothesized to cause autoproteolysis if not controlled. $Alpha_1$ antitrypsin seems to have a major role in
controlling these enzymes which may be released by polymorphonuclear leukocytes. COPD occurs in patients with a deficiency of protease inhibitor as in ATT deficiency. Excessive protease might overwhelm the usual control mechanisms;
this might be expected from patients with chronic bronchial
suppuration as in the proband in this family who had deficiency of secretory antibodies and smoked cigarets heavily.

Previous studies of immunoglobulin levels in COPD are
few and the results are contradictory. In particular, IgA
levels in serum have been reported normal, high, and low.
Falk and coworkers mentioned that one of 6 patients with COPD
had selective IgA deficiency similar to the proband in this
study.

In conclusion, a large family with co-existant selective IgA deficiency and early onset familial COPD is reported. An intermediate pattern of inheritance, although not
proven, seems likely in this family. Possible predisposition to COPD and emphysema in patients with selective IgA
deficiency is suggested.

NOTE ADDED IN PROOF Binding of various proteins including $alpha_1$ antitrypsin to IgA was reported by Tomasi and
others at this symposium. This suggests another mechanism
for COPD in patients with IgA deficiency. If IgA serves a
transport role for AAT, IgA deficient patients may have
relative AAT deficiency at the local lung level despite
normal serum levels.

DISCUSSION

Dr. Cooper - Dr. Mary Ann South will begin the discussion.

Dr. South - The papers yesterday, both Dr. Heremans' and Dr. Brandtzaeg's, which gave evidence for the existence of transport of IgA and presented hypotheses for this transport mechanism, were delightful to me. They called to mind the really incredibly naive little diagram we presented in 1965, in which we postulated that the IgA molecule was made in the plasma cell, the secretory component (which we called "transport piece" then) was made in the epithelial cell, and that the two parts of the secretory IgA molecule then got together in the epithelial cell and were from there secreted onto the mucous surface. This hypothesis, to my knowledge, still has not been adequately tested. It seems that now we have the tools at hand for this kind of testing, and the methods for study of the transport mechanism. This information will be of great clinical importance to those of us who treat patients with IgA deficiency. If we understand exactly what the transport mechanism is, we can plan a rational therapy, presenting the patient with IgA in the correct molecular form to be acceptable to the transport system or by an alternative route, so that the most effective antibody type and concentration can reach the mucosal surface. Infection, especially chronic infection, of these mucous surfaces is still the greatest clinical problem we face in the patients with humoral immune deficiency.

Dr. Cooper - Dr. Smith would like to say a word about local antibody in experimental pyelonephritis.

Dr. Smith - We have shown in experimental pyelonephritis in rabbits a significant synthesis of immunoglobulin in the kidney which is predominantly IgG although in hematogenous pyelonephritis secretory IgA is synthesized. We have shown in previous studies antibody to the somatic antigen of the infecting organism in the IgG class but little or no antibody in the IgA class. I wish to present today studies done in collaboration with Jan Holmgren and Lars Hanson in which we utilized the enzyme linked immuno-absorbant assay (ELISA),

the technique Dr. Hanson showed earlier, to determine if
local antibody in various Ig classes was synthesized in
pyelonephritic kidney. We found that in pyelonephritic
kidneys, local antibody in IgA class was present in a number
of experiments prior to day 20 but after day 20 was present
in only a rare specimen. In contrast, IgG antibody was
present beginning at day 11 and in high titers throughout
the study. Of interest is the fact that IgM antibody is
first noted at day 20 but does persist thereafter. Thus,
these studies indicate that the ELISA technique can be utilized in a study of local antibody at infected sites as well
to detect antibody in urine as shown by Dr. Hanson today and
demonstrates that antibody in all three classes develops to
lipopolysaccharide in infected kidney.

Dr. Cooper - Dr. Ballieux will discuss the kappa/lambda ratio
in the gut.

Dr. Ballieux - Some time ago we presented data at the Bruges
colloquium (Poen et al. Prot. Biol. Fluids 16 (1969) 485) on
the elevated serum levels of IgA in patients with various
diseases of the gastrointestinal tract like Crohn's disease.
In relation to this study we investigated the kappa/lambda
ratio of IgA producing cells in the gut. This study was done
in collaboration with my co-workers Mul, de Boer and Taminiau,
and I will present the results in summary.
       In essence the data were obtained by immunofluorescence
studies on jejunal biopsies using a rhodamine (Tritc) labeled
anti IgA antiserum giving red fluorescence and fluorescein
isothiocyanate (Fitc) labeled anti-kappa and anti-lambda
antisera showing green. The antisera used were prepared and
conjugated in our department. The F/P ratio was within the
limits accepted by the fluorescence standardization committee.
The conjugates were absorbed with rat liver powder, human
ABO erythrocytes and rabbit intestine powder and tested for
specificity and optimal dilution on human myeloma bone marrow
cells. The biopsies were handled according to the method
described by Eidelman and Berschauer in 1969.
       This double staining technique permits three types of
cells to be distinguished on the basis of color. Green ones
are plasma cells containing kappa chains and heavy chains
which are not of the alpha class. The yellow cells show
double staining and contain IgA type kappa, and the red-
brownish cells contain IgA with lambda chains. The following
control-experiments were done on sections of jejunal biopsies:
a. Simultaneous incubation of anti IgA-Tritc (the one we

used throughout the study) and of a different anti IgA-Fitc
conjugate. Except for one cell among several hundreds, all
plasma cells showed double staining, indicating that both
anti IgA antisera had the same specificity and therefore
most probably all IgA containing cells are stained with the
Tritc conjugate. b. Simultaneous incubation of anti-kappa
Fitc (the one we used throughout the study) and of different
anti-kappa-sera conjugated with Tritc. All cells studied
showed double staining, indicating that the anti-kappa-Fitc
conjugate would reveal all kappa-containing cells. c. Simultaneous incubation of anti IgG-Fitc, anti IgM-Fitc and
anti IgA-Tritc. No cells were seen with double staining,
indicating that the anti IgA-conjugate would not be bound
by plasma cells containing IgG or IgM. d. Simultaneous
incubation of the anti IgA-Tritc, anti kappa-Fitc and anti
lambda-Fitc. Not one single cell showing only red fluorescence was detected. This indicated that all cells containing
alpha chains also contained kappa or lambda chains. e. Simultaneous incubation of the anti lambda-Fitc and a Tritc
conjugate of the anti kappa antisera used for this study.
No double staining was seen indicating that no double producers were present and also proving that no cross-reacting
specificity was present in the antisera.

Four to five hundred cells per biopsy were counted
separately by two individuals. From the results of the
independent countings the kappa/lambda ratio of IgA containing cells was determined in 32 patients. An average ratio
of 63:37 was found. A few remarks can be made on the basis
of the results. In the first place no relationship between
the kappa/lambda ratio and the clinical diagnosis could be
made. In the second place the sum of the cells containing
IgA kappa and IgA lambda respectively was always about 100
percent. That means that no or just a very few cells contained only alpha chains or produced both kappa and lambda
chains. And finally, I think the most important conclusion
is that in the jejunum the ratio of IgA kappa and lambda cells
does not significantly differ from the kappa/lambda ratio
of immunoglobulins producing cells in human bone marrow as
determined by Dr. Hijmans. Therefore the kappa/lambda ratio
is not a characteristic parameter of the IgA secreting system
of the small intestine.

Dr. Cooper - Now we go back away from the responding population of cells to what is stimulating them in the first place
and Dr. Bockman would like to elaborate a bit on the flow of
antigens into lymphoid areas along the gut.

Dr. Bockman - We have been studying the specialized epithelium inserted between the luminal pole of lymphoid follicles
in the chicken bursa, rabbit appendix, and mouse Peyer's
patch, and the respective lumina. As studied in embryonic
chick bursa, this specialized follicle-associated epithelium
differentiates after the arrival of lymphoid cells. Follicle-associated epithelium (FAE) is characterized by blunt,
irregular microvilli and numerous pinocytotic vesicles and
vacuoles. Lymphoid cells are frequently observed within the
epithelium. Ferritin and India ink tracers are taken up by
these cells. Some of the tracers are transmitted to the
underlying lymphoid follicles.

Our attention has turned, recently, to FAE in human
appendix. We are currently studying, by electron microscopy,
a series of specimens from fetal appendix and from non-
inflamed appendix of children. In a fetus of approximately
14 weeks, the specialized relationship of lymphoid cells and
FAE has been observed. Some of the lymphoid cells are present within the epithelial layer, in close approximation to
FAE cells filled with pinocytotic vesicles (Figure 1). This
is not a transitory event, as shown by the identical relationship in the appendix from a five-year-old boy.

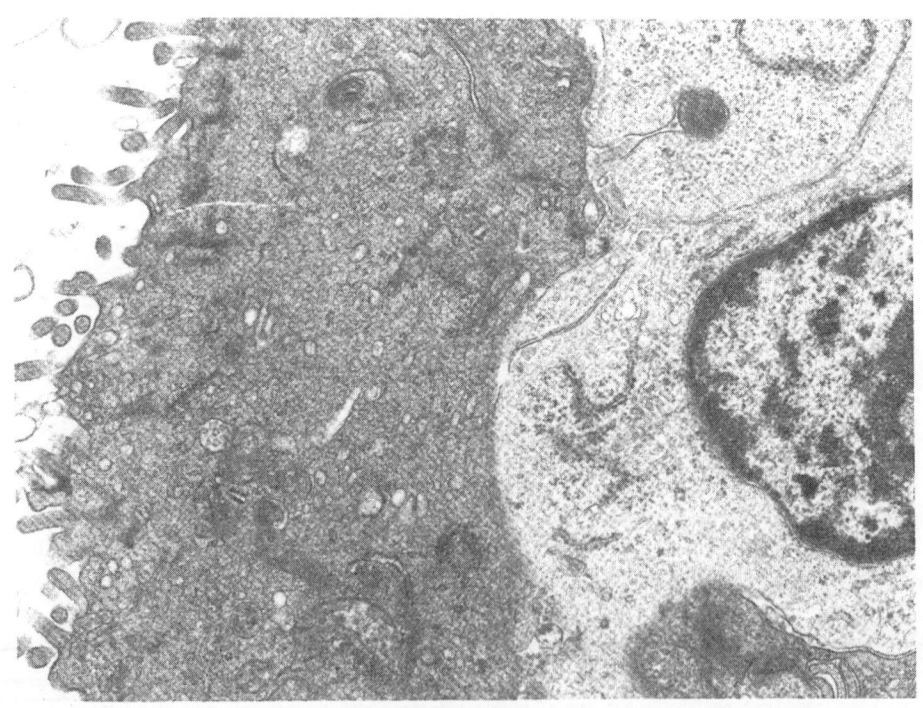

Figure 1

FAE is a logical route for intraluminal antigens to gain access to B cells comprising the underlying follicles, trig-gering a migration of cells to other mucosal surfaces, where IgA may be secreted.

Dr. Cooper - Dr. Moore would like to discuss a dissociation between serum and secretory IgA in an unusual patient.

Dr. Moore - In the majority of patients, levels of serum immunoglobulin A accurately predict levels of secretory A, although in a few cases with serum IgA deficiency, secretory A has been found in apparently normal amounts. We wish to report a case we believe to be the first detected instance of the converse situation. This child had combined immune deficiency in association with deficiency of adenosine dea-minase. From the time of diagnosis until she received a marrow transplant, her serum immunoglobulins M and G were low. Serum IgA, however, was normal to high for her age group. This IgA was largely IgA kappa, and had restricted heterogeneity. Immunoglobulin surface markers for IgA could not be demonstrated on marrow or peripheral lymphocytes, but cytoplasmic immunofluorescence on marrow did identify a small number of cells positive for IgA. Despite normal levels of IgA in serum, small amounts of IgA could be identified in saliva only on 40 fold concentration and only prior to the 17th month of age. No salivary IgM was found and IgG dis-appeared at about the same time that the IgA did. Immuno-electrophoresis and immunodiffusion studies suggested that the IgA in saliva was probably unassociated with secretory component which was present. Stool extracts, in contrast, clearly contained IgA and some IgG. We have not yet esta-blished if this IgA was associated with secretory component. Despite the presence of IgA in stools, a small bowel biopsy and a rectal biopsy revealed very few cells containing IgA. A few cells stained positive for IgM but virtually none for IgG. A lip biopsy showed no evidence for immunoglobulin containing cells. Despite profound peripheral lymphopenia, this patient had lymphonodular hyperplasia by both x-ray and biopsy.

This, then, was an infant with adenosine deaminase deficiency and combined immune deficiency who, despite normal to high levels of IgA in serum, had a marked defi-ciency of IgA in saliva. This was further abnormal in that the traces of IgA in saliva were not complexed to secretory component. She was virtually lacking in immunoglobulin pro-ducing cells in the mucosa, despite the presence of

lymphonodular hyperplasia. Cells with immunoglobulin A
surface markers were not demonstrable in either peripheral
blood or marrow. It may be that the cells of the secretory
immunoglobulin system have increased dependence either
directly or indirectly on the enzyme adenosine deaminase.
The initial colonization of the mucosa with IgA producing
cells may have been deficient, or these cells or their
function may have been lost over time. The small quantities of IgA that we did find in the patient's secretions
may have been transported from serum as discussed earlier
by Dr. Heremans and some of the other people here.

Dr. Capra - Just a comment on Dr. Frommel's paper - really
an extension in a sense to another species. Dr. Hurwitz at
the Animal Medical Center has been collaborating with our
group for some time and with him we have had the opportunity
to study six cases of IgA myeloma in the dog. As Dr. Vaerman
and Dr. Heremans showed several years ago, canine IgA is
almost exclusively dimeric and as you would expect the IgA
myelomas in dogs are polymeric. However, in five out of
the six dogs we have studied it was almost exclusively in
the higher polymer forms with a relatively small amount of
dimeric IgA. However, we have recently seen one **serum in**
which the IgA was exclusively dimeric with no higher polymers.
So at least in another species this tendency to polymerize
is found in the naturally occurring disease. (I should point
out that these canine myelomas are not induced.)
     I would like to ask Dr. Ballieux and Dr. Hijmans if they
have ever looked at the IgA producing cells with light chain
variable region subgroup specific antisera. These antisera
are available now and on the basis of the data that we presented last evening, one would predict that the variable
region subgroups would be markedly different in IgA than they
would be in IgG and IgM producing cells. This would be a
much simpler experiment to do than the time-consuming survey
of several individual myeloma proteins.

Dr. Cooper - The answer from Drs. Ballieux and Hijmans is no.
Dr. Capra, while you are up perhaps you might have some comment on Dr. Moore's observation of serum IgA in abundance
and secretory IgA in very small amounts. Did you not mention
that you had seen similar dissociation?

Dr. Capra - Yes, we have had the opportunity to study two
adults with IgA deficiency. Both these patients had low
serum IgA but had absent salivary IgA. This was most puzzling

if we assume that the cells that are making this are somehow connected. Both these patients are being extensively
studied at the present time. Jejunal biopsies confirm the
absence of IgA producing cells. I do not know if there are
other cases like this around.

Dr. Cooper - We have seen a patient in whom bone marrow contained plasma cells making IgA in numbers consistent with
the serum levels, whereas in the intestines we could find
absolutely no IgA producing cells. I believe Dr. Hijmans
proposed that the cells making some of the circulating IgA
might be entirely different from the ones that were settling
along the intestine. I wonder if this is indeed what we
are seeing in this patient. One of these subgroups may be
present, located at sites other than along the intestine and
making plenty of circulating antibody, while the group that
populates the gut is lacking.

Dr. Hijmans - To answer Dr. Capra's question, no. While I
have the microphone, indeed we find a kappa/lambda ratio
for the cells in the bone marrow of 1.5. If we break down
these data for the classes, the kappa/lambda ratio for IgA
is around 1, so this class has a relative excess of lambda.

Dr. Hong - I was actually very disturbed by Dr. Moore's
paper because it had always been my feeling, based on earlier
observations, that there would not be a dissociation in that
particular direction. I know of four patients who have
normal levels of secretory IgA but virtually undetectable
serum IgA. Some of these have normal numbers of IgA producing cells in the intestine. From the work of Craig and
Cebra, we felt that this might be consistent with the notion
that one of the maturating events necessary to the complete
IgA system was a peripheralization of precursor cells. We
envisioned that there might be some individuals who started
off with a low number of IgA precursor cells. After the
antigen and the clonal expansion steps that you talk about,
Max, there might still be a restricted number of IgA producers. Therefore the amount of peripheralization that occurs
over a period of time would never be enough to produce goodly
levels in the serum. Thus, you could have fairly reasonable
levels of IgA in the secretions as compared to serum, but
not the reverse. That was a good theory until Dr. Moore
presented her case. I really do not know what to do except
to say that theories are put out to be disproven. There is
another case which might be similar to yours that we have

observed recently. This is an adult who had chronic renal
disease of unknown origin. Interestingly enough, this patient had normal levels of serum IgA. He presented with
intractable diarrhea, but unfortunately he died before
fluorescence studies could be performed on his intestine.
His diarrhea was cured completely through the oral administration of colostrum.

Dr. Cooper - Dr. Moore, wasn't there a question of whether
some of this patient's lymphoid cells might have come from
the mother? If so, might not the serum IgA have come from
a subpopulation of cells that did not home to the gut?

Dr. Moore - Originally, we thought that she had received a
maternal transplant transplacentally because of the gamma
G allotypic markers. That theory is still possible in that
there are no data to refute it. However, we now understand
her parental history a little bit better and know that
there is consanguity. The markers can also be explained on
that basis.
    If there are separate precursor cells for serum IgA
and secretory IgA, even though they may have a common ances-
tor, maternal cells acquired transplacentally would probably
be ones that would seed to the lymph nodes or wherever the
circulating IgA comes from, rather than to the gut so as
to produce the situation found in this child. Alternatively,
the effect of her ADA deficiency may have been less delete-
rious to the IgA producers in lymphoid tissues than to her
other immunoglobulin producing cells.

Dr. Ogra - I would like to ask if anyone at the meeting has
looked at the secretory immunoglobulins in Nezelof's syndrome?
In the patient that Dr. Moore presented, do we know the biologic activity of the immunoglobulins? And could this possibly be the Nezelof syndrome?

Dr. Cooper - Can anyone answer that quickly? One of the
problems is that it is hard to define Nezelof's syndrome in
modern terms now that we have got more lymphocyte markers.

Dr. Ballieux - Dr. Stoop in our group studied one patient
with a Nezelof syndrome who was treated with a thymus transplantation. Before this substitution the specific humoral
immunity was found to be undisturbed as far as could be
established: immunoglobulins of all types and classes were
present in adequate amounts in serum and external secretions.

The bone marrow and lymph nodes contained plasma cells. Normal serum titers of antibodies against DPTP, vaccinia virus and the pathogenic microorganisms involved in the infections were found. Specific cellular immune defense was entirely absent.

(Stoop, J.W., Eijsvoogel, V.P., Zegers, B.J.M., van Bekkum, P.W., Ballieux, R.E.: Thymus transplantation in Nezelof's syndrome Folia Med. Neerl. 15 (1972) 135.
Stoop, J.W., Eijsvoogel, V.P., Zegers, B.J.M., van Bekkum, D.W., Ballieux, R.E.: The Nezelof Syndrome. The effect of thymus transplantation and transfer factor administration. In preparation.)

Dr. South - We have studied one patient with what we called Nezelof's syndrome, who had normal, in fact, elevated serum levels of serum IgA and normal salivary levels of IgA.

Dr. Fudenberg - I would like to raise a point and see if I can get a possible explanation in terms of genetic control of IgA synthesis, as regards the possibility that there are two separate systems for IgA production, namely the gut and the bone marrow. Patients with IgA myeloma with tremendous serum levels of IgA never have involvement of the gut. I must have seen a hundred IgA myelomas by now and have never seen one with gut involvement. This must mean that there is something naive in our simple explanation for genetic control of IgA synthesis. Does anyone have any explanations?

Dr. Cooper - We have no volunteers. Thank you all for this discussion.

SESSION F

THE IgA ANTIBODY RESPONSE
IMPLICATIONS FOR ORAL HEALTH

CHAIRMAN: ALEXANDER R. LAWTON

THE INDUCTION AND CHARACTERIZATION OF SECRETORY IgA ANTIBODIES

P. C. Montgomery, J. Cohn and E. T. Lally

Department of Microbiology, School of Dental
Medicine and Center for Oral Health Research
Philadelphia, Pennsylvania 19174

INTRODUCTION

In addition to humoral immunity, which is characterized by the presence of circulating antibody, a second distinct type of immunity involves the localized production of secretory antibodies (reviews 1, 2, 3). Numerous investigators, employing different antigens in a wide variety of animal systems, have been able to stimulate localized antibody production (4-13). The characteristic structural features of secretory IgA (review 3), which allows it to be differentiated from its serum counterpart, make IgA the ideal immunoglobulin class to be used in studies on the inductive process. Of particular relevance to our current studies was the demonstration that local immunization, by the intramammary route, with either dinitrophenylated bovine gamma globulin (6) or group A streptococci (8) could induce specific colostral IgA antibodies. Other evidence strongly suggested that gut associated lymphoid tissue was not only involved in the production of intestinal IgA antibodies (5, 9, 11, 13), but also might play a role in IgA production at remote sites (7, 9, 10, 12) including secretory sites (10, 12, 14).

Our investigations have been directed at developing a system which could be used to assess the immune potential of the secretory antibody response and to gain an insight into the mechanism of secretory antibody induction. We have described a hapten-bacterial conjugate, dinitrophenylated-type III-pneumococcus, which was capable of inducing high titers of serum anti-hapten antibody

(15) and more recently colostral IgA antibodies (16). The present report a. further defines our system for studying the induction of secretory IgA antibodies, b. explores the effect of different types of hapten-carrier conjugates and routes of immunization on the secretory antibody response and c. assesses the immunochemical properties of secretory IgA antibodies. Our results will be discussed in terms of the immune potential of the secretory antibody response and the mechanism of secretory antibody induction.

MATERIALS AND METHODS

Antigen Preparation and Immunization Methods. Dinitrophenylated-bovine gamma globulin, DNP-BGG, (17) and dinitrophenylated-type III-pneumococcal vaccine, DNP-Pn, (15) were prepared as described previously. New Zealand white female rabbits were immunized with DNP-BGG or DNP-Pn according to one of the protocols outlined in Table I. Oral immunization was carried out 3x/week by dispensing 5.0 mg DNP-BGG or 2.5 mg DNP-Pn directly into the rabbit's mouth. Oral immunization was initiated either 2 weeks

TABLE I

IMMUNIZATION PROTOCOL[1]

| Group | Prefeed[2] (p) | Injections[3] | | Feed[4] (f) |
		Mammary (m)	Intravenous (i)	
I		+		
II		+		+
III	+	+		+
IV	+			+
V			+	

[1] Quantities of antigen and immunization methods are detailed in the text. Groups I-IV were identical for both antigens, group V DNP-Pn only.

[2] Oral immunization for 2 weeks prior to impregnation.

[3] Injections for 4 week gestation period.

[4] Oral immunization for 4 week gestation period.

prior to breeding (groups III and IV) or during the week of breeding (group II) and continued through gestation. Intramammary
injections (groups I, II and III) were carried out for 4 weeks with
2.5 mg DNP-BGG or 1.0 mg DNP-Pn distributed equally among the
mammary glands. In this case antigens were emulsified in decreasing concentrations of complete Freund's adjuvant, 25%, 10%,
10%, 0% (total volume-1.0 ml). Intravenous injections of DNP-Pn
(group V) were carried out 3x/week (15): week 1 (0.1); week 2
(0.2); week 3 (0.3) and week 4 (0.5 ml/injection; DNP-Pn concentration 0.5 mg/ml, protein). Three days after the termination
of pregnancy, rabbits were bled and milking was initiated. Milk
fractions from individual rabbits were pooled.

Milk Fractionation. Pooled milk fractions were clarified by
centrifugation (18). Secretory IgA was purified by a two-step
chromatographic procedure employing Sephadex G150 and Sepharose 6B column chromatography (16). The purity of IgA antibodies
was judged by radioimmunoelectrophoresis. IgA concentrations
were determined spectrophotometrically employing an $E_{1cm}^{1\%}$ 280
nm of 13.5 (18).

Radioimmunoelectrophoresis. The details of this technique
are described elsewhere (15). The source and specificity of the
antisera directed against rabbit serum, colostrum and immunoglobulin components have been described previously (16). An
additional antiserum (goat origin) directed against rabbit secretory IgA was kindly provided by Drs. Emmings and Genco. The
ligand, α-N(4-hydroxyphenacetyl)- ϵ -N-(2,4-dinitrophenyl)-L-
lysine, HDL (19) was iodinated to yield [^{131}I] HDL or [^{125}I] HDL
(15) and used to develop the slides.

Hapten Binding Analysis. The hapten binding capacity (HBC)
of sera and secretory IgA samples was measured by the modified
Farr technique (15, 20). One hundred μl serum aliquots were
assayed directly. Purified secretory IgA samples were adjusted
to identical protein concentrations and 50 μl of the purified IgA
sample was added to 50 μl of normal rabbit serum. Normal rabbit serum was employed to provide the carrier protein necessary
for adequate precipitate formation. Fifty μl of 10^{-6}M [^{125}I]HDL
(3mCi/ μmole) was added to 100 μl of test sera or secretory IgA
samples prepared as described above and run in triplicate. After
the ligand reacted for 15 min at 4°C, 300 μl of 75% saturated
ammonium sulfate was added. Incubation for 30 min at 4°C was
followed by centrifugation at 2500 rpm for 2 hr. The precipitates

were washed 2x with 60% saturated ammonium sulfate and counted in a Packard 5212 gamma counter. The HBC was calculated as the % of total ligand bound relative to appropriate control samples. Serum and secretory IgA negative control samples were obtained from a series of 5 unimmunized rabbits and these values were set at 0%. A positive control serum pool was prepared from a series of rabbits hyperimmunized with DNP-BGG (anti-DNP antibody titer- 2.5 mg/ml by quantitative precipitin; K_0 = $8x10^8$ L/M by fluorescence quenching titration of the purified IgG class antibody with ϵ-DNP-lysine). The positive control value was set at 100%. In addition an internal standard possessing an HBC of 50% was run with each test set. HBC's for experimental samples were obtained from at least 4 to 8 separate determinations.

Hapten binding curves were constructed employing a variation of the ammonium sulfate precipitation technique described above. In this case a series of ligand ($[^{125}I]$ HDL) dilutions were employed for each test sample (10^{-5} to 10^{-8}M). The binding data were analyzed by the Sips equation, $\log [r/(n-r)]$= $a \log c + a \log K_0$, in terms of r and c. r represents the moles of ligand bound per mole of tetravalent antibody (n=4, ref. 8 and this study) and c is the free ligand concentration. The molar concentration of antibody was calculated from the binding data (15, 20). Calculations were performed with a Wang 720C calculator using programs written by Ronald Kahn in our laboratory.

RESULTS

Antibody Response to DNP-BGG. In all instances anti-DNP antibodies were studied and no attempt was made to quantitate amounts of carrier specific antibodies present in the samples. Analysis of the serum samples by radioimmunoelectrophoresis revealed that all DNP-BGG immunized rabbits produced IgG class anti-DNP antibodies. No other class of serum antibody was detected. The hapten binding capacity (HBC) data for serum samples, presented in Table II, confirm that all rabbits produced serum antibody. Animals which received intramammary injections (group I) or the combination protocols (groups II and III) displayed substantially higher HBC's than animals stimulated by the oral route (group IV). The HBC's of over half of the rabbits in groups I, II and III (5/9) were greater than 80%.

Radioimmunoelectrophoretic analysis of clarified milk samples revealed that all immunized rabbits possessed IgG class antibodies and that all but one animal (group I) produced antibody of
the IgA class. No IgM class antibodies were demonstrated even
though IgM was detectable with our antisera. HBC's for secretory
IgA samples purified from milk fractions of individual rabbits were
measured; the ranges of these values are listed in Table II. Values for animals in all 4 experimental groups did not exceed 15%,
with the majority of the animals, 8/12, displaying HBC's of less
than 10%.

Antibody Response to DNP-Pn. Analysis of serum samples by
radioimmunoelectrophoresis showed that 10/26 DNP-Pn immunized
rabbits produced IgG class anti-DNP antibodies. As in the DNP-
BGG immunized rabbits, no other serum antibody class was detected. The HBC's for serum samples of the DNP-Pn immunized
rabbits are presented in Table II. Rabbits under either the combination protocols (group II, 3/4 and group III, 3/4) or intravenous injections (group V, 2/2) showed a predominance of serum

TABLE II

HAPTEN BINDING CAPACITY (HBC) OF SERUM AND
PURIFIED SECRETORY IgA

Antigen	Group (protocol)	Number of Rabbits	Hapten Binding Capacity[1]	
			Serum	Secretory IgA
DNP-BGG	I (m)	5	5-89	0-15
	II (m, f)	3	13-95	4
	III (p, m, f)	1	90	4
	IV (f)	3	1-5	3-4
DNP-Pn	I (m)	7	0-4	14-25
	II (m, f)	4	0-10	4-18
	III (p, m, f)	4	0-9	14-21
	IV (f)	9	0	18-25
	V (i)	2	4-11	0

[1] Expressed as % of [125I] HDL bound; range of % values
listed, see Materials and Methods for details of control
samples and calculations.

responses.   The majority of rabbits (5/7) stimulated by intramammary injections (group I) did not mount a serum response, whereas
all animals stimulated by the oral route (group IV, 9/9) failed to
produce serum antibody (in no case did the HBC's of sera positive
rabbits exceed 11%).

Radioimmunoelectrophoretic analysis of clarified milk samples from DNP-Pn immunized rabbits showed that only those rabbits with serum IgG class antibodies possessed IgG class antibodies
in their secretions.   IgA class antibodies were present in all but
the intravenously immunized animals (group V).   The ranges of
HBC's obtained with purified secretory IgA samples are listed in
Table II.   Groups stimulated by the intramammary (group I, 6/7)
and oral route (group IV, 4/8) contained more rabbits with HBC's
in excess of 15% than did those groups exposed to the combination
protocols (group II, 1/4 and group III, 1/4).   Purified IgA samples
from intravenously immunized animals (group V) did not bind
hapten.

Immunochemical Properties of Secretory IgA Antibodies.   Before assessing the binding properties of secretory IgA antibodies,
it was necessary to determine the number of binding sites present
on the IgA molecule.   Figure 1 shows the $\underline{r}$ vs $\underline{c}$ plot for one such
set of binding data obtained with the secretory IgA of rabbit 63
(DNP-Pn, group IV).   Although the points are scattered, it is apparent that the plot reaches a plateau as $\underline{r}$ approaches 4.   This
value agrees with that previously reported for rabbit secretory
IgA (8) and was subsequently used in the binding calculations.

Table III summarizes the binding properties of those secretory IgA anti-DNP antibodies isolated in sufficient quantities to
permit analysis.   All association constants (K_0) ranged between
10^5 and 10^6 L/M.   The K_0 values for the DNP-BGG immunized rabbits, 4/6, were in the 10^6 L/M range, while the K_0 for DNP-Pn
rabbits were more consistently (9/12) in the 10^5 L/M range.   The
route of immunization did not appear to influence these values.
The heterogeneity indices ($\underline{a}$) appeared to be consistently lower for
secretory IgA antibodies obtained from rabbits immunized with
DNP-BGG.   Values approaching 1.0 were consistently attained with
DNP-Pn immunized rabbits (with the exception of rabbit 68), indicating that these secretory IgA antibodies may possess some degree of molecular restriction.   The route of immunization appeared
to have little effect on the $\underline{a}$ values.

Table III also lists the antibody concentrations for a number of

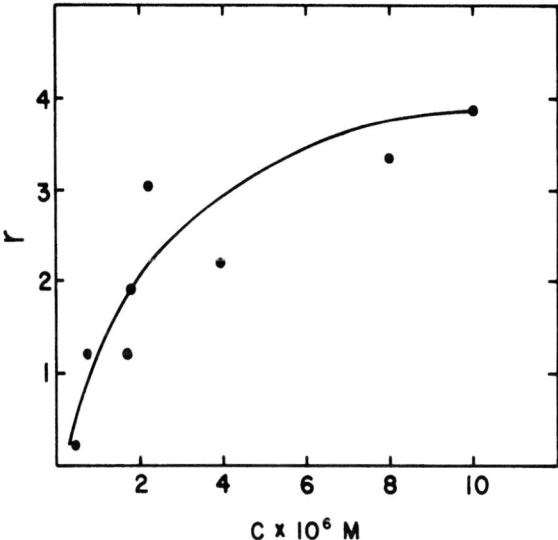

Figure 1. Binding of [^{125}I] HDL by secretory IgA purified from milk of rabbit 63 as determined by the modified Farr technique. The r values, moles of hapten
bound per mole of antibody, were plotted against c,
the molar concentration of free hapten.

secretory IgA samples. Antibody concentrations are expressed in
terms of μg of antibody per original ml of milk. Concentrations
of specific IgA antibodies were consistently higher in the DNP-Pn
immunized rabbits. Animals receiving DNP-Pn antibody by the
oral route appeared to produce quantities of secretory IgA antibody
comparable to animals receiving this antigen by other routes of
immunization.

DISCUSSION

A number of factors are important in the induction of secretory antibodies: a. species and physiological state of the animal,
b. nature of the antigen (structure, physical state: particulate vs
soluble, infectious vs non-infectious), and c. method of immunization (dose, presentation and route of antigen administration).
Our studies were confined to the nature of the antigen and its route
of administration.

DNP substituted on either a soluble protein (BGG) or a particulate bacterial (Pn) carrier is effective at eliciting specific secre-

TABLE III

BINDING PROPERTIES OF SECRETORY IgA ANTI-DNP ANTIBODIES[1]

Antigen	Group (protocol)	Rabbit	K_o (L/Mx10^5)	a	Antibody Concentration[2]
DNP-BGG	I (m)	7	16.0	.6	7.5
		8	3.5	.8	37.5
	II (m, f)	18	53.0	.7	9.6
		L2	98.0	.7	3.0
	III (p, m, f)	L6	6.7	.8	6.9
	IV (f)	L8	50.0	.5	8.1
DNP-Pn	I (m)	45	15.0	.8	5.7
		60	3.6	1.0	62.7
	II (m, f)	30	5.2	.9	16.5
		31	4.5	1.0	25.2
		33	4.3	1.0	12.6
	III (p, m, f)	43	2.5	1.0	57.0
		69	4.5	1.0	21.1
	IV (f)	63	11.0	.8	39.3
		68	3.3	.4	7.5
		N2	38.0	1.0	8.7
		N5	9.9	1.0	25.2
		N8	8.4	.9	13.8

[1] Average intrinsic association constants (K_o) and heterogeneity indices (a) calculated as described in the Materials and Methods.

[2] μg of antibody/original ml of milk. Data obtained directly from binding studies.

tory anti-DNP IgA class antibodies, with the latter inducing antibodies with higher HBC's. Two factors influence the HBC values, antibody concentration and affinity. In general the affinities of all secretory IgA antibodies were low (10^5-10^6 L/M). Secretory IgA antibodies from DNP-BGG animals possessed consistently lower titers and higher affinities than animals immunized with DNP-Pn. The heterogeneity indices (a), which may be used as an initial indication of antibody heterogeneity (21), indicate that secretory

IgA antibodies from animals immunized with DNP-BGG possess more heterogeneity than those immunized with DNP-Pn. These immunochemical data indicate, for the first time, that the secretory IgA antibody response may possess an immune potential analogous to that seen in the serum antibody response.

The effect of the route of antigen administration on the secretory antibody response is difficult to evaluate because of the small number of animals in each group. However, it is readily apparent that oral immunization with either form of hapten-conjugate induces secretory IgA antibody production at a remote site (mammary gland). At least two explanations can account for these data; 1) antigen or some processed form of antigen could pass from the gut into the mammary tissue and induce a local secretory IgA response. It is known that BSA (9) and other soluble proteins (5, 10) are capable of triggering serum responses when administered orally. Our data from animals orally immunized with DNP-BGG show a detectable serum response which may indicate that this antigen gained access to remote secretory tissue. However, in the case of DNP-Pn, no serum antibodies were detected. Although our detection methods measure serum antibodies at the .01 μg level (P.C.M., unpublished observations), it is possible that low level serum responses could have been missed. Our findings are consistent with other studies in which oral immunization with pneumococcus has failed to induce serum antibodies (G. Schiffman, New York Univ., Downstate Med. Ctr., personal communication). Furthermore, studies on the intravenously immunized animals showed that when sufficient quantities of circulating DNP-Pn antigen were present to induce serum antibodies, secretory IgA antibodies were not induced. While the presence of some form of processed antigen which could escape detection or fail to trigger a serum response cannot be ruled out, we feel that a second explanation could account for the data obtained with the DNP-Pn antigen; 2) IgA precursor cells receive an initial stimulation in the gut and these stimulated cells migrate out and seed remote sites including secretory sites. Our data on animals orally immunized with DNP-Pn supports the notion of a preferential seeding of remote secretory sites, but factors influencing this seeding process remain obscure. Our observation that local intramammary immunization was as effective in inducing secretory IgA antibodies as oral immunization indicates that antigen may play a significant role. However, further investigation will be necessary to conclusively establish the existence of such a mechanism for secretory antibody induction.

Acknowledgements. This study was supported by USPHS grant DE-02623. E.T.L. is supported by a grant from the American Fund for Dental Education. We wish to thank C. Campbell and B. Margolis for their excellent technical assistance.

REFERENCES

1.   Tomasi, T.B. and Bienenstock, J., Adv. Immunol., 9:1, 1968.
2.   Tomasi, T.B., in Secretory Immunologic System, edited by
        D. Dayton, P. Small, R. Chanock, H. Kaufman and T.
        Tomasi, U.S. Government Printing Office, 1971.
3.   Tomasi, T.B., New Eng. J. Med., 287:500, 1972.
4.   Ogra, P.L., Karzon, D.T., Righthand, F. and MacGillivray,
        M., New Eng. J. Med., 279:893, 1968.
5.   Crabbe, P.A., Nash, D.R., Bazin, H., Eyssen, H. and
        Heremans, J.F., J. Exp. Med., 130:723, 1969.
6.   Genco, R.J. and Taubman, M.A., Nature, 221:679, 1969.
7.   Bazin, H., Levi, G. and Doria, G., J. Immunol., 105:1049, 1970.
8.   Taubman, M.A. and Genco, R.J., Immunochem., 8:1137, 1971.
9.   Dolezel, J. and Bienenstock, J., Cellular Immunol., 2:458, 1971.
10.   Heremans, J.F. and Bazin, H., Ann. N.Y. Acad. Sci., 190:
        268, 1971.
11.   Eddie, D.S., Schulkind, M.L. and Robbins, J.B., J. Immu-
        nol., 106:181, 1971.
12.   Bohl, E.H., Gupta, R.K.P., Olquin, M.V.F. and Saif, L.J.,
        Infect. Immunity, 6:289, 1972.
13.   Fubara, E.S. and Freter, R., Infect. Immunity, 6:965, 1972.
14.   Craig, S.W. and Cebra, J.J., J. Exp. Med., 134:188, 1971.
15.   Montgomery, P.C. and Pincus, J.H., J. Immunol., 111:42, 1973.
16.   Montgomery, P.C., Rosner, B.P. and Cohn, J., J. Immunol.
        Comm., submitted for publication.
17.   Benacerraf, B. and Levine, B.B., J. Exp. Med., 115:1023, 1962.
18.   Cebra, J.J. and Robbins, J.B., J. Immunol., 97:12, 1966.
19.   Wang, T.-I and Montgomery, P.C., Immunochem., 10:481, 1973.
20.   Stupp, Y., Yoshida, T. and Paul, W.E., J. Immunol., 103:
        625, 1969.
21.   Montgomery, P.C. and Williamson, A.R., J. Immunol., 109:
        1036, 1972.

HUMAN NASAL EXOCRINE IgA ANTIBODY: FORMATION AND SOME ACTIVITIES

Richard W. Newcomb

Children's Asthma Research Institute and
Hospital
Denver, Colorado, 80204

Evidence was sought for anamnestic attributes of exocrine IgA antibody production. A human was immunized with a protein antigen to which prior exposure was unlikely, serum albumin from Alligator mississippiensis (ASA). One mgN of ASA, diluted in saline and delivered repeatedly as nose drops during 5 consecutive days, constituted one "dose". Values for antigen binding by IgG, IgA and IgM were measured separately by radioimmunoprecipitation.

Five doses, given at 2 to 3 week intervals, failed to result in antibody production, but then 3 doses given on consecutive weeks were followed by the appearance of IgG and IgA antibodies in both serum and homogenized, concentrated nasal fluids. Local production and secretion of nasal IgA antibody were indicated by its levels, which were 19 times those in serum IgA, and 20 times those in sputum IgA and by its molecular size and possession of SC. Levels of this exocrine IgA antibody (exIgA-Ab) decreased rapidly, reaching half the initial value in 1 month, and becoming undetectable in 4 months. A single dose of ASA given then resulted in production of nasal exIgA-Ab. Nevertheless, subsequent immunizations, including doses given on 3 consecutive weeks, never resulted in exIgA-Ab values more than half the initial level, suggesting a negative feedback control on exIgA-Ab production.

Evidence for "maturation" of the exIgA-Ab response was sought in measurements of relative avidities of serum

IgG antibodies and exIgA-Ab. Avidities of neither class
of antibody showed any significant increase during the period of time studied, but exIgA-Ab samples had consistently
higher avidities than IgG antibodies.

Counitchansky et al. (1) have reported that trypsin
and chymotrypsin form proteolytically active complexes with
exocrine IgA, raising the possibility that exIgA-Ab, thus
carrying an enzyme molecule, might accelerate digestion of
its specific antigen. However, exIgA-Ab to ASA that had
been pre-incubated with trypsin was no more effective for
the proteolysis of ASA than trypsin alone. Moreover, we
were unable to confirm any effect of exocrine IgA on the
rate of digestion of TAME by trypsin, casting doubt upon
the presence of IgA-enzyme complexes.

Taubman and Genco (2) have observed that rabbit colostral IgA antibodies to group A streptococcal polysaccharide
did not precipitate polyvalent antigen, but in fact inhibited antigen precipitation by IgG antibodies. They suggested that their observations could by explained by a high
degree of monogamous polyvalency of exIgA-Ab. Similarly,
our preparations of exIgA-Ab to ASA did not precipitate radioiodinated ASA at a wide range of antigen-antibody ratios,
at concentrations up to 100 times the precipitating concentration of IgG antibodies, and at pH 8.0 or 5.5. Nevertheless, precipitation of labelled ASA by IgG antibodies (human or rabbit) was only slightly inhibited by prior incubation of antigen with excess exIgA-Ab. The inability of ex-
IgA-Ab to precipitate ASA was not caused by inhibitors of
precipitation that we have described in high molecular-
weight fractions of respiratory fluids (3). Furthermore
the ability of exIgA-Ab to cross-link molecules of ASA was
indicated by three findings: the exIgA-Ab was very effective
in agglutinating passively sensitized red blood cells. When
exIgA-Ab was reacted with an insoluble immunoadsorbent composed of ASA coupled to cellulose, the adsorbed exIgA-Ab
could still react with soluble labelled ASA, effectively
binding labelled ASA to the immunoadsorbent. In the radioimmunoprecipitation test, values of IgG antibodies are augmented by complexes of exIgA-Ab with soluble antigen that
tend to cross-link antigen to the IgG-antibody-antigen complexes (4).

These results clearly show that the failure of exIgA-
Ab to precipitate ASA is not explicable by excessive monogamous polyvalency.

Acknowledgements: Supported by a grant from the John A. Hartford Foundation, Inc.

REFERENCES

1. Counitchansky, Y., Berthillier, G., Got, R., Clin. Chim. Acta, 30:83, 1970.
2. Taubman, N.A., Genco, R.J., Immunochemistry, 8:1137, 1971.
3. Newcomb, R.W.,Immunol. Commun., II:3, 1973.
4. Newcomb, R.W., Ishizaka, K., DeVald, B.L.,J. Immunol. 103:215, 1969.

THE IgA ANTIBODY-FORMING CELL RESPONSE IN THE RABBIT
SUBMANDIBULAR GLAND FOLLOWING SEVERAL DIFFERENT METHODS
OF IMMUNIZATION

Fred G. Emmings and Robert J. Genco

Department of Oral Biology, School of

Dentistry, State University of New York at
Buffalo, 4510 Main Street, Buffalo,N.Y. 14226

INTRODUCTION

Secretory IgA (sIgA) is found in the saliva of humans
and other animals where its principle sources are the major
salivary glands. Taubman and Smith (1) showed that salivary
IgA antibody, induced by vaccination with cariogenic S. mutans, was correlated with a decrease in dental caries in
rats. The practical use of the secretory immune system in
protection against disease in humans depends partly on a
clear understanding of the mechanisms which govern the induction of a secretory immune response. There are numerous
reports showing that topical application of antigen to the
gastrointestinal or respiratory tracts can result in induction of sIgA antibodies (cf. reviews 11,12). It is not clear
however, how best to induce sIgA antibody production in
solid organs such as the salivary and lacrimal glands. In
this study we systematically examined several methods of immunization designed to stimulate a secretory immune response
in the salivary glands of rabbits.

METHODS AND RESULTS

A combined direct and indirect immunofluorescent staining (IFS) technic was developed to evaluate effects of immunization. Purified IgG from immune sera was conjugated with
fluorescein or rhodamine and chromatographed on DEAE-cellu-
lose. Conjugate fractions were absorbed and tested for

specificity by gel diffusion. Tissues fixed in formalin
(13) were frozen, sectioned, and then incubated with a rhodamine conjugate specific for one of the three major Ig
classes diluted in a solution containing 2 mg/ml dinitrophenylated human gamma globulin ($DNP_{17}HGG$). Sections were
washed and incubated with an anti-DNP fluorescein conjugate.
Fluorescence microscopy revealed antibody to DNP and Ig
class simultaneously in the same cell. Specificity of the
staining reactions was confirmed by blocking of immunoglobulin staining with concentrated unconjugated homologous antiserum and by antigen absorption. Blocking of antibody staining was accomplished by adsorption of the anti-DNP conjugate
with insolubilized DNP or by the addition of $10^{-3}M$ DNP-
lysine.

We first determined the response of rabbits to direct
submandibular injection of dinitrophenylated bovine serum
albumin ($DNP_{24}BSA$). After ether anesthesia the submandibular
glands were surgically exposed and injected with $DNP_{24}BSA$ in
saline or in one of several adjuvants (see Table 1). Rabbits
were sacrificed after 16 days, their glands excised and sections from at least 2 parts were evaluated by direct and
combined IFS. Ten fields (480x) were examined in each section and stained cells in at least 40 fields counted from
each gland. From Table 1, it can be seen that adjuvant had
no effect on total numbers of IgA-containing cells in the
gland but the number of IgG-containing cells increased. In
the glands injected with antigen alone 90% of the anti-DNP
cells contained IgA. In the glands injected with adjuvant,
almost all of the anti-DNP cells were located in the wall of
the granuloma and 90% of these contained IgG. Salivary glands
taken from rabbits 6 hr. after injection of $DNP_{24}BSA$ in saline showed, by direct IFS, a uniform distribution of antigen. These experiments showed that immunization of the salivary glands with DNP-BSA in saline resulted in selective
stimulation of an IgA antibody response.

To test the effect of preimmunization on this IgA antibody-forming cell (AFC) response, two groups of rabbits were
preimmunized either by feeding $DNP_{17-24}BSA$ for 28 days, or
by multiple intraperitoneal (IP) injections of $DNP_{17-24}BSA$
over several months. These 2 groups and a third group of
unsensitized rabbits were subsequently immunized by direct
injection of the submandibular glands with $DNP_{24}BSA$ in saline as described above. It can be seen from Fig. 1, that
the group which had **not** been preimmunized prior to local

Table 1. Evaluation of Immunocyte Response in Submandibular
Gland to Local Immunization

Group(a)	Ig-Containing Cells/10 HPF		Anti-DNP Cells		
	IgA(range)(b)	IgG(range)(b)	/10 HPF	%IgA	%IgG
Non-immune	102(60-155)	22(0-54)		0	0
DNP(e) in saline	86(82-90)	21(14-35)	1.6	89.3	10.5
DNP in CFA(d)	83(82-90)	43(0-109)	17.0	4.5	86.7
DNP in alum + B. pert.(g)	76(51-107)	79(39-127)	10.0	0	97.4
DNP in IFA(d)	86(53-109)	34(0-83)		ND(f)	ND
DNP in alum	81(28-128)	57(4-136)		ND	ND
Toxoplasma gondii	81(44-197)	35(3-55)		0	0

(a) 2 rabbits each group; (b) Average at least 40 hi-power
(480x) fields (HPF); (c) Number of cells staining with both
anti-IgA and anti-DNP conjugates as a % of total anti-DNP
staining cells (at least 15 cells); (d) CFA and IFA-complete
and incomplete Freund's adjuvant; (e) $DNP_{24}BSA$; (f) Not Done;
(g) Alum precipitated $DNP_{24}BSA$ with 1.5×10^7 Bordetella
pertussis organisms/ml.

immunization responded with 46% of the anti-DNP cells containing IgA after 8 days and 89% after 16 days. All of the
anti-DNP cells in this group were found to contain either
IgG, IgA, or IgM.

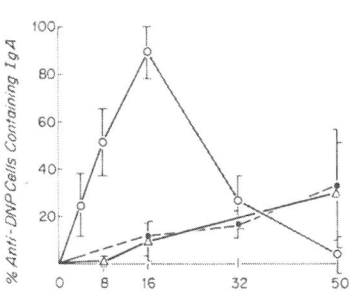

Figure 1. Percent of anti-DNP cells containing IgA in the
submandibular glands of rabbits at intervals following local
immunization of the gland with $DNP_{24}BSA$ in saline. 0-local
immunization only; ● - fed 0.1% $DNP_{17}BSA$ in drinking water
for 28 days prior to local immunization; Δ - extensively intraperitoneally immunized for 6 months prior to local immunization. Vertical bars represent 2 standard errors of
the mean.

This early IgA anti-DNP response was not seen in either pre-immunized group. Total numbers of IgA anti-DNP cells in the non-preimmunized group were greatest at 8 days. At this interval the IP pre-immunized group contained similar total numbers of anti-DNP cells while the fed group contained less than 6% of that number.

No anti-DNP cells were found in submandibular glands of rabbits which had been preimmunized and then sham immunized in the glands. Also, no IgA anti-DNP cells were found in the Peyer's patches, small intestines or mesenteric nodes of rabbits selected from any of the groups. In the IP preimmunized group serum antibodies to BSA were detectable by gel diffusion and antibodies to DNP by radioimmunoprecipitation. Serums of the fed group contained no antibodies to DNP but 40% of the rabbits showed antibody to BSA.

DISCUSSION

We have presented evidence for an early transitory IgA-AFC response following primary immunization of a salivary gland with antigen in saline solution. This is consistent with other studies (3,4) based on appearance of IgA antibodies in serum and secretions which show peak IgA responses 4-9 days after primary immunization. Though the percentage of IgA-AFC peaked at 16 days, we found significant numbers of IgA-AFC as early as 4 days and total numbers of IgA-AFC highest at 8 days. Walters and Jackson(5) immunized mice IP with E. coli lipopolysaccharide and, using a modification of the Jerne plaque technic, found peak numbers of IgA plaque-forming cells in the spleen 5 days after primary immunization.

The early IgA-AFC response to DNP-BSA was depressed by feeding or intraperitoneal injection of this antigen prior to direct submandibular gland immunization. Since the IP group had serum antibody to DNP, we carried out a passive immunization experiment to determine if preexisting serum antibody would depress the early IgA-AFC response. Normal rabbits were injected intravenously with antiserum obtained from rabbits in the IP preimmunized group. The passively immunized rabbits showed an early transitory IgA-AFC response to submandibular injection similar to that seen in normal rabbits. These experiments suggest that there is little effect of serum antibody on the secretory immune response. There is an indication from our data that the rabbits fed DNP-BSA were partially tolerant to DNP since the total numbers of anti-DNP cells, as well as the % of anti-DNP cells which contained IgA, were markedly depressed as compared to the non-preimmunized group. Tolerance to haptens has been induced by feeding (7,8). Tolerance can result from unresponsiveness in either T-cell or B-cell populations or both (10). Since the IgA response appears to be more T-cell dependent than the IgC or IgM responses (9,2), we suggest that depression of the IgA-AFC response seen in our experiments was due to partial T-cell tolerance induced by prior exposure to antigen.

The experiments reported here show that local injection of antigen into a major salivary gland can give rise to an early, transient IgA antibody-forming cell response. This response can be markedly depressed by prior exposure to antigen suggesting an interplay between the secretory immune system and systemic immune systems.

These studies were supported in part by U.S.P.H.S. Grants DE-02814, DE-0167 and United Way Fellowship FTF-10-UB-72 and U.S.P.H.S. Fellowship F3-DE-37,958.

REFERENCES

1. Taubman, M.A. and Smith, D.J., J. Dent. Res. 52:(spec. issue):277, 1973.
2. Perey, D. and Bienenstock, J., J. Immunol. 111:633, 1973.
3. Bandilla, K.K. and McDuffie, F.C., Fed. Proc. 27:563, 1968.
4. Mäkelä, et al., in Nobel Symposium 3, Gamma Globulins, Structure and Control of Biosynthesis, ed. by J. Killander, Almquist and Wiksell, Stockholm, 1967.
5. Walters, C.S. and Jackson, A.L., J. Immunol. 101:541, 1968.
6. Tada, T. and Okumura, K., J. Immunol. 106:1002, 1971.
7. Chase, M.W., Proc. Soc. Exp. Biol. Med. 61:257, 1946.
8. Pomeranz, J.R., J. Immunol. 104:1486, 1970.
9. Clough, et al., J. Immunol. 107:1624, 1971.
10. Chiller, et al., Science 171:813, 1971.
11. Tomasi, T.B., Ann. Rev. Med. 21:281, 1970.
12. Tomasi, T.B. and Grey, H.M., Prog. in Allergy 16:81, 1972.
13. Eidelman, S. and Bershauer, J.A., Stain Technology 44:43, 1969.

THE ESTABLISHMENT OF SYSTEMIC IMMUNITY FOLLOWING ANTIGENIC STIMULATION OF THE LYMPHOID TISSUE OF THE GASTROINTESTINAL MUCOSA

Richard M. Rothberg, Sumner C. Kraft and
Suzanne M. Michalek
Departments of Pediatrics and Medicine
Pritzker School of Medicine
University of Chicago
Chicago, Illinois 60637

Despite a considerable literature about secretory immunoglobulins and their possible exocrine functions (1), the systemic immune responses which follow local immunization at mucosal surfaces have received relatively little attention. This aspect of local immunization is important since this is the way mammals normally become immunized against environmental antigens such as food, bacterial and transplantation antigens (2,3,4). Using a food antigen, systemic aspects of local immunization have been investigated in adult rabbits drinking water containing 0.1% bovine serum albumin (BSA). Such orally immunized animals produce circulating anti-BSA in the absence of circulating immunogenic concentrations of the antigen (2). This antibody appears to recognize only surface antigenic sites rather than new determinants exposed by digestion (5) and a relative absence of circulating antigen reactive lymphocytes has been demonstrated during oral immunization (6).

The preferential circulation of lymphocytes to the lymphoid tissue of origin, with about 10% being sequestered in the spleen (7), suggested the present experiments to learn a) if splenectomy would permit detection of antigen reactive cells in the circulation of orally immunized animals, b) the distribution of active anti-BSA producing cells among the lymphoid tissues of orally immunized animals, and c) if the peripheral lymphoid tissues of such animals have acquired the capacity to produce anti-BSA upon direct stimulation.

Splenectomized or intact rabbits were orally, subcutaneously, or intravenously (i.v.) immunized against BSA. Circulating antibodies were measured by the ammonium sulfate technique (6), circulating antigen-reactive cells (ARC) were detected by ^{3}H-thymidine incorporation into short-term lymphocyte cultures (6), and antibody forming cells (PFC) were detected by a modified Jerne plaque technique (8).

The amounts of antibody detected in the splenectomized and sham-operated orally and parenterally immunized animals were comparable. The effect of splenectomy on the detection of circulating BSA responsive lymphocytes following oral or parenteral immunization is shown in Table I. Splenectomy reduced the detection of ARC after i.v. immunization but did not alter the detectability of ARC in the subcutaneous group. Splenectomy, however, enhanced the capacity to detect ARC in the orally immunized group in that 4 of 15 cultures from splenectomized animals responded to BSA in contrast to only 3 of 61 cultures from intact animals (p <0.01).

Since these data suggested a cellular mechanism for the dissemination of the capacity to produce anti-BSA, from the lamina propria to the systemic lymphoid tissues, the distribution of active PFC was determined. Figure 1 shows that the spleen was the major site of antibody production in the i.v. immunized animals. Despite 3- to 10-fold greater amounts of circulating antibody, lower concentrations of PFC were detected at a later date in the spleens of the subcutaneously and orally immunized animals. The peripheral lymph nodes were the major site of anti-BSA production in

TABLE I

Effect of splenectomy on cellular immune responses following parenteral or oral immunization to BSA.

Immunization route	Splenectomy	Number of animals	Number of positive cultures/ Total	Significance (p value)
Intra-	No	5	5/15	<0.05
venous	Yes	4	0/12	
Subcu-	No	9	23/43	N.S.
taneous	Yes	4	7/11	
Oral	No	14	3/61	<0.01
	Yes	5	4/15	

the subcutaneously immunized animals; the high concentrations of PFC in these lymph nodes are shown by the numbers
above the curve. Essentially no PFC were detected in the
peripheral lymph nodes of the orally immunized group. The
mesenteric lymph nodes from all 3 groups contained no PFC/
10^6 lymphocytes except for small numbers in the subcutaneous group on day 30. To increase the sensitivity of the assay, 10^7 lymphocytes from the mesenteric lymph nodes were
cultured and the results are shown in Figure 2. During the
40-day period, only small numbers of PFC were found in the
mesenteric nodes of the orally immunized group, confirming
that this was not the major site of antibody production in
these animals.

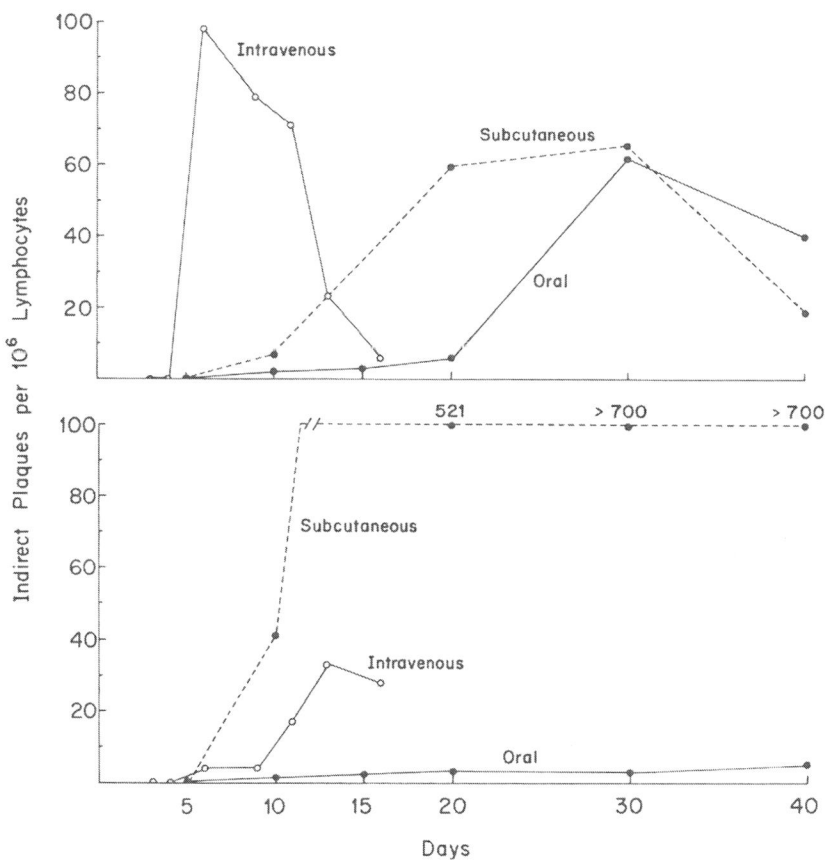

Figure 1. Concentration of anti-BSA producing cells per
10^6 lymphocytes in spleen (top) and peripheral lymph nodes
(bottom). Each point on the oral immunization curves represents the mean response of 4 or more animals.

The lymphoid tissues of the orally immunized animals were also studied by the direct PFC technique at a concentration of 10^7 lymphocytes per culture. The spleen and peripheral nodes contained more than 5 direct PFC during the appearance of detectable circulating antibody (days 10 and 15) but, except for one instance (day 40 in the peripheral nodes), none of the lymphoid tissues contained more than occasional PFC during the remainder of the experiment. The only PFC detected in Peyer's patches or the appendix were found in the latter by the direct technique just prior to the appearance of detectable circulating antibody.

These findings suggested that following low dose antigen ingestion systemic immunization occurs in the absence of significant antibody production by the systemic lymphoid tissues. To demonstrate the presence of cells capable of antibody production in the systemic lymphoid tissues, 3 rabbits drinking 0.1% BSA for 7 weeks were given 50 mg i.v. BSA 24 hours after stopping antigen ingestion. In addition, 4 nonimmunized rabbits were identically injected and 4 animals were only orally immunized for 5 to 7 weeks. Circulating antibody concentrations were measured prior to and 3

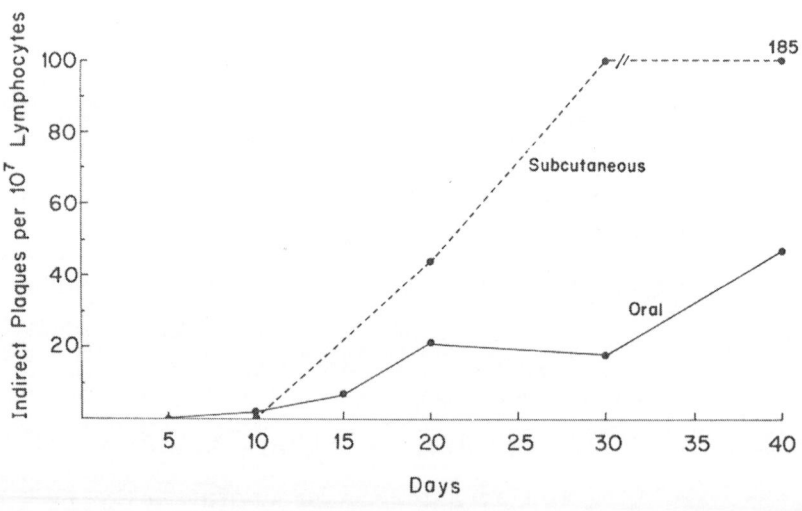

Figure 2. Anti-BSA producing cells per 10^7 lymphocytes in the mesenteric lymph nodes.

days after the injection, and concentrations of PFC were determined on the third day by both indirect and direct techniques. Table II shows that circulating anti-BSA was not
detected in the previously nonimmunized animals and the pre-
injection amounts of circulating antibody were comparable
in the orally immunized groups. Two of the 3 orally immunized animals receiving the i.v. injection had no detectable circulating antibody 3 days later; there was a marked
reduction in the amount detected in the third animal. Indirect PFC were not detectable 3 days after the i.v. injection of nonimmunized animals, while the animals only ingest-
ing BSA had a mean concentration of PFC similar to that previously observed in orally immunized animals. Following
i.v. challenge, orally immunized animals demonstrated a
marked increase in the number of indirect PFC in all 3 lymphoid tissues. This was most striking in the mesenteric
lymph nodes where the concentration of PFC in each of the 3
animals exceeded all previously observed concentrations. A
similar increase in PFC was detected in the peripheral nodes
of 2 of these 3 animals. Direct PFC were found only in the
spleens of the i.v. challenged orally immunized animals:
mean concentration 105 per 10^7 lymphocytes (range 2-289).

The present studies provide additional evidence that
prolonged exposure of intestinal lymphoid tissue to low concentrations of ingested BSA is followed by the local production of antibody and a gradual sensitization of systemic
lymphoid tissues by the dissemination of sensitized lympho-

TABLE II
Circulating anti-BSA and anti-BSA producing cells in orally
immunized rabbits 3 days after 50 mg BSA intravenously

Immuni- zation route	No. of animals	Mean antigen binding capacity[a]		Mean indirect PFC/10^6 lymphocytes		
		Before i.v. BSA	After i.v. BSA	Spleen	Mesen- teric nodes	Peri- pheral nodes
Intraven- ous only	4	0	0	0	0	0
Oral only (7 wks)	4	4.0	-	44	4	4
Oral (7 wks) plus i.v.	3	5.3	0.4	353	243	195

[a]The μg I*BSA N bound by 1.0 ml of antiserum when 0.02 μg
I*BSA N was the amount of antigen added.

cytes. The antigen or its fragment must enter the lamina propria and antigen recognition occur. The ensuing steps in the lamina propria are unknown but they are followed by the appearance of specific antibody. The relative absence of PFC in the spleens and lymph nodes of orally immunized animals confirms that these tissues had not been exposed to immunogenic concentrations of antigen prior to the appearance of circulating antibody. After circulating antibody is present, any antigen entering the lymphatic or systemic circulation should be bound and prevent the sensitization of systemic lymphoid tissues (9). Furthermore, a significant decrease in the intestinal absorption of 0.1% BSA has been demonstrated following oral immunization against this antigen (10).

REFERENCES

1. The Secretory Immunologic System, Edited by D.H. Dayton, P.A. Small, R.M. Chanock, H.E. Kaufman, and T.B. Tomasi, U.S. Government Printing Office, Washington, D.C., 1971.
2. Rothberg, R.M., Kraft, S.C., Farr, R.S., Kriebel, G.W., and Goldberg, S.S., ibid, p. 293.
3. Robbins, J.B., Parke, J.C., Scheerson, R., and Wishnant, J.K., Pediat. Res., 7:103, 1973.
4. Mittal, K.K., Terasaki, P.I., Springer, G.F., Desai, P.R., McIntire, F.C., and Hirata, A.A., Trans. Proc., 5:499, 1973.
5. Wright, R.N. and Rothberg, R.M., J. Immunol., 107:1410, 1971.
6. Goldberg, S.S., Kraft, S.C., Peterson, R.D.A. and Rothberg, R.M., J. Immunol., 107:757, 1971.
7. Griscelli, C., Vassalli, P., and McCluskey, R.T., J. Exp. Med., 130:1427, 1969.
8. Rothberg, R.M., Kraft, S.C., Asquith, P., and Michalek, S.M., Cell. Immunol., 7:124, 1973.
9. Uhr, J.W. and Moller, G., Adv. Immunol., 8:81, 1968.
10. Walker, W.A., Isselbacher, K.J., and Bloch, K.J., Science, 177:608, 1972.

DISCUSSION

Dr. Lawton - Perhaps I can ask a question of Dr. Emmings. Dr. Emmings, you did not show, I don't believe, the total number of cells making DNP antibodies in glands of animals preimmunized with DNP-BSA and then challenged locally. Were there fewer IgG antibody forming cells, as well as IgA producers?

Dr. Emmings - Are you asking whether the remainder of the anti-DNP cells contain IgG?

Dr. Lawton - I am asking whether, when you preimmunized the animals and then stimulated them locally in the submandibular glands, the total number of anti-DNP cells was suppressed, or only that fraction making IgA anti-DNP?

Dr. Emmings - There were many anti-DNP cells of other classes than IgA in the intraperitoneal preimmunized group but not in the fed group.

Dr. John Butler - I would like to ask Dr. Montgomery if he has looked at the binding affinity of either local or serum IgG or IgM antibodies. Do these antibodies have similar affinities and heterogeneity indices as you reported for the IgA response?

Dr. Montgomery - No, we have not. We could look at the IgG antibodies, but no IgM production was detected. In other rabbits immunized with DNP-Pn the affinities of anti-DNP serum antibodies are usually low, on the order of 10^5 liters/mole (see J. Immunol. $\underline{111}$:42, 1973). At any rate the affinities to DNP on bovine gamma globulin as carrier are usually much higher, around 10^8 liters/mole. But we have not looked at affinity of serum antibodies in rabbits used in this study.

Dr. Genco - I have been deferring enough questions; I would like to respond to that. Dr. Taubman and I have data comparing IgG and IgA secretory IgA antibodies to N-acetylglucosamine purified from the same colostrum. The IgG antibodies are about a log higher in affinity than the IgA antibodies.

Dr. Cebra - The apparent monogamous polyvalency that Dr. Newcomb showed for rabbit secretory IgA need not mean that

this dimeric IgA may differ in conformation in solution or
on an E.M. grid from the conformation of human IgA. It
could actually reflect a difference in segmental flexibility
or ability say, for the molecule to bend. It is of interest
that the sensitive phage assay for antibody seems to require,
for the phage inactivation, cross linking of tail fibers.
In our lab, Dr. Cordele has shown that guinea pig gamma 1
and gamma 2 antibodies differ and that gamma 1 antibodies
do not seem to inactivate haptenated phage. You can correlate this by fluorescence polarization decay measurements
with diminished segmental flexibility of the gamma 1 molecule. Ray and Makala, looking at IgA from the mouse which
they raised in vitro, showed that this dimeric IgA does
inactivate haptenated phage. It would be very interesting
to look at whether secretory IgA from the rabbit would or
would not, and to do segmental flexibility studies on this
molecule.

I have a question for Dr. Montgomery. Leaving aside
the Farr binding assay which reflects affinities as well as
amounts and what have you, he must have isolated his antibodies in order to do equilibrium dialysis and site counting.
I would like to know with absolute values whether group 4
which were the orally immunized animals had more or less
antibody than could be isolated than those animals that were
injected directly into the mammary tissue.

Dr. Montgomery - The answer to your question is that they
were comparable. We have had few animals with sufficient
antibody to isolate, but the numbers on that last slide
reflect absolute concentrations. We could see no difference
in the injected and fed groups. In both we had some high and
some low responders. The higher responses seemed to occur
with the DNP-Pn immunized animals rather than in the DNP-BGG
group.

Dr. Hijmans - I have a question for Dr. Rothberg. Does he
or anybody else have data on the contribution of the bone
marrow to the antibody pool? The reason I am asking this
question is that we have found evidence that in man the bone
marrow can be considered a major source of circulating
immunoglobulins. Dr. Benner and his colleagues have now
shown that this also can be true under certain conditions in
mice. Do you have any information concerning this source or
the role of the bone marrow under these experimental conditions?

Dr. Lawton - Dr. Rothberg says no. Dr. Heremans?

Dr. Heremans - I have three remarks. Firstly, as to the
hypothesis presented by Dr. Newcomb that the internal linkage could occur in an antigen molecule exposed to secretory
IgA antibodies. I find this difficult to believe because
that would mean that the same antigeneic determinant should
occur twice at least in a single polypeptide chain, and
usually polypeptide chains are not repetitive in their
sequence. Now, of course, the alligator albumin may be somewhat unusual. I know nothing about it, but still I think it
is a dangerous hypothesis to work on. My second remark
concerns the tolerance effect reported by Dr. Emmings. Two
days ago I showed you a slide in which it could be seen that
after oral feeding of sheep red blood cells for four days
the animals went into a prolonged state of tolerance, as far
as the plaque forming cell response in the spleen was concerned, to repeated administration of the same antigen. This
is obviously the same phenomenon that has been shown today
by Dr. Emmings and also by, I think, Dr. Newcomb. It is
fairly pleasing to see that other people can reproduce a
finding and gain information that it is not only a matter
of secretory antibody preventing the further uptake of
antigen as we show, but that there must be a real tolerance
phenomenon behind it in addition. Now the third remark concerns the data presented by the group of Dr. Rothberg and
Dr. Kraft. You will have noticed that there is a consistent
discrepancy between their findings on oral immunization and
those of several other groups including our own. We in
general find that oral immunization leads to an early immune
response of systemic nature which is, however, selectively
addressed to the IgA class, whereas they cannot find this.
We have found this for mice, for rats and for guinea pigs,
and believe it to be a rather general phenomenon. I am very
surprised that their rabbits will not obey that law. Perhaps
genetic or species factors are at play because we know that
certain strains of mice refuse to mount an IgA response
following oral immunization.

Dr. Bohl - In regard to the paper by Dr. Montgomery, I would
like to say that to those of us who are interested in providing passive immunity against intestinal infections, this
paper is quite meaningful. It gives additional data on the
relationship between an antigeneic stimulation of the gastrointestinal tract and the presence of IgA antibodies in
mammary secretions, suggesting that if one wants to provide

passive immunity against intestinal infections to suckling
animals, an obvious approach is to orally vaccinate females.
I think this has already been shown in the case of transmissible gastroenteritis (TGE) viral infection in swine. Also,
Dr. Kohler and I have some preliminary information that this
approach is effective in enteric colibacillosis in suckling
newborn pigs. Dr. Ogra made a statement yesterday to the
effect that if serologically negative women were vaccinated
intramuscularly with killed polio vaccine, IgA polio antibodies were found in mammary secretions. I think this is
essentially what he has stated. Now, this is at first
glance in contradiction to what Montgomery and I have indicated might happen in the case of rabbits and swine, respectively; but there is one point that should be considered
as a possible explanation. It could very well be that the
serologically negative women have been previously infected
with polio virus but, perhaps, sufficiently long ago that
they no longer had detectable antibodies in their sera.
Thus, it would be very interesting to examine the colostrum
of so-called serologically negative women to see if antibodies against polio could be detected. Examination of
colostrum for antibodies might be a much more sensitive
method for indicating past infections with enteric pathogens
than screening for the presence of serum antibodies. We
have found this to be true in the case of swine.

Dr. Bienenstock - I am intrigued by some of the consistent
discrepancies which appear in the type of work presented
today, as evidenced by Drs. Emmings and Rothberg, and I
would like to ask a general question. One of the differences
appears to relate to methodology. Can one compare the Jerne
plaque technique, either direct or indirect, with methods for
detecting specific antibody in cells using radiolabeled or
fluorescinated antigens? The question that I have is whether
or not, in fact, the appearance of antibody containing cells
has to be necessarily correlated with antibody producing
cells. In other words, could there be an essential difference between antibody containing cells and antibody producing
cells and is there potentially a mechanism which switches
the cell from simply synthesis to synthesis for export?

Dr. Rothberg - I would like to respond to both comments. I
think that technique has a great deal to do with these results. In our studies we have been using the indirect Jerne
technique which would include IgA cells as well as IgG cells.
We have had great difficulty with rabbits, or at least our

rabbit strain, in getting specific IgA plaques, so we are
reporting only 7S antibody production, and not whether it is
IgG or IgA. In the newborn human, as well as in other animals,
IgA cells are present along the gut but IgA is not generally
found in serum for a few weeks. I think this may be the case
in our studies; we may indeed have local IgA producers in
the gut which export antibodies into the secretions for
several weeks before serum antibodies are found. Antigen
dose is another important consideration. We have stuck to
our 0.1% BSA immunization schedule in the rabbit because we
are sure that this produces a local immune response. In
studies done with Dr. Bienenstock, similar immunization of
rats failed to induce systemic antibodies at all.

THE RELATIONSHIP BETWEEN SERUM AND SALIVARY ANTIBODIES
AND CELL-MEDIATED IMMUNITY IN ORAL DISEASE IN MAN

T. Lehner, S.J. Challacombe, L. Ivanyi and
J.M.A. Wilton
Department of Oral Immunology and Microbiology
Guy's Hospital Medical and Dental Schools
London, SE1 9RT

INTRODUCTION

Immunity to diseases of the mouth shows considerable
complexity, as the three principal immune systems, secretory
and serum antibodies and cell mediated immunity, can be involved in the development and course of the diseases. Humoral and cellular immune responses to the commensal organisms,
as well as to the aggregation of bacteria and their products
on the tooth surface (bacterial plaque), have been studied
recently. The immune responses to fungal, viral, Gram-
positive and Gram-negative organisms in normal subjects, and
in patients with the disease these organisms may cause, are
worthy of analysis, as they may clarify the factors responsible for protection.

The findings in normal subjects suggest that in some
oral diseases effective protection from infection requires
an intact immune response of secretory and serum antibodies,
as well as cell-mediated immunity. Recent sequential studies
with bacterial plaque accumulation in man revealed that
immunization through the gingiva may take place under relatively normal conditions (1). Whilst serum haemagglutinating
antibody titres remain constant, cell-mediated immune responses are increased both to related antigens, Veillonella
alcalescnes, Actinomyces viscosus and autologous plaque soni-
cates, and to apparently unrelated antigens, PPD and Proteus
mirabilis. This investigation was designed to explore the
possibility that gingival immunization by means of bacterial

plaque accumulation might induce secretory antibodies and
changes in serum and salivary immunoglobulin concentration.
A further aim was to analyse the changes in B and T lymphocyte responses, using endotoxin to stimulate lymphocytes and
the mixed leucocyte reaction, and to test for salivary and
serum antibodies and cell-mediated immune responses to
Streptococcus mutans.

MATERIALS AND METHODS

The investigation was carried out in 6 male and 4
female subjects, 21-23 years old. They were instructed to
stop using a toothbrush, mouthwash or any other cleansing
aid for 28 days (2). Samples of venous blood were with-
drawn from all subjects and unstimulated whole saliva was
collected for 5 minutes from 4 subjects before and then at
weekly intervals during the period of abstention from oral
hygiene, between 9:00 and 9:30 a.m. After the blood and
saliva samples were taken on day 28, most of the plaque was
removed mechanically and the subjects started cleaning their
teeth; any remaining plaque was carefully removed a week
later. Blood and saliva samples were then collected at about
monthly intervals up to day 98; after separation of the serum
and centrifuging the saliva at 2,000g for 20 minutes the samples were stored at -20°C. The gingival index (3) was also
recorded throughout the period of study.

Leucocyte cultures from all subjects were prepared in
duplicate or triplicate with each antigen and without antigen,
in the presence of 15% autologous serum, and were harvested
and assayed by methods described previously (4). However,
the mixed leucocyte culture MLC (5) and stimulation of
lymphocytes with endotoxin were carried out only in 4 subjects. In the MLC 0.5ml (5 x 10^5) of mitomycin treated
lymphocytes were added to a culture of 0.5ml (5 x 10^5) of
lymphocytes. The results were expressed in terms of the
stimulation index (SI), as the ratio of ^{14}C thymidine uptake
in antigen stimulated and control cultures.

Macrophage migration inhibition test (MMI) (6) was performed by the indirect method (7). The migration index (MI)
was calculated as the ratio between the migration area of
macrophages in antigen-stimulated and control culture supernatants.

Haemagglutination test (8) was used for serum antibodies
(9) and salivary antibodies were estimated by a modified

micromethod (10). The results were expressed as the mean
$\log_2$ reciprocal titre of 2 separate estimations.

Complement fixation test was performed (11) in WHO trays,
using 3 HC50 of guinea pig complement and 2% Alsever preserved sheep red cells, sensitized with 1:400 rabbit haemo-
lytic serum (Wellcome Reagents). The results were expressed
as in the haemagglutination test.

Immunoglobulin estimation: Serum IgG, IgM and IgA and
salivary IgA were estimated (12). The MRC serum standards
were used for both serum and saliva and the specific antisera to the heavy chains were supplied by Wellcome Laboratories. The MRC standards were converted from units to
mg/100ml by the following factors: x 10 for IgG, x 2 for IgA
and x 0.7 for IgM.

Antigens: Streptococcus mutans (S. mutans; Ingbritt)
and Veillonella alcalescens (V. alcalescens) were cultured
and disintegrated by ultrasonication and used in dilutions
of 1:10, 1:20 and 1:4, 1:8 as described previously (4).
Purified cell wall antigen was prepared from S. mutans (13)
and used at an optimal concentration of 10mg/ml (14). Lipopolysaccharide from V. alcalescens was prepared by the phenol-
water extraction procedure (15) and used at a previously determined optimal concentration of 100µg/ml.

RESULTS

Basic response of serum and salivary immunoglobulins
and T and B lymphocytes to accumulation of bacterial plaque:
Accumulation of bacterial plaque was associated with a rise
in the gingival index of inflammation from a mean value of
0.23 (+ standard error of 0.04) to that of 1.22 (+ 0.06) from
day 0 to 28 and then dropped rapidly to 0.46 (+ 0.08) by day
35 and to the pre-experimental value by day 49 (Fig. 1).
Salivary IgA concentration showed only an increase from a
mean value of 5.0mg/100ml to 7.4mg/100ml by day 7 and then
stayed between 6 and 7mg/100ml up to day 35, after which it
fell to a baseline level by day 56. Serum IgA concentration
was increased from a mean level of 150mg on day 0 to 178mg/
100ml by day 21, and after falling to the baseline level on
day 28 it increased to 183mg/100ml by day 49 to 56. Serum
IgM showed only a small increase from 86mg/100ml to 101mg/
100ml by day 14 and it further increased to 120mg/100ml by
day 77-98. Serum IgG was increased from a mean concentration

of 1060mg/100ml to 1200mg/100ml by day 14 and an elevated
level was maintained throughout the period of observation.
The standard errors of the mean immunoglobulin concentrations
were rather large so that the changes failed to reach the 5%
level of significance. The large standard errors reflect
the wide variation in immunological indices from one subject
to another; the results are therefore also given for a single subject, as an illustration of the comparative changes
in the immunological indices (Fig. 2). The gingival index
of inflammation increased from 0.25 to 0.67 by day 14 and
reached a peak value of 0.82 by day 28. Salivary IgA and
serum IgA and IgG concentrations increased, but the time
course was different from those of the mean values.

Stimulation of lymphocytes by endotoxin was negative
before (1.0 $\pm$ 0.2) and during the initial 14 days of bacterial plaque accumulation (Fig. 1). A significant level was
reached by day 21 (2.0 $\pm$ 0.06) and maximum lymphocyte transformation of 3.6 ($\pm$ 1.35) was found by day 28, with low levels being maintained up to day 98 (2.1 $\pm$ 0.09). The MLC
reaction was enhanced, increasing from 8.4 ($\pm$ 2.9) on day 0
to a peak value of 31.8 ($\pm$ 13.2) by day 21 and falling to a
baseline level by day 35 (6.9 $\pm$ 1.0), but showing a further
rise by day 77-98 to 21.8 ($\pm$ 5.3). Profiles for the MLC
and endotoxin stimulation are also given for the single subject (Fig. 2), and these are comparable with the mean values
of the group.

Specific serum and salivary antibodies and cell-mediated
immune response to Streptococcus mutans: Secretory IgA
haemagglutinating antibodies to cell walls of S. mutans were
found in whole saliva but showed little variation in the
titre which remained between $\log_2$ 2 and 3 (Fig. 3). Serum
haemagglutinating and complement fixing antibodies also remained constant, with only minor fluctuation between $\log_2$
3-4 and 1-2, respectively. However, cell-mediated immunity
to the sonicate of S. mutans was not detectable before bacterial accumulation began, though lymphocyte transformation
and MMI were significantly increased 7 to 14 days after the
start of the experimental period (Fig. 3). Both indices
showed a remittant pattern; lymphocyte transformation
yielded two peaks at days 14 and 28, but MMI preceded lymphocyte transformation by 7 days and both reached negative
values by day 77. The results in the single subject (Fig. 2)
also showed only minor variations in salivary and serum
antibody titres, but the stimulation index of lymphocytes

to S. mutans increased from 0.75 on day 0 to 8.0 by day 28.
The sequential serum and salivary antibody titres and CMI
to V. alcalescens were comparable to those shown for S.
mutans but due to limitations of space are not given here.

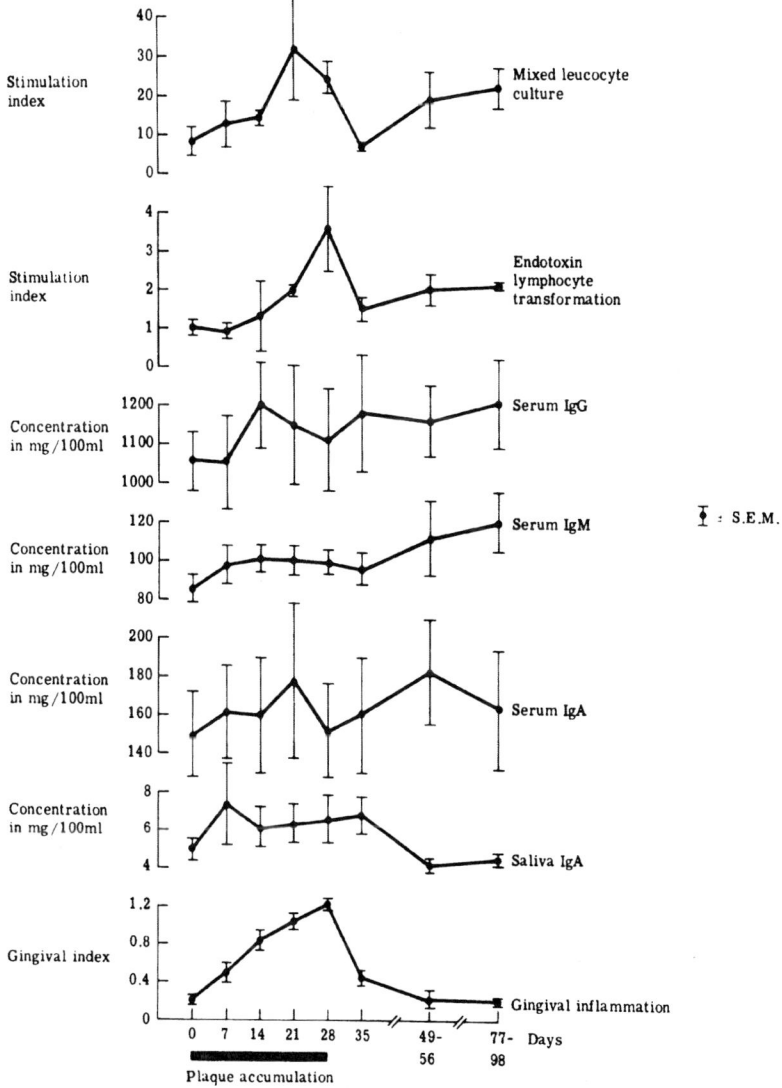

Figure 1. Sequential serum and salivary immunoglobulin
concentrations, T and B lymphocyte responses and gingival
inflammation to accumulation of bacterial plaque.

DISCUSSION

The striking feature of plaque accumulation was its
effect on cell-mediated immunity. Both T and B lymphocyte

functions were enhanced, as tested by MLC reaction for T
lymphocytes (16) and endotoxin activation for B lymphocytes
(17,18). Lymphocytes were also stimulated by S. mutans,
plaque, V. alcalescens, Actinomyces viscosus, Proteus mirabilis and PPD to increased DNA synthesis and to release
migration inhibition factor (1). These findings suggest
that dental bacterial plaque may have an adjuvant effect on
T and B lymphocytes, enhancing their responses for a limited
period of time which is dependent on the duration of plaque
accumulation. The adjuvant effect might function on a T to
T in addition to T to B lymphocyte level, possibly by the

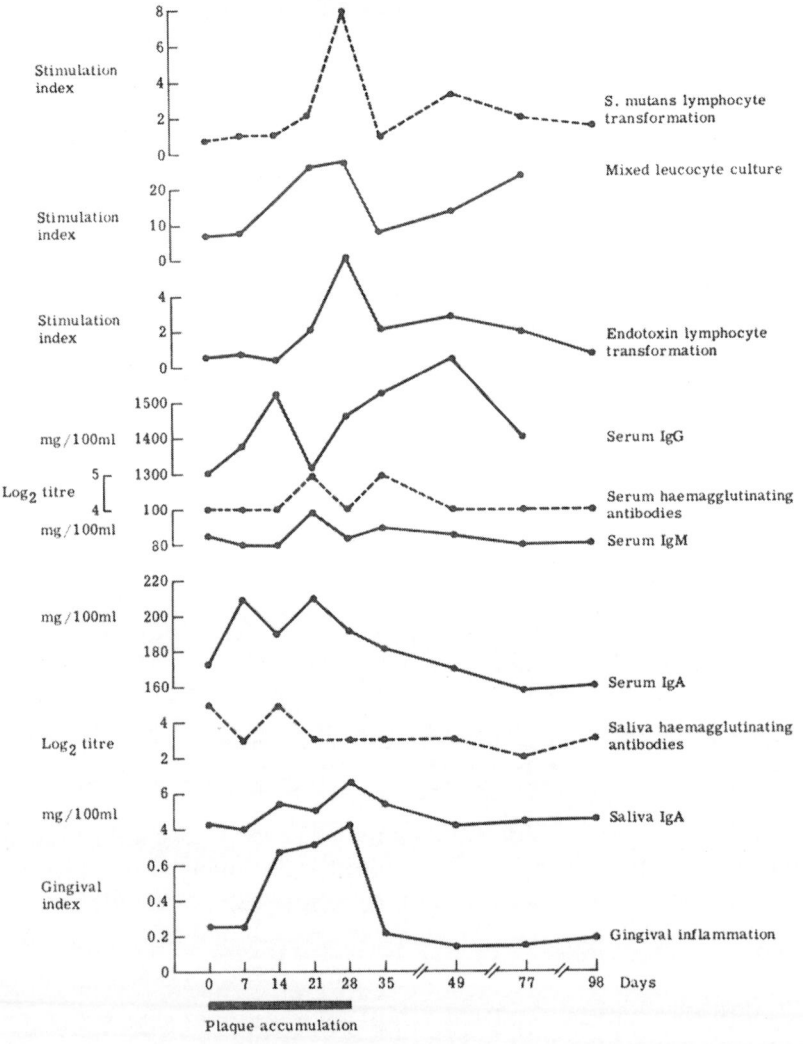

Figure 2. Sequential serum and salivary immunoglobulins,
antibodies and cell-mediated immunity in one subject.

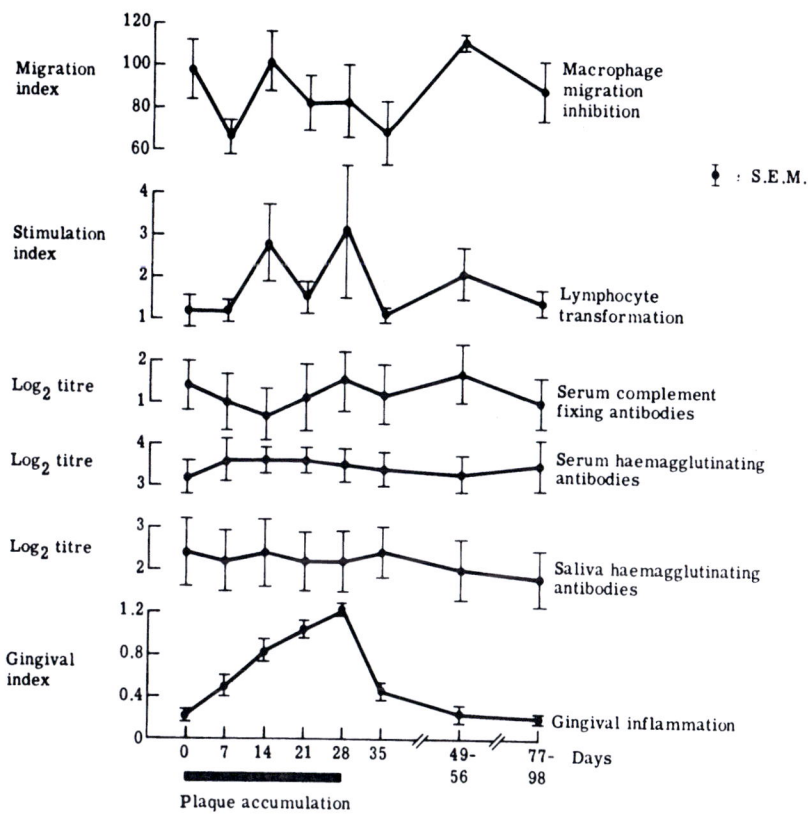

Figure 3.   Sequential serum and salivary antibodies and cell-
mediated immunity to Streptococcus mutans, induced by accumulation of bacterial plaque.

release of mitogenic (19) or other factors which may mediate
lymphocyte transformation. However, if the thymus independent antigens in plaque (endotoxin, dextran and levan) parti-
cipate in the reaction, then cellular cooperation might occur
on a B to T lymphocyte level. It is especially relevant that
potent adjuvant effects have been shown for endotoxin (20)
and dextran (21) so that the immune responses induced by
plaque might be governed by the collective adjuvant effects
of these substances. The local immune responses may therefore be modulated by plaque lipopolysaccharides and dextrans
and seem to be directed to both T and B lymphocytes. However,
these have been shown to influence predominantly T lymphocyte
functions, in that lymphocyte transformation and macrophage
migration inhibition are enhanced with only minor changes to
antibody titres. This is consistent with the findings that
low doses of antigens, as is the case with dental plaque,
preferentially induce CMI (22).

Although salivary IgA and serum IgA, IgG and IgM concentrations increased during plaque accumulation, a corresponding increase in salivary and serum antibodies to a variety
of microorganisms was not detected. This could be a measure
of sensitivity of the tests used, or the bacteriological
nature of the plaque and accessibility of its various components to the immune system. However, the discrepancy is
consistent with the findings that with an increase in the
number of antigens in a secondary immune response, there will
be an increase in non-specific immunoglobulin containing
plasma cells, but a relative decrease in specific antibody
containing cells (23).

An analysis of the immune responses to some of the oral
microorganisms (Table 1) suggests that in normal subjects
serum and salivary antibodies to a selected fungal, viral,
Gram-positive and Gram-negative organism are commonly elicited directly, but that the CMI responses may be induced only
with the fungal and viral agents. However, the apparently
negative CMI responses to the two bacteria can be augmented
by bacterial plaque so as to convert these to positive reactions. Hence, all 4 microbial agents can be made to elicit
in normal subjects an intact serum, salivary and CMI response
(Table 1). In 4 chronic or recurrent oral diseases there is
a selective immunodeficiency in which salivary antibodies and
CMI seem to be related, but both show an inverse relationship
to serum antibodies. There is evidence that an inverse relationship may be induced between CMI and antibody formation
(24). An independent relationship between serum and salivary
antibodies has been found in dental caries in man (25,8). A
raised serum antibody level and impaired CMI to the specific
or related microorganisms has been found in recurrent herpetic infection (26), juvenile periodontitis (27) and some
patients with chronic candidosis, whilst others showed a depressed serum antibody but intact CMI in chronic candidosis
(28,29). Furthermore, an impaired CMI in chronic mucocuta-
neous candidosis is associated with a decreased salivary IgA
class of antibodies in the presence of increased serum IgG
and IgM antibodies (28,29). In recurrent herpetic infections
an impaired CMI (26) seems to be associated with decreased
serum IgA antibodies to Herpes simplex (30) and a lack of
demonstrable secretory IgA antibodies in saliva (31).

An inverse relationship between serum antibodies on the
one hand and CMI and secretory antibodies on the other, as
well as an association between IgA antibodies and CMI seems

Table 1. The Relationship Between Serum and Salivary Antibodies and Cell-Mediated Immunity in Oral Disease and Controls.

	Microorganism	Serum Antibodies	Salivary IgA Antibodies	Cell-mediated Immunity	LT	MMI
I. Normal Immune Responses						
1. Controls with past exposure to the organisms	Candida albicans	+	+	+	+	+
	Herpes simplex 1	+	-*	+	+	+
	Streptococcus mutans	+	+	-	-	-
	Veillonella alcalescens	+	±	-	-	-
2. Controls exposed to the adjuvant effect of plaque	Streptococcus mutans	+	+	+	+	+
	Veillonella alcalescens	+	+	+	+	+
II. Impaired Immune Responses						
1. Recurrent herpetic infections	Herpes simplex 1	++	-*	→	‡	-
2. Chronic candidosis	Candida albicans	{ ++ / - }	±‡	- / +	- / +	- / +
3. Juvenile periodontitis	Veillonella alcalescens	+	±	→	-	+
4. Dental caries	Streptococcus mutans	++	±	-**	-**	-

* = IgG antibodies reported
→ = Impaired
** = Converted to + with plaque accumulation

LT = Lymphocyte transformation
MMI = Macrophage migration inhibition

to emerge from an analysis of selected oral diseases. The
interpretation of these relationships is not clear, but one
important factor might be antigenic access and presentation
to local lymphoid tissue; antigens favouring T cell stimulation may induce CMI, whereas antigens which favour T-B cell
interaction may induce antibody formation (24).

SUMMARY

Sequential changes in serum and salivary immunoglobulins, antibodies and cell-mediated immunity were studied in
subjects who accumulated dental bacterial plaque over 28
days. Although in individual subjects the salivary IgA concentration increased by up to 33% and serum immunoglobulins
by up to 20%, the mean increases in concentrations failed to
reach the 5% level of significance because of wide variations
between individual subjects. There was no detectable increase in the serum or salivary antibodies tested. However,
T lymphocytes tested by the mixed leucocyte reaction and
stimulation of B lymphocytes by endotoxin showed enhanced
responses. An increase in lymphocyte transformation and macrophage migration inhibition was recorded with antigens from
related organisms, Streptococcus mutans and Veillonella
alcalescens, as well as unrelated antigens, such as PPD and
Proteus mirabilis. These results suggest that dental bacterial plaque may have an adjuvant effect on T and B lymphocytes.
An analysis of some chronic or recurrent oral diseases revealed an independence of serum antibodies from salivary
antibodies and cell-mediated immunity, but a relationship
between the latter and salivary antibodies.

Acknowledgements: This work was carried out under a project
grant from the Medical Research Council. We are indebted to
the volunteers who took part in the investigation and for
the expert technical assistance given by Mr. R.G. Ward, Mrs.
J. Caldwell and Mrs. S. Bennett.

REFERENCES

1. Lehner, T., Wilton, J.M.A., Challacombe, S.J. and
    Ivanyi, L., Clin. exp. Immunol. (in press), 1973.
2. Löe, H., Theilade, E. and Jensen, S.B., J. Periodont.
    36:177, 1965.
3. Löe, H. and Silness, J., Acta Odont. Scand. 21:533, 1963.
4. Ivanyi, L. and Lehner, T., Arch. oral Biol. 15:1089, 1970.
5. Lemmel, E.M. and Good, R.A., Nature 221:1164, 1969.

6. Ivanyi, L., Wilton, J.M.A. and Lehner, T., Immunology
    22:141, 1972.
7. Thor, D.E., Jurizez, R.E., Veach, S.R., Miller, E. and
    Dray, S., Nature 219:755, 1968.
8. Challacombe, S.J., Guggenheim, B. and Lehner, T.,
    Arch. oral Biol. 18:657, 1973.
9. Hammarström, S., Lagercrantz, R., Petmann, P. and
    Gustafsson, B.E., J. exp. Med. 122:1075, 1965.
10. Sever, J.L., J. Immun. 88:320, 1962.
11. Bradstreet, C.M.P. and Taylor, C.E.D., Month. Bull.
    Min. Hlth. 21:96, 1962.
12. Mancini, G., Vaerman, J.P., Carbonara, A.O. and
    Heremans, J.F., in Protides of the Biological Fluids,
    Vol. XI, Edited by H. Peeters, Elsevier, Amsterdam, 1963.
13. Schuster, G.S., Hayashi, J.A. and Bahn, A.N., J.
    Bacteriol. 93:47, 1967.
14. Challacombe, S.J., Caries Res. (in press), 1973.
15. Westphal, O., Lüderitz, O. and Bister, F., Z.
    Naturforsch. 7:148, 1952.
16. Johnston, J.M. and Wilson, D.B., Cell. Immunol. 1:430,
    1970.
17. Anderson, J., Möller, G. and Sjöberg, O., Cell. Immunol.
    4:381, 1972.
18. Ivanyi, L., Lehner, T. and Burry, H.C., Immunology
    (in press), 1973.
19. Dumonde, D.C., Wolstencroft, R.A., Panayi, G.S., Matthew,
    N., Morley, J. and Howson, W.T., Nature 224:38, 1969.
20. Johnson, A.G., Gaines, S. and Landy, M., J. exp. Med.
    103:225, 1956.
21. Battisto, J.R. and Pappas, F., J. exp. Med. 138:176,
    1973.
22. Salvin, S.B., J. exp. Med. 107:109, 1958.
23. De Vos-Cloetens, C., Minsart-Baleriaux, V. and
    Urbain-Vansanten, G., Immunology 20:955, 1971.
24. Parish, C.R., Transplant. Rev. 13:36, 1972.
25. Lehner, T., Cardwell, J.E. and Clarry, E.D., Lancet 1:
    1294, 1967.
26. Wilton, J.M.A., Ivanyi, L. and Lehner, T., Brit. med.
    J. 1:723, 1972.
27. Lehner, T., Wilton, J.M.A. and Manson, D. (in preparation)
28. Chilgren, R.A., Quie, P.G., Meuwissen, H.J. and Hong, R.,
    Lancet 2:688, 1967.
29. Lehner, T., Wilton, J.M.A. and Ivanyi, L., Immunology 22:
    775, 1972.
30. Tokumaru, T., J. Immun. 97:248, 1966.
31. Douglas, R.G. and Couch, R.B., J. Immun. 104:289, 1970.

ORAL MANIFESTATIONS OF IgA DEFICIENCY

Paul B. Robertson and Max D. Cooper

Institute of Dental Research
Departments of Pediatrics and Microbiology
University of Alabama in Birmingham
Birmingham, Alabama 35294

The IgA system is viewed as a major local defense
mechanism of mucous membranes, and IgA deficiency seems to
be a significant predisposing factor to a variety of sinopulmonary infections and intestinal disorders (1-6). Since
IgA is the predominant immunoglobulin in secretions (7-10),
including saliva, a protective role for this class of
immunoglobulins in dental caries and periodontal disease has
been suggested. Indeed, results of one investigation
suggested that a deficient secretion of IgA in saliva might
be associated with increased caries incidence (11). At
present, however, the concept of immunity in dental caries is
speculative and no conclusive evidence is available regarding
the capacity of the IgA system to protect the periodontium
(12-14). In addition, no description of the oral status of
IgA deficient patients is available in the literature.

The present investigations were designed to assess
oral manifestations of isolated IgA deficiency in children.
This report is concerned with preliminary clinical findings
of particular interest to the practitioner.

METHODS

A population of patients manifesting isolated IgA
deficiency with the clinical profile shown in Table I was
evaluated. Serum IgA was undetectable in all but three of
the patients (B,D,E) who had very low serum IgA levels
(<11mg/100ml). Thymus system development was evaluated by

497

TABLE I

Patient	Age (Yrs)	Sex	Primary Diagnosis	Clinical Observations
A	5	M	"Sporadic"* IgA deficiency	Rhinitis, otitis, media, occasional diarrhea
B	5	F	"Sporadic"IgA deficiency	Rhinitis, otitis media
C	5	F	Congenital rubella	Rhinitis, otitis media, pneumonia
D	5	M	Familial IgA deficiency	Rhinitis, otitis media
E	6	F	Familial IgA deficiency	Bronchitis, pneumonia
F	7	M	Familial IgA deficiency	Rhinitis, otitis media, septic arthritis
G	9	M	"Sporadic" IgA deficiency	Rhinitis, otitis media, pneumonia, pulmonary tuberculosis, intestinal malabsorption
H	11	M	Familial IgA deficeincy	Rhinitis, otitis media
I	19	F	"Sporadic" IgA deficiency	Rhinitis, otitis media

* "Sporadic" IgA deficiency is used to refer to those patients in whom the defect is neither clearly familial, nor associated with known environmental factors.

skin testing for delayed allergy, lymphocyte responsiveness to PHA, proportion of blood lymphocytes killed by an anti-T lymphocyte antiserum, and, in some patients, population of thymus-dependent areas of lymph nodes. Gross impairment in T cell development was not found in any of the IgA deficient patients.

Each patient received a complete oral examination which included a detailed dental history. Teeth decayed, filled, and extracted due to caries were recorded. A soft tissue exam was performed with particular attention to lips, tongue, and buccal mucosa. The Gingival Index (15) and Periodontal Disease Index (16) were recorded for each patient. Plaque retention was evaluated with 1% fast green as disclosant by the method of Podshadley and Haley (17).

Panorex radiographic surveys were accomplished when indicated. Non-affected siblings served as controls and received comparable examinations. Information regarding diet, medical histories, dental experience, and oral hygiene practices was obtained in interviews with parents, usually the mother.

RESULTS

A summary of clinical findings is presented in Table II. The past medical histories of these patients were extensive and the majority of patients were extremely apprehensive during initial dental examinations. Complete lapses of oral hygiene were observed during periods of acute illness, particularly during upper respiratory infections. This observation was most pronounced in those cases where the parent was unaware of the importance of plaque control in maintaining oral health. During such periods, gingivitis (described below) became more severe and was occasionally accompanied by hemorrhage.

A frequent finding in these patients was so-called "bottle caries". The pattern of decay was typical and affected primarily the labial surfaces of maxillary anteriors. The surfaces of cusps were often affected. Proximal and lingual surfaces were severely involved in one case (C) with destruction of entire crowns. The mandibular incisors appeared to escape attack entirely, and few lesions were observed in mandibular posterior teeth. The high caries incidence recorded in these patients was almost entirely within the maxillary dentition, particularly the incisors. Interviews with mothers of IgA deficient children exhibiting this pattern of decay disclosed nocturnal bottle feeding and long term use of syrup-base oral medications. Two of the children (B,C) were bottle fed commercial formulae and formulae mixed with cereal up to the age of 30 months. Mothers utilized the bottle in an effort to calm the child at night during frequent periods of upper respiratory distress and to ease associated nightly coughing.

It is noteworthy that several of the IgA deficient patients were totally free of caries. A study of caries incidence in matched controls and IgA deficient patients is in progress.

A prevalent finding in IgA deficient individuals was mouth-breathing. This observation is consistent with the

TABLE II

Patient	Decayed & Filled Teeth	Extracted (Caries) Teeth	Habitual Mouth-Breathing	Tetra-cycline Banding
A	0	0	+	
B	11*	1	+	
C	15*	2	+	
D	0	0	+	
E	10*	0		+
F	4	0	+	+
G	0	0		
H	10*	0		+
I	18	6	+	

* "Bottle" pattern of caries (See text for description).

chronic rhinitis, sinusitis, and recurrent naso-pharyngeal infections exhibited by these patients. Children with habitual mouth-breathing (A,B,C,D,F,I) also manifested varying degrees of gingival hyperplasia in anterior-maxillary interproximal areas. The marginal palatal gingiva of the maxillary six anterior teeth in three patients (B,D,F) were moderately inflamed.

While eruption of gingivitis (18) was noted in several of the IgA deficient patients, its severity appeared not to differ from that observed in immunocompetent controls. Chronic gingivitis was usually associated with the extensive carious involvement of maxillary anterior teeth previously described.

One case of acute necrotizing ulcerative gingivitis was encountered. The patient (I) had a history of recurrent gingival ulceration with hemorrhage, odor, and pain. The characteristic lesions involved both the interdental papilla and marginal gingiva. No other oral tissues were affected. Smears taken of the lesions demonstrated many spirochetes, fusiform bacilli, and desquamated epithelial cells. Initial daily treatment included removal of pseudomembranes, debris, and supra-gingival calculus. The patient was placed on strict oral hygiene procedures and rinses with 3% hydrogen peroxide. During the first week, little improvement in the acute condition was noted. Deep scaling and curettage were

instituted, and the patient's condition slowly improved
over a five week period. The condition recurred four
months later and exhibited the same resistance to local
therapy. The patient had some interproximal alveolar bone
loss as a result of the recurrent acute ulcerative gingivitis.

The remainder of the patients showed no clinical or
radiographic signs of early periodontitis.

Three patients exhibited moderate to severe dis-
coloration of teeth which was particularly prominent on the
maxillary and mandibular incisors and was due to the
administration of tetracycline.

DISCUSSION

Observations on the present group of IgA deficient
patients suggests that the incidence of caries and
periodontal disease may be related in part to lapses of
oral hygiene, long term feeding by bottle, and mouth-
breathing.

Caries and periodontal disease in this report on the
oral status of the IgA deficient patient are probably
related in some part to the high plaque scores observed
during frequent periods of sinopulmonary infection. Fox (19)
has suggested that the family becomes so deeply involved
with caring for the total medical problems of the
chronically ill child that dental care is overlooked.
Indeed, plaque scores were substantially higher when
patients were seen while hospitalized. In addition,
interviews with parents revealed all but total lack of home
oral care during periods of upper respiratory infection.
In view of the fact that the etiology of caries and
periodontal disease is directly related to microbial plaque,
the observation is significant both in terms of studies
relating dental pathology to immunological deficiencies
and in terms of the treatment of these patients by the
general practitioner.

There is substantial evidence to indicate that certain
commercial milk formulae containing high percentages of
carbohydrate produce a characteristic pattern of caries if
placed in the mouth of the child during sleeping hours,
particularly if continued over many years (20-23). In
addition, Finn (24) has observed a similar pattern of caries

produced by nightly ingestion of a spoonful of medication in sucrose-syrup just prior to retiring. The syrup tended to bathe the maxillary teeth, and decreased salivary flow appeared to allow a syrup film to remain for lengthy periods of time. Both practices could account for the dramatic carious involvement of the maxillary incisors in these patients.

There is general agreement that habitual mouth-breathing can substantially modify an existing gingivitis (25). Erythema and hyperplasia affecting primarily the maxillary labial and palatal gingiva have been described by a number of investigators (26,27). In addition, it has been suggested that mouth-breathing may modify the progression of dental caries, particularly in the anterior maxillary dentition (25).

Overall evaluation of the role of IgA deficiency in caries and periodontal disease is exceedingly complex, but present incomplete data would suggest that IgA deficiency does not necessarily lead in any direct way to destruction of the teeth or their supporting structures. In those cases where oral hygiene and dietary control were evident, no significant pathology was observed. Our experience emphasizes, however, that IgA deficient children may have a considerable amount of dental pathology as indirect consequences of their increased susceptibility to infections of the respiratory tract.

REFERENCES

1. Pierce, A.E., Vet. Rev. Annot. 5:17, 1959.
2. South, M.A., Cooper, M.D., Wollheim, F.A. and Good, R.A. Amer. J. Med. 44:168, 1968.
3. South, M.A., Cooper, M.D., Hong, R., Wollheim, F.A. and Good, R.A. in Birth Defects Original Article Series, Vol. IV, No. 1 (Immunologic Deficiency Diseases in Man) p. 283, D. Bergsma and R.A. Good, eds., University of Florida Press, Gainesville, Florida, 1968.
4. Heremans, J.F. and Crabbe, P.A. in Birth Defects Original Article Series, Vol. IV, No. 1, (Immunologic Deficiency Diseases in Man) p. 298, University of Florida Press, Gainesville, Florida, 1968.
5. Hobbs, J.R., Lancet, 1:110, 1968.
6. Huntley, C.C. and Stephenson, R.L., North Car. Med. J., 29:325, 1968.
7. Tomasi, T.B., Jr. and Ziegelbaum, S. J. Clin. Invest. 42:1552, 1963.

8. Chodirker, W.B. and Tomasi, T.B., Jr. Science, 142:1080, 1963.
9. Remington, J.S., Vosti, K.L., Lietze, A., and Zimmerman, A.L. J. Clin. Invest. 43:1613, 1964.
10. Keimowitz, R.I. J. Lab. Clin. Med. 63:54, 1964.
11. Lehner, T., Cardwell, J.E. and Clarry, E.D. Lancet, 1:1294, 1967.
12. Genco, R.J. J. Periodont. 41:196, 1970.
13. Brandtzaeg, P., Fjellanger, I. and Gjeruldsen, S.T. Scan. J. Haemat. Supplementum No. 12, 1970.
14. Sims, W. Oral Surg. 34:69, 1972.
15. Löe, H. and Silness, J. Acta. Odont. Scand. 21:532, 1963.
16. Ramfjord, S.P. J. Periodont. 30:51, 1959.
17. Podshadley, A.G. and Haley, J.V. Public Health Reports 83:259,1968.
18. McDonald, R.E. Dentistry for the Child and Adolescent, C.V. Mosby, Saint Louis, 1969.
19. Fox, L.A. Pediat. Clin. N. Amer. 20:245, 1973.
20. Syrrist, A. and Selander, P. Odont. Tidskr 61:237, 1953.
21. Winter, G.B., Hamilton, M.C. and James, P.M.C. Arch. Dis. Child 41:207, 1966.
22. Robinson, S. and Naylor, S.R. Brit. Dent. J. 115, 1963.
23. Kroll, R.G. and Stone, J.H. J. Dent. Child, 34:454, 1967.
24. Finn, S.B. Current Dental Comment 1:35, 1969.
25. Emslie, R.D., Massler, M. and Zwemer, J.D. J. Amer. Dent. Assoc. 44:506, 1952.
26. Lite, T., DiMaio, D.J. and Burman, L.R. Oral Surg. 38:382, 1955.
27. Alexander, A.G. Paradontologie 24:49, 1970.

DISCUSSION

Dr. Anthony Rizzo, Initial Discussant - Thank you very much,
Dr. Lawton. I can say, as Dr. Robertson said, I am very glad
to be back in Birmingham. I graduated from this Dental School
and I am very proud of that. I have had occasion several
times before to serve as discussant. Usually I get manuscripts
a few days before the meeting to use in preparing my own discussion. What invariably happens, however, is that speakers
either do not say what they intended to say, or what is worse,
they say what I intended to say. In either case I end up with
something that is more or less an extemporaneous rendition.
I recall Dr. Freter's remarks of yesterday when he was the
initial, initial speaker. He said the color of the ribbon on
his badge was green and that was a color of hope. So I have
been looking at the badge in a hopeful manner to see what
would come forth.

What I hope to do here is to try to bring a little perspective to the oral disease picture in relationship to Dr.
Lehner's presentation mostly, and also to Dr. Robertson's presentation. I think we ought to recognize that we have a peculiar kind of situation in periodontal disease where the bacterial plaque sits on the tooth in close relationship to the
gingival tissues and causes disease, apparently not by whole-
sale invasion, but by elaborating antigens and other products
that lead to chronic inflammation of the gingival tissues.
Over a long period of time the adjacent collagen fibers and
bone are destroyed, and the teeth finally fall out. This process is no respector of persons: witness what happened to George
Washington. Dr. Lehner's laboratory has been a principle
source of evidence that cell mediated immunity stimulated by
oral organisms in the plaque is an important part of the disease
process. His case for the role of cell mediated immunity in
this disease has been considerably strengthened in the last
few years by work at Alabama, Seattle, and the National Institute of Dental Research which has tied in cell mediated immune
reactions to tissue destruction. For example, it has been shown
recently that cell mediated immune responses of lymphocytes
sensitized to oral organisms can produce substances which turn
on collagenase in macrophages, which inhibit protein synthesis,
which kill connective tissue cells, and which cause bone resorp-
tion. So the picture is sort of coming together. In his past

experiments, Dr. Lehner has made a case for cell mediated
immunity in cross sectional studies in which patients with
disease and without disease were compared. Today he has gone
a step further and presented longitudinal studies in which he
produced the early signs of disease, and then showed that cell
mediated immunity accompanies it. This he did in patients who
showed neither cell mediated immunity nor the disease before
the experiment. Thus we recognize yet another contribution
from this productive laboratory.

I think the situation we have in periodontal disease is
somewhat like that described in Dr. Rothberg's presentation on
antigenic stimulation through the gastrointestinal mucosa. I
think we are dealing with a topical system and if we are
going to design models that are meaningful in human disease
process we will have to make our models accordingly. To supplement, to amplify, and to be able to really interpret human
experiments, we need model systems like those Dr. Rothberg used.
Several years ago, in attempting to develop some animal experiments meaningful in periodontal disease, we employed topical
methods to expose the gingival tissues of rabbits to antigens
for prolonged periods. In these experiments we first irri-
gated the gingival tissues with solutions of different antigens, and then examined the gingival tissue that was absorbing
antigen, the regional lymph nodes, the spleen, the systemic
circulation for an immune response. We found that high concentrations of antigen over a relatively long exposure time
produced responses in all of those areas: a strong cellular
response in the gum and in the regional lymph nodes, plaque
forming antibody cells in the regional lymph nodes and in the
spleen, and also circulating antibody. But when a low concentration of an antigen (10^{-3} ug/ml) was bathed over the gum
tissues for about four hours, a response occurred only in the
regional lymph nodes, where specific antibody-forming cells
were demonstrable. There was no cellular response either in
the gingival tissue itself or in any other place in the body.
(This work was done with Steve Berglund.) What I would like to
suggest is that we have to bring into the picture of interpretation the quantitative aspects of the concentration of antigen and the exposure time if we are going to make any sense
out of periodontal disease, and perhaps some other GI diseases.

In regard to Dr. Robertson's paper, I think that he said
about everything that should be said. I would simply like to
add that I was struck by the fact that the one patient who
was old enough to really show signs of destructive periodontal disease did so in this study. I think with the con-
tinuation of this study, with the appropriate controls for
the respiratory disease that accompanies IgA deficiency,

I am sure that some meaningful results will be obtained. I would like to thank the chairman for allowing me to comment on these interesting papers. Thank you very much.

Dr. Genco - I have a question for Dr. Robertson. It was not clear to me whether the IgA deficient patients had compensatory IgM in the saliva.

Dr. Cooper - Most of them were not examined, but the parotid secretions in most of the IgA deficient patients we have looked at, some of them included here, did not have remarkable increases in IgM. They were no different than normal when concentrated and measured by serum standards.

Dr. Good - A technical question for Dr. Lehner. The concern that I have is linking the endotoxin stimulation in man to the B cells. We have struggled very hard with this, not using, of course, the Veilonella endotoxin which you used, but have been unable to do the sort of things with endotoxin in in vitro antibody producing systems with human cells that we can do in mice. I would like to know the details of your identification of this responsiveness to the Veilonella endotoxin as a B cell response.

Dr. Lehner - I think there is little doubt, as shown by Oppenheim and Perry, that in man the response of lymphocytes to endotoxin is poor. Most workers have used the Difco preparation of E. coli endotoxin which is not a particularly well purified antigen. Now, the endotoxin that we have used from Veilonella alcalescens has been prepared by the phenol method of extraction of Westphal's and it was pronase-treated as well. On the other hand, we have not used lipid A polysaccharide or protein fractions, so that the possibility of stimulation by other antigens cannot be excluded. The evidence that this is a B lymphocyte stimulating mitogen or antigen in man is from using synovial fluid lymphocytes. These are effectively stimulated by putative B cell mitogens, such as pokeweed mitogen and endotoxin, but their response to T cell mitogen (PHA) was poor and to PPD was negative (Ivanyi, L., Lehner T. and Burry, H.C. Immunology 25:905, 1973). At the moment Dr. Ivanyi is separating B and T lymphocytes from peripheral blood to test the validity of endotoxin being a B cell mitogen in man.

Dr. Cassell - My question is directed to either Dr. Robertson or Dr. Cooper. I am curious to know if there was a predominant or a common etiologic agent responsible for the respiratory infections that were observed in your nine patients.

Dr. Cooper - None that we were able to detect by clinical patterns or by routine bacteriological cultures. Many of the infections that these children have seem to be viral infections; at least they occur at times when epidemic upper respiratory tract infections are occurring.

Dr. Cassell - Were they by any chance cultured for myco-plasma or were any serological diagnostic tests made for mycoplasma infections?

Dr. Cooper - No, they were not.

Dr. Dawes - I would like to ask Dr. Robertson a question. Several of the papers we have heard so far have implied that salivary IgA can influence the type of bacteria in the dental plaque and in the oral cavity. I would like to ask whether any attempt has been made to see whether there is an unusual distribution of microorganisms in the dental plaque in those patients with IgA deficiency.

Dr. Robertson - The answer is: I don't know. We did not try to quantitate numbers or types of bacteria.

Dr. Jukka Koistinen - I would like to ask Dr. Robertson about this familial IgA deficiency. What is meant by that? How were the index cases selected? Were they the patients pre-sented in the paper and what was the physical condition of the other family members who were lacking IgA? Were they totally healthy or did they have any illness?

Dr. Cooper - Familial just means that there were other members of the family, either siblings or parents, with IgA defici-ency. What were the manifestations in family members? One of these children's father, I believe, had total IgA deficiency. He and one other individual are the only pati-ents from a group of about 40 IgA deficient patients that we have seen, including mainly children but adults as well, who have not had recurring infection. He has had absolutely no problems except for some arthritic complaints that have just begun over the last few years. In terms of organisms in the mouth, we have not looked at the distribution of these. However, in the intestine we did look a few years back at

some of our IgA deficient patients and compared the numbers
and kinds of bacterial flora in a weighed sample of feces
with their siblings. We found no differences in the types
and numbers of organisms in these children. This seemed all
the more remarkable because of the repeated disturbance of
their microintestinal flora through the use of antibiotics
given for their respiratory infections.

Dr. Fudenberg - I have a couple of questions and comments
intermixed. These data are indeed very striking but as I
gathered you have used only patients with IgA deficiency
that turned up because of clinical problems. Now since the
incidence of IgA deficiency in random blood donors who are
healthy by history is about one in five to seven hundred
in Caucasian populations, one in three thousand in Japanese
populations, one in three hundred in Finnish populations, I
wonder if you have done any mass screening in your blood
bank, for example, to see how many IgA deficients you have
and go look to see what their dental history is in terms of
caries. That is question one.

Dr. Robertson - It is a good idea but we have not done it.

Dr. Fudenberg - Now the second comment is that if one has
recurrent infections of the oral mucosa or the respiratory
tract and associated IgA deficiency, I would caution against
concluding that these are cause and effect. Two of our
eight patients with chronic granulomatous disease came to
us because of recurrent infections and IgA deficiency. We
think that their phagocytic dysfunction is much more important in causing disease than is the IgA deficiency. And
lastly, I gather that collagens are components of both the
gingiva and the tooth. As you perhaps know, Dr. Wells in
our lab has shown a strikingly high incidence of anticol-
lagen antibodies in IgA deficiency. I wonder if you have
had a chance to look at the people who developed caries or
other dental manifestations and those that do not, for such
antibodies. If you have looked at them I would appreciate
the answer; if you have not looked perhaps Dr. Rizzo might
be interested in having the National Institute of Dental
Research provide the funds for such a study.

Dr. Sigel - There are some reports, the most recent one from
Phil Glade, suggesting that MIF may not be a truly immunologic manifestation of lymphocyte reaction, but that various
cells can produce substances that inhibit migration of macro-

phages. I therefore question specificity of the reactions reported by Dr. Lehner, in so many instances being generated by antigens which are not related to the plaque. I am not questioning blastogenesis so much as MIF.

Dr. Lehner - May I answer Dr. Sigel's question about the specificity of the macrophage migration inhibition test? One can produce a long list of papers by David and other workers showing a very significant association between migration inhibition and delayed hypersensitivity to specific antigens. However, I should like to draw attention to the fact that we carried out longitudinal studies, starting from a negative baseline and becoming positive as a result of plaque accumulation and gingival inflammation. In our controls we have used the serum alone, fetal calf serum, and we usually reconstituted the supernatant from unstimulated lymphocytes with the particular antigen tested; from these results we are inclined to think that this is a specific response. On the other hand, we have not isolated the migration inhibition factor and there are other lymphokines almost certainly present in the supernatant, so that there might be some nonspecific reactivity. By and large, our controls behaved quite differently to those in which we have used the specifically stimulated lymphocyte supernatants.

Dr. Lawton - At this time I would like to turn over the meeting to Dr. Frederick Kraus and, if I may, for the members of the committee I would like to extend my thanks to Dr. Kraus for doing the vast bulk of the work in organizing this very excellent meeting.

Dr. Kraus - Thank you, Dr. Lawton. Thank you, everybody. We have heard some fifty major presentations and several hours of discussion. Who is the man to clear out weary minds, to point out what has been achieved by this Symposium and what vistas have been opened? A computer might be adequate for space travel but it takes a great human mind to analyze such a wealth of material while it is being presented and to offer conclusions. All of us know the one man who is capable of making such an immediate summation. We are honored, indeed, that he has accepted the task. Dr. Robert Good.

CONCLUSION

IMPRESSIONS, SUMMARY AND QUESTIONS RAISED BY THE IgA
SYMPOSIUM

Robert A. Good

Memorial Sloan-Kettering Cancer Center

1275 York Avenue   New York, New York 10021

During this conference, Dr. Richard Hong has referred
to the IgA immunity system as an adolescent. By this, he
implies that the IgA system is beginning to show signs of
maturity, while at the same time being hard to understand
and certainly difficult to contain. I am sure all of us
can agree with him as we grapple with the huge amount of
new information and attempt to sort this into a manageable
understanding of IgA and its relationship to immunity in
general.

I would like to begin my analysis of this conference
at the very beginning by thinking back briefly about the
opening remarks made by President Volker. He told us that
with the first $100,000 budget for the dental school whose
birthday we are celebrating with this conference, he saw
to it that $10,000 - one part in ten, was set aside for
research. This I am sure was done to launch the development
of this magnificent school in a climate of true scholarship.
One of the most important aspects of true scholarship is
the recognition of what is unknown. Real teaching must
involve induction of scholarly behavior on the part of the
students, and the only way this can be accomplished is to
make sure the teachers or inducers can behave as true
scholars, and as such contribute to the inquiry into what
is not known. Scholars must try to organize our chaotic
universe according to formats which they can see and to set
patterns that will challenge their best students to attempt
to develop, through scholarly efforts, organizations and

513

patterns of their own. In this framework, research into the
unknown is absolutely essential, as is the recognition of the
fact that there is a constantly evolving, constantly developing framework that must be manipulated and fashioned in the
light of new information. Thus, assessing in a conference
such as this the very frontier of developing knowledge on
IgA is an essential function of a great institute of
learning like the Dental School of the University of
Alabama and as such, a most important part of the life of
this institution. It is good to celebrate the quadricen-
tennial birthday of such an institute with a conference
exploring an area of science that must be, as is implied
in Hong's words, incomplete, difficult to master, hard to
understand, and still capable of following a number of
directions many of us cannot at this moment foresee.

An appropriate first question to ask as we begin
considering our conference is "Are we still true to our
beginnings and can this great center of learning honestly
say today that one-tenth, a tithing of all its resources, is
being devoted to that most essential ingredient of
scholarship research?" I hope this is the case, but somehow I wonder.

Such cost accounting might be appropriate to consider
in relationship to the endeavors of our culture in every
sphere. I do not think the research establishment would
feel so oppressed, for example, if 5 to 10% of the entire
cost of biomedical enterprise in our land were being devoted
to the research and scientific development which could
assure its maximum effectiveness in years to come.

In a personal way I realized the impact of scholarly
endeavor on the body of knowledge from my own attempt to
encompass the body of knowledge in medicine when I was a
medical student. I sat in the front row of every class.
I took down everything the professor said, complemented this
body of knowledge with the information I learned from my
instructors in the laboratory, from relevant information I
would glean from reading and digesting the best textbooks
on each subject, and even from extracting the substance
of the most relevant articles in contemporary scientific
journals. All this I included in my notes for study
in beautiful Morocco-bound notebooks. The scheme seemed
to work because it gave me very high grades in school,
top scores in state and national board examinations

and my choice of training spots and fellowships. I closed
my notebooks, however, for 10 years. When I opened them
again and studied them 10 years after so carefully
completing them, I was astonished to find that they were
almost entirely filled with lies. Except for a few
descriptions, such as well-established anatomy, everything
that seemed so orderly and beautiful with the rather
comprehensive treatment I had given it for one moment in
history had changed, grown and been reordered by the
scholarship of the intervening 10 years. That is why it
is important so frequently to take stock as we have done
in this conference and to consider what has been happening
in the research laboratories and in our thinking on so
many subjects. Thus, the most impressive thing to me about
the first day of our conference is that as a celebration in
a dental school we were having such a conference and that
this conference was occurring in a school launched under
the philosophy that 10% of the budget for teaching should
be devoted from the very outset to research.

    I had, on that first day, to reflect also on the very
origins of this discourse and to consider just where it was
that the beginnings of a discourse must have come from that
could occupy several days plus several evenings of intensive
scientific exchange. It was easy because of the participants in this conference to think back on how we all came
to work on IgA as a special immunity system. Surely we all
owe much to Pierre Grabar and his associates and the others
who first recognized that gammaglobulins were complex,
that antibodies were located in several separable components
of Tiselius' gammablobulins, and that the β2A was a real
entity. Heremans was into this game very early and has
been making frequent contributions to the subject for many
years. Very early, however, being the excellent chemist
he is, he developed a method for isolating IgA. When he
came to Kunkel's laboratory at the Rockefeller University,
he had already perfected such a method. Wanting to obtain
some purified IgA, he selected one of the huskies of the
lab, obtained a large amount of blood and isolated, isolated
and isolated with his fine new method and obtained no IgA.
Anyone but Heremans would have suspected his method of
being faulty and perhaps returned home to correct the
method. Not Heremans. He concluded that there was something wrong with the husky, healthy subject and proceeded
to isolate and purify his IgA from another donor and

succeeded without trouble. Later, when Lars Hanson was also
found while in Kunkel's laboratory to lack IgA, Heremans,
Rockey, Lars Hanson and Kunkel reported on the isolated
absence of IgA in healthy young men. This was an important
paper for many reasons, but perhaps mostly because it showed
that IgA could be completely lacking from blood, yet this
absence might be associated with quite good health. It
led, however, to numerous subsequent studies by Heremans,
Lars Hanson, South, Hong, Cassidy, Buckley, Amman, and
many others, of persons having a selective absence of IgA.
These studies indicated that people born without the capacity
to produce this antibody as a population are not healthy.
We have heard in this conference that they may experience
with inordinate frequency, respiratory diseases, gastrointestinal disease, autoimmunities and mesenchymal diseases,
and certain kinds of oral pathology. As much as anything,
from studying people who lack the IgA system, we can
realize that the system plays a great importance in the
body economy.

The IgA system plays a major role in defending the
body against development of respiratory infection,
respiratory allergy, sprue, autoimmune and mesenchymal
diseases. We know this because as a population patients
lacking the IgA local antibody system have such diseases
far more frequently than do members of the population who
possess the local and systemic immunity system represented
by IgA. Thus, we can carry out our studies of this IgA
system with the firm conviction that we are studying an
interesting and challenging system that plays a most
important role in the body economy.

There is another way to be sure that a subject is of
major importance in human biology. That is to see whether
the scientists associated with Henry Kunkel have considered
it important enough to study and work with. Here again the
very makeup of our conference says that the IgA system
passes a crucial test. At this conference we have a near
army of trainees, associates and former students of Kunkel,
and Kunkel himself. One only has to realize that Heremans,
Lars Hanson, Tomasi, Grey, Fudenberg, Franklin and Jerry,
and even I studied with Kunkel in his little laboratories
at the Rockefeller University. These are but a small part
of that extraordinary group of scientists Kunkel has trained
and helped develop who have contributed so very much to

current understanding of immunobiology in genetic, molecular
and biologic terms.

Here a brief anecdote might help put my interpretation
in proper perspective. Max Cooper, one of the major
organizers of this conference, had recently come to study
with me in Minnesota. We were always very short of space
in our laboratories. Since I always left it to the research
fellows to select their own project and gave them no technical help and very little space, Max had been confined for
several months to a couple of drawers and two square feet
of table top space in which to work. Very late one night
he confided to Henry Gewurz, who was a late night worker,
that he had not done much yet but a lot of people-watching.
He was, however, sure of one thing; there wasn't a single
person he had seen in that laboratory, whom he would accept
as one who could fit under a bell-shaped curve. Henry,
being very loyal, tried briefly to defend his colleagues
in this strange laboratory, and failing to be convincing,
just walked away. After several weeks, when Max Cooper had
made his discovery about how regularly to produce agammaglobulinemia, absence of plasma cells and absence of
germinal centers in chickens, using bursectomy and irradiation in newly hatched chickens, his behavior changed
dramatically. He kicked and shoved his way into adequate
bench space, he marshalled technical help, he worked day
and night at his discovery, he fought with his so-called
superiors, he disagreed every day with the boss, he
neglected his family. In short, he took on the characteristics of the usual, really working scientist. Henry Gewurz
met him one day and recognizing the change in his behavior,
he said, "Indeed not a single one." It was this line that
came to mind as I contemplated the many contributions made
to this and other subjects in immunology from a single
laboratory, that of Henry Kunkel at the Rockefeller University. There certainly must have been, through the years,
very few in that laboratory who could be found to fit under
a bell-shaped curve.

Thus, we know that the IgA system does have real
importance because we have seen what happens in the form of
disease to humans who lack the system. We are, however, not
at all sure how it exerts its major role in the body economy.
It may be important simply in preventing, in a major way,

the application of antigenic stimulation to the other
immunity systems. In the talks today, we heard that a
local immunity system, which may in large part be the IgA
local antibody system, interferes with absorption or
adherence of antigens from the absorbing surfaces of the
GI tract. Perhaps this is why the IgA system, unlike the
other immunity systems, seems, as Heremans stated, to be
associated with a kind of negative memory. Perhaps this is
because the IgA system protects the T-cell system, IgM,
IgG, systemic IgA, and IgE from stimulation by combining
with antigens, which in the absence of an IgA system,
might stimulate locally the IgE antibody and produce
allergy, autoimmunity, and mesenchymal disease. I doubt,
however, that when studied locally the IgA system lacks
memory. I believe we will find, with proper experiments,
that it possesses memory based on cell proliferation and
rapid differentiation like all the other immunity systems
but that it seems to impose inhibition of memory by becoming
very efficient in keeping antigenic stimuli out of the body.

It is becoming very important to think in terms of
domains. Dr. Jurg Mueller and I have been much impressed
recently with the evidence that there exists an entero-
enteric domain. According to this concept, antigens,
especially particulate antigens, can stimulate in the Peyer's
patches lymphoid cells of both T and B-cell classes because
the particles are allowed to enter through the specialized
epithelium overlying this specialized lymphoid site, to
stimulate lymphoid cells in this location, which can then
be disseminated to the lamina propria along the gut tract
as a local antibody system. Even a special local cell-
mediated immunity provided by T-lymphocytes of this origin
can be provided for the epithelium of the gut. Henney
and Waldman surely have shown such a local cellular immunity
for the respiratory tract. We thought our concept a great
one, and one quite consistent with the earlier important
studies of Cebra and his students that dealt with the
origin of the IgA system, both systemically distributed
and distributed along the GI tract from the cells of appendix
sacculus rotundus and Peyer's patches of the rabbit. Now
we discover from this conference that such a beautiful
organization may indeed be a pack of lies because it is
incomplete. From the work of Bienenstock and Perry, it has
become evident that one need think of an entero-pulmono-
enteric-pulmonic system, and to make matters still

more complicated, the studies of Bohl suggest that this local
antibody system generated by gastrointestinal stimulation
may selectively involve a component that resides in the
mammary gland. This appropriate antigenic stimulation via
the gastrointestinal tract can have consequences reflected
in local immunity and resistance of the mammary gland and
vice versa. This is, indeed, a most exciting concept that
requires extensive and critical experimental attention.

To think critically about a local immunity system, one
must think about how the special form of IgA gains the
locations where it can be effective and maintain itself
in a molecular form in which it can be most effective. This
seems to be a function of the secretory or transport piece.
In our laboratory we always talked about this as a transport
rather than a secretory piece because to me secretion is
getting from the inside of a cell to the outside and
transport is getting from one side of a membrane to another.
These may be semantic differences and I think it unwise to
arouse differences that my colleagues deem to have been
settled by a "peace corps." From this meeting, further
evidence complementary to that obtained earlier by Hong in
his studies of bladder sweat, indicate that the dimeric IgA
held together by J chains and joined to the secretory
component resists enzymatic degradation. Thus, Kobayashi
has convinced us that the secretory IgA really is resistant
to enzymatic digestion. The resistance to enzymatic
digestion, he tells us, has nothing to do with any really
enzymatically resistant components of the secretory IgA
molecule, but with the molecular conformational characteristics that relate to the combination with the secretory
component. Thus the resistance of secretory IgA to
enzymatic digestion is a function of the way the molecule
is tightly packaged so that it is hard to interpose enzymes
that can launch hydrolysis.

The two-cell production of separate components to make
up a final molecule with important biologic action is also
interesting to contemplate. We used to think this relationship of plasma cell product to product of epithelial cell
was quite unique. But how unique was it? I think more and
more as we learn of the molecular interactions we begin
to see many examples of such interactions. The relatively
specific attachment of Clq to the Fc portion of the IgG and
IgM molecules to launch the classical complement cascade may
be an example. The activation of the alternate complement

pathway through the properdin or C3PA mechanism by cobra
venom factor may be another. Perhaps more and more as we
learn about the molecular recognition and receptor mechanisms
in biology, we will see that not only cells, but molecules
utilize a relatively simple recognition and attachment
mechanism based on complementarity of structure to do what
they must do and to get where they must go. These thoughts,
provoked by the reports in this conference, raise fundamental questions that can soon be addressed with our
increasing knowledge of the molecular biology of IgA and
its associates. Does the secretory component have a
phylogenetic history of its own? What is its basic role in
the body economy? Similar questions can be raised about
J chains. Will we encounter diseases based on inability
to produce J chains or secretory component? The biologic
link between the J chain and secretory component on the one
hand and the IgA molecule on the other may be quite different, especially since the J chain is produced by the very
same cell that produces the dimeric IgA or the pentameric
IgM. By contrast the secretory component is produced by the
epithelial cell, and the dimeric IgA, with its J chain, by
the plasma cell which may arise even from a different germ
layer.

It was pointed out very clearly by the early presentations of the conference that dimeric IgA is not only a
product of the GI tract or other epithelial surface. Dimeric
IgA was shown by Radl to be produced and found in bone marrow
and lymphoid tissues. Where cells are preferentially located
may have little to do with the basic functions of these cells
in the body economy. For example, red blood cells so inex-
tricably linked to bone marrow of mammals and man, in more
primitive forms, are not located in the marrow because there
is no marrow, but in fishes and amphibians to gonads and
hematopoietic sites in the anterior kidney. Shifts during
development permit us to see this in another way. Stem
cells for the B-cell system that seem entirely to be located
in the bursa of Fabricius, shift upon involution of the
bursa to the marrow and spleen, as the studies of the
Toivanens show. Thus, in this new information, I am not
sure we have learned anything fundamental about the
appropriate location of cells producing secretory IgA.
Tomasi has shown us that isolated bladder segments do
synthesize dimeric IgA.

Another way to phrase the question, it seems to me, is

the following: If a clinician wishes to achieve the
selective advantage of the IgA system for his patient, must
he give monomeric IgA, dimeric IgA, dimeric IgA combined
with transport piece, or can he only gain the desired end by
transplanting appropriate precursor cells that will set up
the dimeric IgA-producing system in the proper locations
within the body? Long ago, Max Cooper carried out experiments in my laboratory that convinced me that to get IgA
across the barrier into saliva, one had to give something
other than IgA as it exists, for the most part, in human
serum. This observation provokes an even more general
conclusion. The immunoglobulins we must use in efforts
at replacement therapy in the immunodeficient patient are
very poor. Even IgG as it is given intramuscularly in
standard medical treatment is a very poor product for replacement therapy. By the time it gets into the circulation
it is in large part broken down enzymatically, so that it
is spoiled as an opsonin. It may be even more of a problem
to obtain and deliver just the right molecular form of IgA
for substitution therapy. Dr. Brandtzaeg, however, addressed fundamental issues in this regard in his studies of the
activation kinetics involved in transport of dimeric IgA
across cellular barriers. He suggested that specificity for
transport of dimeric IgA and polymeric IgM, and binding of
secretory piece are indeed a function of the presence in
the molecules of the J chain. The transport or secretory
piece then may act as a receptor for the right kind of IgA
or IgM molecule. As I indicated above, such a mechanism
involving appropriate receptors may be important in many
biologic processes. Leu et al showed that M.I.F. uses
surface receptors to talk to peritoneal macrophages, and
Brambel and others may have presented evidence that the
Fc portion of the IgG molecule uses a similar mechanism
selectively to get across the placental or yolk sac barriers
into the fetus. I was, however, a bit surprised by the
demonstration by Brandtzaeg that the affinity of IgA for
the secretory component was not so specific and really even
weaker than the affinity expressed for secretory component
by polymeric IgM. This may be an important contribution.

The Molecular Analysis

One had to be impressed with the molecular analysis of
IgA. We can now talk about the details of IgA structure in
impressive terms that reflect our ability to take the
molecule apart and analyze it piece by piece. We now see

that several different laboratories have well defined
purified preparations of J chains. We can agree on a
molecular weight and we are quite a way toward completing
the amino acid sequencing. In addition, we see that several
have purified the secretory piece and it is just a matter
of time before complete analysis of the structure of this
part is at hand.

Mestecky taught us not only about the proper molecular
weights of the J chains but just exactly how IgA attaches
to the secretory piece and how this involves the J chain.
Thus, although J chain is essential in some way to the
attachment of secretory IgA, it is the penultimate cysteine
residue isolated from cyanogen bromide cleaved material
that yields the octapeptide of the alpha chain that really
combines with the J chain. The role of the J chain, although clearly involved in some way in the attachment, must
still be resolved.

Franklin confirmed this very nice contribution and
then gave us the sequence of amino acids around the crucial
cysteine fragment. Koshland, who with her students discovered J chains just a few years ago, showed us that J
chain is associated only with polymeric and absent from
monomeric IgA. She gave us in this conference a very nice
stoichiometric chemical analysis by which she was able to
show that J chains have to be associated with IgA and IgM
in a relationship that involves one J chain per appropriate
polymer. Thus, we see that the J chains somehow or other
determine the polymer size. As her feminist interpretation
would have it, the J chain acts as a clasp and not as a
bracelet to complete the polymer. I wonder if a male
scientist could have made that discovery.

I can see a beautiful testing ground for this view.
Michael Sigel, Gary Litman, Acton, and others have found
different polymer sizes of IgM to be a basis of phylogenetic
play with the IgM molecule. Do we see in each different
form of IgM, the dimeric, tetrameric, pentameric, and hexameric IgM of the stingray, amphibia, horned shark, and other
elasmo-branchii and clawed toad respectively, the appropriate
amount of J chain? Indeed, is J chain essential to the
polymeric construction of the molecule in these several
phylogenetically distinct forms of primitive fish? This
is a neat problem which should test Bunny Koshland's

predictions that an oxidation step coupled with secretion
is involved in closing the polymer. Parkhouse contributed
to this analysis by showing that J chain really imposes a
rate limiting step in determining the amount of immunoglobulin being secreted. This might be essential if the
J chain closes the polymer. His findings were based, I
think, on a beautiful analysis utilizing models of various
pool sizes that revealed that J chains are always in short
supply and thus rate limiting. Using Anfinsen's scram-
blease he helped with a direct demonstration that the
J chains are essential to the process of polymerization.

Tomasi contributed a nice new wrinkle. Even though
I did not like Tomasi's model nearly as much as our feminist
model, I was impressed with his isolation of 8 10S IgA
proteins and found that all 8 contained bands that had
rapid electrophoretic mobility which he showed to be alpha-
1 - trypsin inhibitor and/or albumin. Now, I don't know
what IgA is doing associating with albumin, but I can think
of important consequences of its being associated with
alpha - 1 - trypsin inhibitor. Indeed, only yesterday afternoon we were presented with a fascinating case of emphysema
associated with absence of IgA. Could such a relationship
of IgA deficiency and certain forms of pulmonary disease
relate not only to inability to resist infection, but to a
deficiency of alpha - 1 - trypsin inhibitor because the
latter cannot be properly delivered to the respiratory
apparatus in association with IgA? Conversely, could the
obscure role of genetically determined alpha - 1 - trypsin
inhibitor deficiency and progressive pulmonary disease be
associated with anomalous delivery of IgA and deficient
local immunity when the alpha - 1 - trypsin inhibitor is
lacking? Stranger associations have been found.

I like the contribution of Jerry and Kunkel, particularly the evidence for a fascinating mechanism relating
stabilization of the molecule, actually even to its SS
bonding, to the secretory component. That is, changes that
were induced by combination of the secretory component
seemed after binding to be related to the induction of
process involving SS bonding where this had not previously
existed. This to me is a new mechanism and one that we
need to think about a great deal.

The sequencing of the molecule is coming along very
well, 40 to 50% finished. It looks to me as though the

sequence is following Vince Lombardi's admonitions. As I
remember them, these included - go to their strengths, run
for daylight, don't let them catch their breath. From what
Putnam told us, that is exactly what is happening in the
molecular analysis of the immunoglobulins. We are down to
the last of the big 5. First light chains λ, κ, then γ and
μ and now α. The strategy for all the rest seems straightforward. We already see in the data very great differences
in the phylogenetic conservation in different segments of
the molecule. This holds both for the V-region, and from
component to component in the different parts of the C-
regions. One has to wonder just how these molecules are
assembled, how they have been put together. Do these long
stretches that show the fantastic conservation have to be
distinguished functionally and phylogenetically from the
regions where there is much more variability? Capra, in
looking at the V-region, found something that I think needs
to be brought out and emphasized. He found VHIII dominant
in the alpha chain and proposed a number of explanations.
The one I like best relates to the possibility that the kinds
of antigens to which the IgA system is being exposed may
really have to do with the selection of a particular type of
variability, a particular type of combining region. The
prediction from this, of course, is that IgE might also have
VHIII predominance because IgE, being of the local type of
immunity system, may be more like IgA in the antigens to
which exposure occurs and quite different from the IgG and
IgM. I hope that in the next conference we will have information on this point. There is another area where the
great phylogenetic play has occurred. Let us think about
phylogenetic play for a second. The early phylogenetic play
with immunoglobulin molecules was the polymer structure and
for this conference it is very important to realize the
tremendous variability that occurred in polymer size during
early phylogeny. Thus, extant primitive forms show great
differences from one another, having, for example, IgM of
hexameric, pentameric, tetrameric, dimeric and monomeric
form. Then play occurred with respect to the nature of the
heavy chain. Multiple heavy chains began to appear with the
lung fishes and the amphibia and there has since been a great
play in this regard. Just look at man with IgM, IgA monomeric and dimeric forms, two subclasses, IgG four subclasses,
IgD and IgE.

Also play has taken place in phylogeny with respect to
domains in the constant region. We have seen evidence for

such play in the IgG type of immunoglobulin of the turtle
and the duck where domains of the constant region of the
H chain seem to have been left out.

In the case Grey described, he seemed to find that the
CH3 region was missing and thus polymerization of the molecule could not occur. If, as I have proposed before, pathology can recapitulate phylogeny, we should see a lot more of
this kind of deficit in pathology. Indeed, I am not at all
sure that Seligmann's so-called alpha chain disease is not
another special example of this. Here it was shown that a
tremendous stretch of the H chain of IgA molecule was
essentially missing. It makes little sense to have a
disease with no light chains and a big gap in the primary
sequence of the heavy chain. There must be something wrong
with the assembly of the molecule because an important part
of the H chain that is involved in molecular assembly has
been left out. I wonder whether or not internal degradation
of light chains might not occur under such circumstances,
rather than that the lack of light chain is not in itself the
fundamental abnormality of that disease. Seligmann will be
with me on the plane going back and he can straighten me out
on that one. We have also clear evidence from all of these
studies that special things happen in the hinge region and
we have known this, I think, from work with the turtle and
the duck in phylogenetic analysis, but we now have much, much
better molecular information on this from the human material.
The secretory and the circulating molecules of dimeric IgA
certainly have very great conformity and I think that this
probably is what is to be expected, if what is being secreted
or transported really is a product of a special set of cells
that are fairly widely distributed. We are well along the
way, as I said, to understanding the primary structure of
the transport or secretory component. This seems to be a
unique molecule at least with respect to the sequences
that are known, and it does not appear to relate in its
sequence structure to any known immunoglobulin. Let us think
just for a half second again about that extraordinary
evidence that Koshland presented. She could make an antibody
against J chains of man in the rabbit and this antibody
would react with phylogenetic forms ranging from the shark
to the human, including a number of intermediate forms.
The only worry that I have about that is that the basic
immunogenic preparation was made in such a fashion that
haptenic component was being detected. It is easy to get
into trouble with cross-reactions to haptenic derivatives,

so I would really like to see the evidence that J chains all through phylogeny relate immunologically to one another, performed with purified J chains and antisera made against them without using adjuvants that can act like haptens.

The only place where I know that a kind of conservation has been exercised so as to ensure immunologic cross-reactivity over such a wide range is with nucleic acids and histones. If it is real, it indicates that J chains have had both a relatively small size coupled with great survival advantage of a major part of the molecule. Perhaps that is why we have not seen patients born with absence of the J chains. Such an event might be an early lethal and you just would not see it. We must keep looking because such a patient could tell us so much about the role of J chains in the body economy.

Clinical Implications

Yesterday afternoon and today we have considered aspects of the IgA system that have important clinical implications. Because of my own special interest I could talk for a long, long time on this part of the meeting but I will try to limit myself to a few highlights.

One thing struck me and that was that we are still struggling to establish the fact that the local immunity system really is primarily dependent on the IgA immuno-globulin molecule. When the local immunity experts get something that really works, it seems to me it is too often IgG or IgM that is being studied. That was true at least until this morning. We heard some pretty good evidence this morning that I may be wrong in this. Walker and those fol-lowing presented evidence that the operation of a local immunity system may involve very much an inhibition of attachment and consequent inhibition of absorption. Thus, defense against a receptor mechanism may be a major function of IgA. The contributions of Polmar and more recently of Soothill, that indicate that immunodeficiency in the IgA system may lead to excessive stimulation of the IgE system, seem very important clinically. Polmar showed very clearly in his earlier work with Terry that patients who lack IgA but possess IgE have more manifestations of respiratory symptoms than do patients who lack IgA and IgE as well. Hobbs put this in an interesting way when he mused, if you can't say A you are likely to say E. Now Soothill comes

along and shows that if the IgA system is even slow to
develop, severe atrophy may be a consequence. A nice
generalization comes from this perspective that we see
clinically manifest in many immunodeficiencies. If one
system is left out in this immunobiologic symphony, others
are likely to play too vigorously and disease can be the
consequence. For example, the excessive autoimmunity
thought so often to be attributable to forbidden clones or
immunologic excesses is in reality attributable often to
lack of ability to produce IgA.

With respect to mechanism of action of the IgA antibodies, we encountered a bit of controversy in relationship
to complement. Like all other controversies this will stir
up new studies that will give, I am sure, vital information
on the point. But Dalmasso's data and Bienenstock's data,
although counterposed, certainly do not refute one another.
There may be quantitative factors involved here that are
related to whether or not the IgA system can address the
complement system. We like the idea that it can, from
Bibi Day's recent studies, on Dr. Alfred Michael's patient,
which showed that there was a possibility of developing
a C' dependent renal disease associated with an IgA
product. This has now been confirmed by Peters et al.

Butler brought us a fascinating finding. Patients
lacking IgA seemed to be responding to a glycocalyx structure that otherwise was not responded to, unless malignancy
was present in the gastrointestinal tract, or in a deriva-
tive of the gastrointestinal tract. I found that a very
exciting and important contribution. Certainly, too, the
concepts and observations of Gibbons paralleling those of
Walker but in relationship to much more immediate issues
perhaps, the issues of whether organisms can even stay
around, whether they colonize in the gastrointestinal tract
and I presume, also, from his data, in the mouth. He
presented evidence that such events may very well relate to
the functions of the local immunity system, if not in a
predominant way to the secretory IgA system. I think that
again needs much more work. We have also seen a beginning
analysis of an association of the local immunity system with
the receptor mechanisms, how these organisms attach to
particular receptors, and how the antibodies of this system
and other systems can interfere. One of the things, of all
the things presented in the conference, that struck me most
was the finding that if you immunize by the gastrointestinal

route, the breast may be immunized. This is terribly important and because it was so unexpected. In the face of
this information it seems rather foolish to be impressed
that some persons lacking IgA may be quite healthy. It
might be much more relevant to look to see what happens to
the offspring of IgA deficient women in Africa or South
America or those in circumstances where they can be
challenged in the appropriate way to really test the system.
The proper experiment might be a bit hard to get at but I
think that it deserves serious consideration. The controversy between Waldman and Lawton is interesting; Lawton,
Cooper and that group have shown so clearly that patients
who lack IgA lack the IgA secreting cells. Such patients
do have plenty of lymphocytes in circulation that produce
but do not secrete IgA, and have IgA at their surface. With
Wu they found that pokeweed mitogen seems to transform or
differentiate such IgA producing B-lymphocytes to IgA
secreting cells. This most exciting finding Waldman told
us he could not confirm, and then presented evidence that
he could get such B-cells producing but not secreting IgA
to differentiate to secretory cells by exposing the cells to
transformed T-lymphocytes from patients with Sezary's
syndrome. I think the whole issue is so important that it
must be thought through carefully to gain the important
components. Whenever we have been engaged in such controversy, we have found that the conditions of the experiments
are crucial and when everything is worked out everybody is
right. As I look at what has been said, I wonder if the
essence of the Waldman, Cooper and Lawton experiments is
not that pokeweed mitogen can stimulate the T-lymphocytes
to transformation and that a product of those T-lymphocytes
is what provokes the differentiation of the IgA producing
but not secreting B-lymphocytes. With the discovery by
Katz, Benacerraf and others that stimulated T-lymphocytes
can produce something that can turn on B-lymphocytes to
respond to certain antigens, for example, many have been
looking for the B-activating factor produced by stimulated
T-cells. Hoffman and Oettgen, for example, have been
substituting for T-lymphocytes in synthesis of antibody
to SRBC in vitro with a peptide released by T-lymphocytes.
Could such a factor provoke differentiation of IgA producing
to IgA secreting B-lymphocytes in patients with selective
absence of IgA? If it could, it might be a marvelous way
to achieve a cellular engineering based on macromolecular
manipulation of an apparent blocked differentiation of
B-lymphocytes - WOW!!

Waldman's experiments with Sezary cells are of real interest. This is particularly true since Prunieras, with Seligmann, Griscelli and Flandrin, have shown that Sezary cells may be malignant cells with several markings of T-lymphocytes. Could they be malignant blasts related to T-lymphocytes? If so, then they might be producers of factors liberated by blast-transformed normal T-lymphocytes.

I am having much difficulty making sense of Hijmans' finding. Hijmans tells us that he has IgA at the surface of all sorts of secretory B-lymphocytes and plasma cells. One surely must worry about cross-reacting antibody, e.g. an antibody to a CHO constituent in IgA, but I doubt this explanation. Hijmans is very, very clever in this kind of work and his finding may be asking us to face again the stickiness of IgA. It seems to attach to so many different things. The work that Cebra presented on the first day of the conference may very well be related, so the crucial experiment would be the stripping experiments to see whether the IgA on the surface is really something synthesized by the cell or something that goes on board for other reasons. The question of cytophilic antibodies has been repeatedly raised. The association of IgA deficiency with all sorts of apparent immunological excesses I handle in a general framework, that is, if there is a deficiency of the immunity system, in any one of its component parts, whether it be in the complement system as an amplification process, whether it be one of the effector mechanisms, or whether it be any one of the specific systems or its interacting components that are deficient, you are likely to see excessive stimulation of the remaining systems. I think within the next few years we will come to quite a precise definition of segmental immunologic deficiencies and excesses.

The T-cell relationship to the IgA system repeatedly came up in this conference and I guess it is becoming a real thing. Still stuck in my craw, however, are those patients with the diGeorge syndrome because they really are so T-cell deficient. We have seen some with more than 95% of their circulating cells that are definable as B-lymphocytes, no cells definable as T. The 5% gap needs to be better defined. And they remain like this for long, long periods of time. If they are a special case, we have got to find in them evidence that once this thing has happened, the T-cell-IgA producing cell relationship does not need to continue. I am still wondering about this

relationship, even though the T-cell-IgA relationship shows
up in T-less nude mice and even in ataxia telangiectasia
of man.

I would like to conclude my paper with a set of
questions:

1. What really is the secretory or transport piece?
Does it have a receptor role or transport role for anything
other than polymerized IgA and IgM immunoglobulins possessing J chains?

2. What is the fundamental role of the J chain?

3. Is there a major survival role for these extraordinary molecules we did not even know existed as late as
three years ago?

4. Is it dimeric IgA or dimeric IgA with J chain and
T-piece that we must give to get injected IgA across the
barriers into secretions in patients lacking IgA?

5. What are the major amplification mechanisms used
by the IgA system?

6. Can the alternate pathway or shunt pathway of the
complement system be the major amplification mechanism
for IgA?

7. Alternatively, is Dr. Spiegelberg's more direct
pathway to cellular activation a primary means of addres-
sing inflammatory cells as a major amplification system
for IgA?

8. What is it that controls the many different polymer
sizes that are employed throughout phylogeny?

9. Will IgE like IgA have a predominance of the VHIII
that Capra has found so impressive in the IgA system?

10. Can we complete the entire molecular definition
of IgA by the time of the next conference similarly with
the complete structure of J chains and S-piece?

11. Will this extraordinary molecular understanding
give us any better understanding of the biology of the local

immunity system than we have right now? I want these molecular analyses to go forward as rapidly as possible, but I
wonder whether I will not again be disappointed by the
contributions to be derived from the complete molecular
analysis to the pragmatic questions of clinical medicine.

12. Does the major function of the IgA immunity system
really equate with the local immunity system? I doubt this
very much.

13. Is it possible that the local immunity system
relates less to IgA than IgG, IgM or cell-mediated T-cell
immunity?

14. If so, what is the major raison d'etre of the IgA
immunity system?

15. Does the real function of the IgA system have to
do with the interfering with absorption of antigens that
cross-react with body constituents? Thus, is the IgA
system a major defense against autoimmunity?

16. What is the function of the association of the IgA
system with constant turnover in the organisms we associate
most intimately? Could it be that to keep our flora in constant change prevents our most intimate neighbors from using
their genetic potential for rapid change to develop means
of dominating their hosts - us?

17. Could it be that the real major advantage of the IgA
system relates to the entero-mammaric system that could provide real protection to offspring feeding at the breast from
enteric infection?

There can be no question that from this conference we
take many fundamental and practical questions with us as we
return to our clinics and laboratories throughout the world.
I for one, and I believe for all of us, want to express deep
appreciation to the organizers and supporters of this conference. To Dr. Kraus, who challenged us to work, to Drs.
Mestecky, Cooper, Lawton, Volker, and all our hosts, many
thanks. We return to our homes enthusiastic about our
experiences and the special experiments we have ready to
go as a consequence of this interaction. As a form of
scholarly behavior, the conference has been a real success.

PROGRAM PARTICIPANTS, INCLUDING CO-AUTHORS

ABEL, C.A., Department of Medicine, National Jewish Hospital
    and Research Center, Denver, Colorado, U.S.A.

ABRAHAM, G.N., Department of Medicine & Microbiology,
    University of Rochester School of Medicine, Rochester,
    New York, U.S.A.

AHLSTEDT, S., Department of Immunology, University of
    Goteborg, Goteborg, Sweden

ALBRIGHT, E.L., Veterans Administration Hospital, Albuquerque,
    New Mexico, U.S.A.

ASVAPAKA, C., Department of Microbiology, Mahidol University
    Faculty of Science, Bangkok, Thailand

BALLIEUX, R.E., Department of Immunology, University Hospital,
    Utrecht, The Netherlands

BENNETT, J.C., Department of Microbiology, University of
    Alabama in Birmingham, Birmingham, Alabama, U.S.A.

BIENENSTOCK, J., Department of Medicine, McMaster University,
    Hamilton, Ontario, Canada

BLOCH, K.J., Department of Medicine, Harvard Medical School,
    Boston, Massachusetts, U.S.A.

BOACKLE, R.J., Department of Molecular Biology, University of
    Alabama in Birmingham, Birmingham, Alabama, U.S.A.

BOCKMAN, D.E., Department of Anatomy, Medical College of
    Ohio, Toledo, Ohio

BOHL, E.H., Department of Veterinary Science, Ohio Agriculture
    Research & Developmental Center, Wooster, Ohio, U.S.A.

BRANDTZAEG, P., Institute of Pathology, Rikshopitalet, Oslo, Norway

BUTLER, J.E., Department of Microbiology, University of Iowa College of Medicine, Iowa City, Iowa, U.S.A.

CAPRA, J.D., Department of Microbiology, Mt. Sinai School of Medicine, New York, New York, U.S.A.

CARLSSON, B., Department of Immunology, University of Goteborg, Goteborg, Sweden

CASSELL, G., Department of Comparative Medicine, University of Alabama in Birmingham, Birmingham, Alabama, U.S.A.

CEBRA, J.J., Department of Biology, The John Hopkins University, Baltimore, Maryland, U.S.A.

CHALLACOMBE, S.J., Department of Oral Immunology and Microbiology, Guy's Hospital Medical & Dental School, London, England

CHUANG, C.-Y., Department of Microbiology, Mt. Sinai School of Medicine, New York, New York, U.S.A.

CLAMP, J.R., Department of Medicine, University of Bristol, Bristol, England

CLANCY, R.L., Department of Medicine, McMaster University, Hamilton, Ontario, Canada

COHN, J., Department of Microbiology, School of Dental Medicine and Center for Oral Health Research, Philadelphia, Pennsylvania, U.S.A.

COLTEN, H.R., Children's Hospital Medical Center, Boston, Massachusetts, U.S.A.

COOPER, M.D., Department of Pediatrics & Microbiology, University of Alabama in Birmingham, Birmingham, Alabama, U.S.A.

CRAIG, S.W.., Department of Biology, The John Hopkins University, Baltimore, Maryland, U.S.A.

CUNNINGHAM-RUNDLES, C., Department of Pathology, New York
    University Medical Center, New York, New York, U.S.A.

DALMASSO, A.P., Veterans Administration Hospital, Minneapolis,
    Minnessota, U.S.A.

DAWE, D., Department of Veterinary Medicine, University of
    Georgia, Athens, Georgia, U.S.A.

DAWES, C., Univeristy of Manitoba, Winnipeg, Manitoba, Canada

DELLA CORTE, E., National Institute for Medical Research,
    London, England

DESPONT, J.-P. J., Department of Medicine, National Jewish
    Hospital & Research Center, Denver, Colorado, U.S.A.

EDELMAN, R., Department of Microbiology, Mahidol University
    Faculty of Science, Bangkok, Thailand

EMMINGS, F.G., Department of Oral Biology, State University
    of New York at Buffalo, Buffalo, New York, U.S.A.

EVANS, R.T., Department of Oral Biology, State University
    of New York at Buffalo, Buffalo, New York, U.S.A.

FINE, J.M., Centre National de Transfusion, Paris, France

FRANGIONE, B., Department of Medicine, New York Univeristy
    Medical Center, New York, New York, U.S.A.

FRANKLIN, E.C., Department of Medicine, New York University
    Medical Center, New York, New York, U.S.A.

FREDERICK, G.T., Department of Veterinary Science, Ohio
    Agricultural Research & Development Center, Wooster,
    Ohio, U.S.A.

FRETER, R., Department of Microbiology, University of Michigan
    Medical School, Ann Arbor, Michigan, U.S.A.

FROMMEL, D., Centre National de Transfusion, Paris, France

FUDENBERG, H.H., Department of Medicine & Immunology,
    University of California Medical Center, San Francisco,
    California, U.S.A.

GANGULY, R., Department of Medicine, University of Florida, Gainsville, Florida, U.S.A.

GENCO, R.J., Department of Oral Biology, State University of New York at Buffalo, Buffalo, New York, U.S.A.

GIBBONS, R.J., Forsyth Dental Center, Boston, Mass., U.S.A.

GOOD, R.A., Sloan Kettering Institute, New York, N.Y., U.S.A.

GREY, H.M., Department of Medicine, National Jewish Hospital and Research Center, Denver, Colorado, U.S.A.

GRISCELLI, C., Department of Pathology, University of Geneva, Geneva, Switzerland

GUGGENHEIM, B., Dental Institute, University of Zurich, Zurich, Switzerland

GUPTA, R.K.P., Department of Veterinary Science, Ohio Agricultural Research & Development Center, Wooster, Ohio, U.S.A.

GUY-GRAND, D., Department of Pathology, University of Geneva, Geneva, Switzerland

HANSON, L.A., Department of Immunology, University of Goteborg, Goteborg, Sweden

HAUPTMAN, S., Department of Immunology, Mayo Medical School, Rochester, Minnesota, U.S.A.

HENSON, P., Department of Experimental Pathology, Scripps Clinic & Research Foundation, La Jolla, Ca., U.S.A.

HEREMANS, J.F., Department of Experimental Medicine, University of Louvain, Brussels, Belgium

HIJMANS, W., Institute for Experimental Gerontology, TNO, Rijswijk, The Netherlands

HONG, R., Department of Pediatrics & Medical Microbiology, University of Wisconsin, Madison, Wisconsin, U.S.A.

HUSER, H., Department of Zoology, Indiana University, Bloomington, Indiana, U.S.A.

INMAN, F.P., Department of Microbiology, University of
Georgia, Athens, Georgia

ISSELBACHER, K.J., Department of Medicine, Massachusetts
General Hospital, Boston, Massachusetts, U.S.A.

IVANYI, L., Department of Oral Immunology & Microbiology,
Guy's Hospital Medical & Dental School, London, England

JACOX, R.F., University of Rochester, Rochester, N.Y., U.S.A.

JERRY, L.M., Department of Experimental Medicine, McGill
University, Montreal, Canada

JODAL, U., Department of Immunology, University of
Goteborg, Goteborg, Sweden

JONES, P.P., Department of Biology, The John Hopkins
University, Baltimore, Maryland, U.S.A.

KAPLAN, R.D., Department of Microbiology, Mt. Sinai School
of Medicine, New York, New York, U.S.A.

KEHOE, J.M., Department of Microbiology, Mt. Sinai School
of Medicine, New York, New York, U.S.A.

KERR-GRANT, D., Department of Pediatrics, State University
of New York at Buffalo, Buffalo, New York, U.S.A.

KINCADE, P.W., Department of Pediatrics & Microbiology,
University of Alabama in Birmingham, Birmingham,
Alabama, U.S.A.

KOBAYASHI, K., Department of Biochemistry, Hokkaido
University, Sapparo, Hokkaido, Japan

KOISTINEN, J., Finnish Red Cross Blood Transfusion Service,
Helsinki, Finland

KOSHLAND, M.E., Department of Bacteriology & Immunology,
University of California, Berkeley, California, U.S.A.

KRAFT, S.C., Department of Pediatrics & Medicine, University
of Chicago, Chicago, Illinois, U.S.A.

KRAUS, F.W., Department of Microbiology, University of
    Alabama in Birmingham, Birmingham, Alabama, U.S.A.

KULHAVY, R., Institute of Dental Research, University of
    Alabama in Birmingham, Birmingham, Alabama, U.S.A.

KUNKEL, H.G., Rockefeller University, New York, N.Y., U.S.A.

LALLY, E.T., Department of Microbiology, School of Dental
    Medicine & Center for Oral Health Research, Philadelphia,
    Pennsylvania, U.S.A.

LAMBIN, P., Centre National de Transfusion, Paris, France

LAMM, M.E., Department of Pathology, New York University
    Medical Center, New York, New York, U.S.A.

LAWRENCE, D.A., Department of Experimental Pathology, Scripps
    Clinic & Research Foundation, La Jolla, Ca., U.S.A.

LAWTON, A.R., Department of Pediatrics & Microbiology,
    University of Alabama in Birmingham, Birmingham,
    Alabama, U.S.A.

LEHNER, T., Department of Oral Immunology & Microbiology,
    Guy's Hospital Medical & Dental School, London, England

LESLIE, G.A., Department of Microbiology, Tulane University
    School of Medicine, New Orleans, Louisiana, U.S.A.

LINDBERG, U., Department of Immunology, University of
    Goteborg, Goteborg, Sweden

LIU, V., Department of Zoology, Indiana University,
    Bloomington, Indiana, U.S.A.

LOW, T., Department of Zoology, Indiana University,
    Bloomington, Indiana, U.S.A.

MCGHEE, J., Department of Microbiology, University of
    Alabama in Birmingham, Birmingham, Alabama, U.S.A.

MCNAMARA, T.F., Department of Microbiology, State University
    of New York at Stonybrook, Stonybrook, N.Y., U.S.A.

MENDEZ, E., Department of Medicine, New York University
    Medical Center, New York, New York, U.S.A.

MESTECKY, J., Department of Microbiology, University of
    Alabama in Birmingham, Birmingham, Alabama, U.S.A.

MICHALEK, S.M., Department of Microbiology, University of
    Alabama in Birmingham, Birmingham, Alabama, U.S.A.

MIGLIERINA, R., Laboratory of Immunochemistry, Hopital
    Saint-Louis, Paris, France

MIHAESCO, E., Laboratory of Immunochemistry, Hopital
    Saint-Louis, Paris, France

MONTGOMERY, P.C., Department of Microbiology, School of
    Dental Medicine & Center for Oral Health Research,
    Philadelphia, Pennsylvania, U.S.A.

MOORE, E.C., Department of Pediatrics, Albany Medical
    College, Albany, New York, U.S.A.

MORAG, A., Department of Pediatrics, State University of
    New York at Buffalo, Buffalo, New York, U.S.A.

MORELL, A., Institute for Clinical & Experimental Cancer
    Research, University of Berne, Berne, Switzerland

MUSHINSKI, J.F., Laboratory of Cell Biology, National
    Cancer Institute, Bethesda, Maryland, U.S.A.

NEWCOMB, R.W., Children's Asthma Research Institute &
    Hospital, Denver, Colorado, U.S.A.

NIEDERMEIER, W., Department of Medicine, University of
    Alabama in Birmingham, Birmingham, Alabama, U.S.A.

OGRA, P.L., Department of Pediatrics & Microbiology, State
    University of New York at Buffalo, Buffalo, N.Y., U.S.A.

OGRA, S.S., Department of Medicine & OB-GYN, State University
    of New York at Buffalo, Buffalo, New York, U.S.A.

OLSON, R.E., Department of Microbiology, Mahidol University
    Faculty of Science, Bangkok, Thailand

ØRSTAVIK, D.S., Institute for Oral Pathology, University
    of Oslo, Oslo, Norway

PARKHOUSE, R.M.E., National Institute for Medical Research,
    London, England

PENN, G.A., Children's Hospital, Columbus, Ohio, U.S.A.

PEREY, D.Y.E., Department of Medicine, McMaster University,
    Hamilton, Ontario, Canada

PLAUT, A.G., Clinical Unit, New England Medical Center
    Hospital, Boston, Massachusetts, U.S.A.

PRELLI, F., Department of Medicine, New York University
    Medical Center, New York, New York, U.S.A.

PRUITT, K.M., Department of Molecular Biology, University of
    Alabama in Birmingham, Birmingham, Alabama, U.S.A.

PUTNAM, F.W., Department of Zoology, Indiana University,
    Bloomington, Indiana, U.S.A.

RADL, J., Institute for Experimental Gerontology, TNO,
    Rijswijk, The Netherlands

RAFF, E., Department of Zoology, Indiana University,
    Bloomington, Indiana, U.S.A.

REED, W.P., Veterans Administration Hospital, Albuquerque,
    New Mexico, U.S.A.

REYNOLDS, H.Y., Laboratory of Clinical Investigation, NIAID,
    NIH, Bethesda, Maryland, U.S.A.

RIZZO, A.A., National Institute of Dental Research, National
    Institute of Health, Bethesda, Maryland, U.S.A.

ROBERTSON, P.B., Dental Branch, University of Texas, Houston,
    Texas, U.S.A.

ROTHBERG, R.M., Department of Pediatrics & Medicine,
    University of Chicago, Chicago, Illinois, U.S.A.

ROWE, D.S., WHO Immunology Research & Training Center,
    Lausanne, Switzerland

RUDZIK, O., Department of Medicine, McMaster University,
    Hamilton, Ontario, Canada

SAIF, L.J., Department of Veterinary Science, Ohio
    Agricultural Research & Development Center, Wooster,
    Ohio, U.S.A.

SANTUCCI, E., University of Rochester, Rochester, N.Y., U.S.A.

SCHROHENLOHER, R.E., Department of Medicine, University
    of Alabama in Birmingham, Birmingham, Alabama, U.S.A.

SCHUIT, H.R.E., Institute for Experimental Gerontology, TNO,
    Rijswijk, The Netherlands

SELIGMANN, M., Laboratory of Immunochemistry, Hopital
    Saint-Louis, Paris, France

SIGEL, M.M., Department of Microbiology, University of
    Miami School of Medicine, Miami, Florida, U.S.A.

SIRISINHA, S., Department of Microbiology, Mahidol University
    Faculty of Science, Bangkok, Thailand

SKVARIL, F., Institute for Clinical & Experimental Cancer
    Research, University of Berne, Berne, Switzerland

SMITH, J., Infectious Diseases, Veterans Administration
    Hospital, Dallas, Texas, U.S.A.

SOHL, A., Department of Immunology, University of Goteborg,
    Goteborg, Sweden

SOUTH, M.A., Department of Pediatric Immunology, University
    of Pennsylvania & Children's Hospital, Philadelphia,
    Pennsylvania, U.S.A.

SPIEGELBERG, H.L., Department of Experimental Pathology,
    Scripps Clinic and Research Foundation, La Jolla,
    California, U.S.A.

STONE, S.S., National Animal Disease Laboratory, U.S.
    Agricultural Research Service, Ames, Iowa, U.S.A.

STROBER, W., Metabolish Branch, National Cancer Institute,
    NIH, Bethesda, Maryland, U.S.A.

SUSKIND, R., Department of Microbiology, Mahidol University
    Faculty of Science, Bangkok, Thailand

TAUBMAN, M.A., Department of Immunology, Forsyth Dental
    Center, Boston, Massachusetts, U.S.A.

TOMANA, M., Department of Medicine, University of Alabama
    in Birmingham, Birmingham, Alabama, U.S.A.

TOMASI, T.B., Jr., Department of Immunology, Mayo Medical
    School, Rochester, Minnesota, U.S.A.

UMANA, G., Department of Psychiatry, West Seneca State
    School, West Seneca, New York, U.S.A.

VAERMAN, J.P., Department of Experimental Medicine,
    University Catholique de Louvain, Brussels, Belgium

VASSALLI, P., Department of Pathology, University of Geneva,
    Geneva, Switzerland

VOSSEN, J.M.J.J., Organization for Health Research, TNO,
    Rijswijk, The Netherlands

WALDMAN, R.H., Department of Medicine & Microbiology,
    University of Florida, Gainsville, Florida, U.S.A.

WALKER, W.A., Pediatric Gastrointestinal Unit, Massachusetts
    General Hospital, Boston, Massachusetts, U.S.A.

WALLACE, R.B., Department of Public Health & Preventive
    Medicine, University of Iowa, Iowa City, Iowa, U.S.A.

WANG, A.-C., Department of Medicine, University of California
    Medical Center, San Francisco, California, U.S.A.

WEBB, D.R., The Mason Clinic, Seattle, Wisconsin, U.S.A.

WILDE, C.E., III, Department of Bacteriology & Immunology,
    University of California, Berkeley, California, U.S.A.

WILTON, J.M.A., Department of Oral Immunology & Microbiology,
    Guy's Hospital Medical & Dental School, London, England

WOLFENSTEIN-TODEL, C., Department of Medicine, New York
    University Medical Center, New York, New York, U.S.A.

WONG, F.C., Department of Zoology, Indiana University,
    Bloomington, Indiana, U.S.A.

WRIGHT, G.P., Institute of Dental Research, University of
    Alabama in Birmingham, Birmingham, Alabama, U.S.A.

WU, L.Y.F., Department of Pediatrics & Microbiology,
    University of Alabama in Birmingham, Birmingham,
    Alabama, U.S.A.

INDEX

545